AF094594

New Therapies of Liver Diseases

New Therapies of Liver Diseases

Editor

Pierluigi Toniutto

MDPI • Basel • Beijing • Wuhan • Barcelona • Belgrade • Manchester • Tokyo • Cluj • Tianjin

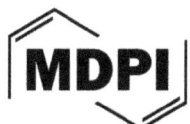

Editor
Pierluigi Toniutto
Hepatology and Liver
Transplantation Unit,
University of Udine
Italy

Editorial Office
MDPI
St. Alban-Anlage 66
4052 Basel, Switzerland

This is a reprint of articles from the Special Issue published online in the open access journal *Journal of Clinical Medicine* (ISSN 2077-0383) (available at: https://www.mdpi.com/journal/jcm/special_issues/new_therapies_liver_diseases).

For citation purposes, cite each article independently as indicated on the article page online and as indicated below:

LastName, A.A.; LastName, B.B.; LastName, C.C. Article Title. *Journal Name* **Year**, *Volume Number*, Page Range.

ISBN 978-3-0365-3859-4 (Hbk)
ISBN 978-3-0365-3860-0 (PDF)

Contents

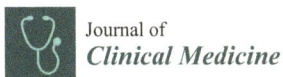

Journal of
Clinical Medicine

MDPI

Editorial

Special Issue "New Therapies of Liver Diseases"

Pierluigi Toniutto

Hepatology and Liver Transplantation Unit, Academic Hospital, University of Udine, 33100 Udine, Italy;
pierluigi.toniutto@uniud.it

Citation: Toniutto, P. Special Issue
"New Therapies of Liver Diseases". *J.
Clin. Med.* **2022**, *11*, 1798. https://
doi.org/10.3390/jcm11071798

Received: 17 March 2022
Accepted: 19 March 2022
Published: 24 March 2022

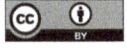
Medical and surgical treatments aimed at curing severe liver diseases and prolonging the survival of patients have improved dramatically in recent years. These advances have mainly been achieved by obtaining a better understanding of the pathophysiology of liver diseases [1]. New and old pharmacological therapies have been applied in a better way based on the new insights obtained in the pathophysiological studies. Moreover, the increased application of technology innovations, both in diagnostic imaging [2] and in surgery [3], enable the cure rate to be increased in patients with advanced liver diseases.

A Special Issue in the *Journal of Clinical Medicine (JCM)* has been dedicated to collecting high-quality scientific contributions from leading experts by focusing on updating the horizon of new pharmacological therapies and new surgical approaches that can be applied to cure several types of liver diseases as a method to address this challenging topic in greater detail.

Two studies investigated the current and future management of cholestatic liver diseases [4,5]. The first study retrospectively evaluated the real-world clinical management of patients with primary biliary cholangitis (PBC), according to the indications of the recent updated clinical guidelines. A study conducted in a large cohort of European patients revealed that biochemical response rates adopting the standard first-line treatment with ursodeoxycholic acid (UDCA) were achieved in a large proportion of patients, depending on the response criteria adopted. In UDCA nonresponders, second-line treatment regimens in which obeticholic acid or bezafibrate were added were promptly applied, leading to significantly increased response rates. These results confirm in real clinical practice that UDCA first-line standard treatment is largely effective in patients with PBC, but highlight the need to detect high-risk patients with an insufficient response to UDCA early in life, since early treatment modification significantly increases subsequent response rates. In addition to obeticholic acid and fibrates, several other molecules are currently under evaluation as potential new therapies both for patients with PBC and with primary sclerosing cholangitis (PSC). This issue has been extensively discussed in a subsequent study [5]. Given the complex nature of PBC and PSC, future treatments for these diseases will probably be based on a combination of drugs, aimed at influencing specific pathophysiological mechanisms in different stages of disease severity.

The current therapeutic strategies for the management of patients with cirrhosis are focused on the prevention or treatment of specific clinical complications such as ascites, gastrointestinal bleeding and hepatic encephalopathy [6]. "Etiologic therapy", which is designed to remove the causative agents of the disease (i.e., viruses or alcohol), prevents clinical decompensation in most patients with cirrhosis. In contrast, a significant proportion of patients with decompensated cirrhosis remain at risk of further disease progression despite the application of etiologic treatments. Thus, the identification of new therapies targeting specific key points in the complex pathophysiological cascade of decompensated cirrhosis is urgently needed. These therapies are presented in updated detail in this Special Issue of *JCM* [7]. Poorly absorbable oral antibiotics, statins, and albumin have been proposed as potential disease-modifying agents for cirrhosis (DMAC), since clinical studies have shown their capacity to prolong survival. The ideal DMACs candidate should be

1

directed to modify the key mechanisms in the pathogenetic network of the gut-liver axis, such systemic inflammation, and immune dysfunction.

The development of ascites is one of the typical complications of advanced cirrhosis. Treatment of non-tense ascites comprises the assumption of a combination of furosemide and anti-aldosterone diuretics, accompanied by a restrictive sodium and water diet [6]. Tolvaptan, a selective vasopressin type 2 receptor antagonist, was approved in some countries for treating ascites in patients who responded insufficiently to conventional diuretics. Several still unresolved questions persist regarding both the long-term efficacy of tolvaptan and its effect on the survival of patients with cirrhotic ascites. A recent Japanese retrospective study presented in this issue of *JCM* seems to show that the addition of tolvaptan prolongs the survival of patients with cirrhotic ascites compared to standard diuretic drug combination alone, especially when tolvaptan is started before high-dose furosemide administration [8]. Although these results are encouraging, further prospective studies in different countries must be performed to standardize the use of aquaretic drugs in treating cirrhotic ascites.

More challenging is the treatment of ascites when it reaches the stage of refractoriness. An updated and exhaustive analysis of this topic has been reported in this issue of *JCM*, including the more recent data regarding the placement of a transjugular intrahepatic portosystemic shunt (TIPS) and chronic albumin administration [9]. TIPS reduces portal hypertension, allows greater control of ascites, and in some cases improves the clinical course of the disease. Some concerns persist regarding both the correct selection of patients with ascites who may truly benefit from TIPS and the prevention of cardiac and neurologic complications after TIPS placement in the long term. The effect of long-term human albumin administration in treating grade 2–3 ascites has been studied in the ANSWER [10] and MATCH [11] randomized clinical trials, producing contradictory results. The different results might be at least partially explained by differences in disease severity of the patients enrolled (slightly less severe in the ANSWER trial) and dosage and duration of albumin treatment (higher and longer, respectively, in the ANSWER trial). Regardless, the long-term albumin administration in patients with persistent ascites remains not systematically used in various parts of the world, despite proved effectiveness both in ascites control and long-term survival. The placement of implantable ascites drainage devices has been experimented with contradictory results. To date, there is no clear indication to use these devices except as part of controlled clinical trials.

In addition to ascites, gastrointestinal bleeding and the development of hepatic encephalopathy (HE) represent the other key determinants of the transition from clinically compensated to decompensated liver cirrhosis. Two contributions to the present issue of *JCM* are devoted to exploring these clinical complications of cirrhosis. The most recent advances in the management of esophageal variceal hemorrhage in cirrhotic patients have been updated [12]. These guidelines were derived from the applications of specific treatment algorithms involving the use of indirect measurement of portal pressure (HVPG) and the rescue placement of TIPS, in addition to vasoconstrictors, endoscopic band ligation of esophageal varices and antibiotic prophylaxis. Patients who may benefit more from early rescue TIPS placement are active bleeders with poor predictors of the response to standard medical treatment (Child C class, portal vein thrombosis, HVPG > 20 mmHg, and systolic blood pressure < 100 mmHg at admission). Although the use of preemptive TIPS in these patients has been recommended since the Baveno V consensus [13], only a minority of potential candidates finally undergo a preemptive TIPS. This finding indicates that preemptive TIPS is largely underutilized in real-life practice. This is a topic where it is probably necessary to implement scientific information in the community of hepatologists, in order not to lose the clinical and survival advantages that the correct indication of the positioning of the preemptive TIPS can bring to patients.

HE in cirrhosis has profound implications in terms of the patients' ability to fulfil their family and social roles, to drive and to provide for themselves. The past few years have been characterized by significantly more attention to HE and its implications. Its definition has been refined, and a small number of new drugs or alternative management strategies have become available, while others are underway [14]. Currently, overt HE is generally managed by the correction of any identified precipitating factors and institution of ammonia-lowering treatment with nonabsorbable disaccharides and nonabsorbable antibiotics [15]. Many therapies other than nonabsorbable disaccharides and nonabsorbable antibiotics have been studied. Among them, L-Ornithine L-Aspartate (LOLA), which is a substrate for the urea cycle and increases urea production in peri-portal hepatocytes, has been extensively studied. Despite promising results, a recent review and meta-analysis suggests that the effect of LOLA is comparable to other ammonia-lowering agents in treating HE regardless of clinical severity. The use of nonurea nitrogen scavengers (sodium benzoate, sodium, glycerol phenylbutyrate, and ornithine phenylacetate) has not been shown to be superior to placebo or to standard treatment in clinically improving HE. Muscle loss impacts nitrogen and ammonia metabolism and is associated with an increased risk of HE. Thus, the maintenance of adequate daily energy (35–40 kcal/kg ideal body weight) and protein intake (1.2–1.5 g/kg ideal body weight) has been associated with the improvement of psychometric performance and quality of life and with the reduction in the risk of overt HE development. In addition to small meals consumed throughout the day, a late evening snack comprising complex carbohydrates should be strongly recommended, as they reduce protein catabolism and interrupt the long fast between dinner and breakfast. The postulated efficacy of branched chain amino acids (BCAAs) administration in treating HE is probably a surrogate for an increase in the intake of proteins containing BCAAs, particularly in patients consuming vegetable diets.

If the development of ascites, gastrointestinal bleeding, HE or any combination of these conditions are the distinct features of acute decompensation of liver cirrhosis, acute-on-chronic liver failure (ACLF) is a distinct syndrome that develops in patients with acutely decompensated chronic liver disease and is characterized by a high 28-day mortality rate. Thus, a special article dedicated to ACLF has been presented in this issue of *JCM* [16]. The key elements identifying the appearance of ACLF are the strong association with precipitating factor(s), the development of single- or multiple organ failures (OFs) and an intense systemic inflammation. Excessive inflammation is responsible for tissue damage and for necrotic cell death, leading to the release of damage-associated molecular patterns (DAMPs) that maintain inflammation by binding to pattern-recognition receptors (PRRs). Although many of the pathophysiological mechanisms responsible for the development of ACLF have been elucidated, additional knowledge is needed to develop treatments besides supportive measures for OFs. To date, early liver transplantation (LT) produces good outcomes in a subset of patients presenting grade 3 ACLF, thus these patients must be early referred to a liver transplant center to verify the feasibility of liver transplant.

Due to the availability of direct antiviral agents (DAAs) for curing hepatitis C virus infection [17], the only two major hepatitis viruses are still awaiting a definitive cure are hepatitis B (HBV) and hepatitis D (HDV). More recent advances in treating these viruses have been highlighted in another article presented in this issue of *JCM* [18]. The main endpoint of all current treatment strategies for these chronic infections is the suppression of HBV DNA and HDV RNA for those patients coinfected with HDV. Unfortunately, the profound suppression of viral replication does not translate to an effective and complete cure of HBV or HBV/HDV coinfection. Among the known barriers to achieve a "functional cure", the most worrisome is HBV covalently closed circular DNA (cccDNA), which allows the virus to permanently persist in hepatocytes and against which nucleot(s)ide analogs have little effect. Regarding HDV infection, the ideal goal of treatment is to obtain simultaneously the clearance of HBsAg and a sustained HDV virological suppression, at least 6 months after stopping the treatment. Unfortunately, both aims are still not reachable. Improving knowledge of the structure and replication cycle of both HBV and HDV has facilitated the development of novel antivirals directly targeting multiple steps in virus replication and preventing the synthesis of new cccDNA. Furthermore, immunomodulators may also be needed to reverse the state of tolerance typical of the chronic phase of viral infection and subsequently promote the immune-induced death of infected hepatocytes, which is crucial for the neutralization of circulating virions. New nucleotide analogs in advanced phase of development are besifovir, metacavir and two prodrugs of tenofovir (tenofovir exalidex and tenofovir disoproxil orotate). Other drugs in development are the attachment/entry inhibitors, such as bulevirtide, which acts upon the sodium taurocholate co-transporting polypeptide (NTCP), a receptor of both HBV and HDV. Therefore, this new drug blocks both HBV and HDV entry in the hepatocytes. Bulevirtide was approved in the European Union in July 2020 as the first effective drug for the treatment of chronic HDV in patients with compensated liver disease. In addition to bulevirtide, a further new drug is lonafarnib (LNF), a farnesyl transferase inhibitor that blocks the assembly and secretion of virions in the cell through HDV antigen prenylation. Preliminary data seem to support the combined use of LNF with ritonavir (RTV). Nucleic acid polymers (NAPs), such REP 2139, are under clinical evaluation and produced promising results, as among 12 enrolled patients 7 have become HDV RNA- and 5 hepatitis B surface antigen (HBsAg)-negative, respectively, after a follow-up of 1 year.

Three contributions presented in this issue of *JCM* have been devoted to providing the main updated knowledge regarding the approach to treat patients with hepatocellular carcinoma (HCC) and cholangiocarcinoma (CCA). One article focused on CCA [19], and two focused on HCC [20,21]. CCA is anatomically classified in intrahepatic (iCCA), perihilar (pCCA) and distal (dCCA) CCA. Surgical resection, obtaining negative margins, represents the best curative therapy for CCA. Systemic treatment with cisplatin plus gemcitabine (GEMCIS) is the first-line approach for patients with advanced-stage CCA, but the results are unsatisfactory, with a 5-year survival rate of approximately 5–15%. Targeted therapies, specific molecular profiling and biomarkers are needed to select new effective therapies for each patient with CCA. For example, approximately 15–20% of iCCAs have been observed to contain FGRF2 translocations, which are implicated in promoting cell proliferation and angiogenesis. Thus, several FGFR 1–3 inhibitors (i.e., pemigatinib and infigratinib) are being evaluated in phase III trials involving patients with advanced CCA, and the preliminary results seem to be encouraging. Mutations in epidermal growth factor receptor (EGFR) have a great importance in guiding treatments in different cancers, nevertheless, no evidence of their efficacy against CCA has been demonstrated. Immune checkpoint inhibitors (ICIs), peptide- and dendritic cell-based vaccines, and adoptive cell therapy, are under investigation to treat patients with CCA. Although the use of immunotherapy in patients with CCA is still limited, several clinical trials are currently evaluating the therapeutic properties of anti-CTLA-4 monoclonal antibodies, the targeting of PD-L1 or its receptor, PD-1, as well as chimeric antigen receptor T (CAR-T) cell immunotherapy. Unfortunately, ICI monotherapy has shown insufficient efficacy in patients with CCA. However, a better understanding of immunologically based therapeutic strategies should be reached, before to design a real precision medicine strategy allowing to reduce clinical aggressiveness of the tumor and to improve the prognosis of patients with CCA.

Compared to patients with CCA, very different treatment scenarios are on the horizon for patients with HCC. In addition to the well-known therapeutic options referring to surgical resection or to locoregional treatments of the tumor, a very large quantity of data is expected from new systemic treatments based on the use of ICIs in combination with other agents, among which vascular endothelial growth factor (VEGFR)-targeted therapies generated very encouraging results. Therefore, atezolizumab (a monoclonal antibody against PD-L1) plus bevacizumab (a monoclonal antibody against VEGF) has been approved as the first-line treatment option for advanced HCC, becoming the standard of care for these patients. Immunotherapy-based treatments will increase the landscape of HCC therapy soon. A very attractive first-line treatment modality in patients with intermediate-stage HCC is to combine locoregional treatments with ICIs, since ablative and intraarterial techniques indirectly induce a peripheral immune response that may enhance the effect of ICIs. Both radiofrequency ablation and transarterial chemoembolization induce necrosis of tumor cells, promoting the release of tumor antigens and the activation of immune-mediated death of tumor cells, which in turn stimulates a peripheral systemic immune response that is potentially amplified by the administration of ICIs. In contrast, the survival benefit for patients' candidates for second-line treatment options (regorafenib/cabozantinib or ramucirumab), although significant, is still modest. Thus, nivolumab with or without ipilimumab and pembrolizumab received FDA approval as second-line treatments.

In addition to locoregional and systemic treatments, liver transplantation (LT) remains the better treatment option for a subset of patients with HCC, since the surgical procedure removes both the tumor and the liver at the same time, which remains the potential source of new neoplastic clones. The Milan criteria (MC) were developed more than 25 years ago and are still considered the benchmark for LT in patients with HCC. However, the strict application of MC might exclude some patients who may receive a clinical benefit from LT. Several expanded criteria have been proposed. Some consider pretransplant morphological and biological variables of the tumor, others consider post-LT variables such as the histology of the tumor, and others combine pre- and post-LT variables. More recently, the HCC response to locoregional treatments before transplantation emerged as a surrogate marker of the biological aggressiveness of the tumor to be used as a better selection criterion for LT in patients beyond the MC at presentation. These issues have been comprehensively updated in this *JCM* Special Issue [21] to present new policies that may be applied to better select patients with HCC for LT. The main innovative approach to select patients for LT presenting at baseline beyond the MC is to evaluate the characteristics and the duration of tumor response after locoregional (or systemic) therapies (downstaging treatment) and consider it a surrogate marker of biological HCC aggressiveness and of the risk of recurrence. It is mandatory to assess the success of downstaging treatments, to confirm the absence of tumor progression during an observation period of at least 3 months after treatment. Patients experiencing a successful downstaging are those eligible for LT as they present a less aggressive tumor biology and a better post-LT survival. Thus, the American and European associations for the study of the liver guidelines are concordant in recommending the adoption of locoregional (systemic) treatment procedures in patients with HCC beyond MC at baseline and the consideration of those who achieved successful downstaging for at least 3–6 months as suitable candidates for LT [22,23].

HCC represents approximately 50% of the indications for LT in Europe and the US. Constant indications for LT are decompensated liver cirrhosis due to cholestatic and autoimmune liver diseases, as well as chronic HBV infection. Decompensated cirrhosis due to chronic HCV infection is declining as an indication for LT, while alcohol- and non-alcoholic steato-hepatitis (NASH)-related liver diseases have increased progressively as indications for LT in recent years. In addition to the established indications for LT, clinical conditions historically considered exclusion criteria for LT, such as severe alcoholic hepatitis (AH), acute-on-chronic liver failure (ACLF), colorectal cancer metastases and cholangiocarcinoma, have been considered new indications for LT in recent years, producing promising survival advantages for patients. This topic has been highlighted in a very updated review [24] presented in this issue of *JCM*, where pros and cons for every new potential indication for LT have been critically discussed. Importantly, all newer indications for LT increase the pressure in an already difficult context of organ shortage. Strategies are therefore needed to increase the pool of transplantable organs, aiming to ensure a better balance between new candidate patients and available resources (organs). Moreover, a very challenging issue will be to optimize the patient selection criteria to ensure a clear gain in life expectancy for those who undergo LT, avoiding the increase in waiting list mortality for those patients who continue to await LT. A multidisciplinary transplant team is needed soon to face and solve this very delicate problem. Furthermore, the new scenario of transplants makes it essential to review and standardize ethical considerations across countries to ensure the same treatment options for all patients.

The COVID-19 pandemic has completely disrupted the global landscape of health systems. The repercussions have been highlighted in all sectors and in that of liver diseases. Data regarding the effect of COVID-19 on LT recipients are still scarce and often contradictory. A recent systematic review [25] presented in this issue of *JCM* showed that the COVID-19 clinical outcome of the LT population was not per se worse than that of the general population, although careful management of immunosuppressive therapy may be needed. In this regard, complete therapy discontinuation is not encouraged, but caution is needed in the use of mycophenolate mofetil (MMF), favoring tacrolimus (TAC) use. Anti-SARS-CoV-2 mRNA vaccine immunogenicity appeared to be low in LT patients, despite a booster dose being strongly recommended by the main scientific societies. The newest SARS-CoV-2 variants, such as Omicron, may further reduce vaccine-induced immunogenicity, suggesting that the level of surveillance should remain very high in this population.

A large body of new insights are derived from the collective work presented in this Special Issue of *JCM* entitled "New therapies for liver diseases". All of them should be considered the beginning of a new era in exploring the pathophysiology of liver diseases and the mechanisms inducing cancer transformation of the liver with the help of technology, artificial intelligence and human perspectives. These new insights will promote the development of new and more effective treatments for several liver diseases that will improve quality of life and patient survival. As the Guest Editor of this Special Issue of *JCM*, I would like to express special thanks to the authors for their remarkable contributions and the reviewers for their professional comments. Furthermore, I would like to thank the *JCM* team for their professional and exceptional support that enabled the project to be achieved.

Funding: This research received no external funding.

Conflicts of Interest: The author declares no conflict of interest.

References

1. Arroyo, V.; Angeli, P.; Moreau, R.; Jalan, R.; Claria, J.; Trebicka, J.; Fernandez, J.; Gustot, T.; Caraceni, P.; Bernardi, M.; et al. The systemic inflammation hypothesis: Towards a new paradigm of acute decompensation and multiorgan failure in cirrhosis. *J. Hepatol.* **2021**, *74*, 670–685. [PubMed]
2. Renzulli, M.; Tovoli, F.; Clemente, A.; Ierardi, A.M.; Pettinari, I.; Peta, G.; Marasco, G.; Festi, D.; Piscaglia, F.; Cappabianca, S.; et al. Ablation for hepatocellular carcinoma: Beyond the standard indications. *Med. Oncol.* **2020**, *37*, 23. [PubMed]
3. Cozzi, E.; Schneeberger, S.; Bellini, M.I.; Berglund, E.; Bohmig, G.; Fowler, K.; Hoogduijn, M.; Jochmans, I.; Marckmann, G.; Marson, L.; et al. Organ transplants of the future: Planning for innovations including xenotransplantation. *Transpl. Int.* **2021**, *34*, 2006–2018.
4. Wilde, A.B.; Lieb, C.; Leicht, E.; Greverath, L.M.; Steinhagen, L.M.; Chamorro, N.W.D.; Petersen, J.; Hofmann, W.P.; Hinrichsen, H.; Heyne, R.; et al. Real-World Clinical Management of Patients with Primary Biliary Cholangitis-A Retrospective Multicenter Study from Germany. *J. Clin. Med.* **2021**, *10*, 1061.
5. Mazzetti, M.; Marconi, G.; Mancinelli, M.; Benedetti, A.; Marzioni, M.; Maroni, L. The Management of Cholestatic Liver Diseases: Current Therapies and Emerging New Possibilities. *J. Clin. Med.* **2021**, *10*, 1763.
6. European Association for the Study of the Liver. EASL Clinical Practice Guidelines: The diagnosis and management of patients with primary biliary cholangitis. *J. Hepatol.* **2018**, *69*, 406–460.
7. Zaccherini, G.; Tufoni, M.; Bernardi, M.; Caraceni, P. Prevention of Cirrhosis Complications: Looking for Potential Disease Modifying Agents. *J. Clin. Med.* **2021**, *10*, 4590.
8. Hosui, A.; Tanimoto, T.; Okahara, T.; Ashida, M.; Ohnishi, K.; Wakahara, Y.; Kusumoto, Y.; Yamaguchi, T.; Sueyoshi, Y.; Hirao, M.; et al. Early Administration of Tolvaptan Can Improve Survival in Patients with Cirrhotic Ascites. *J. Clin. Med.* **2021**, *10*, 294.
9. Zaccherini, G.; Tufoni, M.; Iannone, G.; Caraceni, P. Management of Ascites in Patients with Cirrhosis: An Update. *J. Clin. Med.* **2021**, *10*, 5226.
10. Caraceni, P.; Riggio, O.; Angeli, P.; Alessandria, C.; Neri, S.; Foschi, F.G.; Levantesi, F.; Airoldi, A.; Boccia, S.; Svegliati-Baroni, G.; et al. Long-term albumin administration in decompensated cirrhosis (ANSWER): An open-label randomised trial. *Lancet.* **2018**, *391*, 2417–2429.
11. Sola, E.; Sole, C.; Simon-Talero, M.; Martin-Llahi, M.; Castellote, J.; Garcia-Martinez, R.; Moreira, R.; Torrens, M.; Marquez, F.; Fabrellas, N.; et al. Midodrine and albumin for prevention of complications in patients with cirrhosis awaiting liver transplantation. A randomized placebo-controlled trial. *J. Hepatol.* **2018**, *69*, 1250–1259. [PubMed]
12. Zanetto, A.; Shalaby, S.; Feltracco, P.; Gambato, M.; Germani, G.; Russo, F.P.; Burra, P.; Senzolo, M. Recent Advances in the Management of Acute Variceal Hemorrhage. *J. Clin. Med.* **2021**, *10*, 3818. [PubMed]
13. de Franchis, R.; Baveno, V.F. Revising consensus in portal hypertension: Report of the Baveno V consensus workshop on methodology of diagnosis and therapy in portal hypertension. *J. Hepatol.* **2010**, *53*, 762–768. [PubMed]
14. Mangini, C.; Montagnese, S. New Therapies of Liver Diseases: Hepatic Encephalopathy. *J. Clin. Med.* **2021**, *10*, 4050. [PubMed]

15. Vilstrup, H.; Amodio, P.; Bajaj, J.; Cordoba, J.; Ferenci, P.; Mullen, K.D.; Weissenborn, K.; Wong, P. Hepatic encephalopathy in chronic liver disease: 2014 Practice Guideline by the American Association for the Study of Liver Diseases and the European Association for the Study of the Liver. *Hepatology* **2014**, *60*, 715–735. [PubMed]
16. Gambino, C.; Piano, S.; Angeli, P. Acute-on-Chronic Liver Failure in Cirrhosis. *J. Clin. Med.* **2021**, *10*, 4406.
17. Houghton, M. Hepatitis C Virus: 30 Years after Its Discovery. *Cold. Spring. Harb. Perspect. Med.* **2019**, *9*, a037096.
18. Zuccaro, V.; Asperges, E.; Colaneri, M.; Marvulli, L.N.; Bruno, R. HBV and HDV: New Treatments on the Horizon. *J. Clin. Med.* **2021**, *10*, 4054.
19. Vignone, A.; Biancaniello, F.; Casadio, M.; Pesci, L.; Cardinale, V.; Ridola, L.; Alvaro, D. Emerging Therapies for Advanced Cholangiocarcinoma: An Updated Literature Review. *J. Clin. Med.* **2021**, *10*, 4901.
20. Plaz Torres, M.C.; Lai, Q.; Piscaglia, F.; Caturelli, E.; Cabibbo, G.; Biasini, E.; Pelizzaro, F.; Marra, F.; Trevisani, F.; Giannini, E.G. Treatment of Hepatocellular Carcinoma with Immune Checkpoint Inhibitors and Applicability of First-Line Atezolizumab/Bevacizumab in a Real-Life Setting. *J. Clin. Med.* **2021**, *10*, 3021.
21. Toniutto, P.; Fumolo, E.; Fornasiere, E.; Bitetto, D. Liver Transplantation in Patients with Hepatocellular Carcinoma beyond the Milan Criteria: A Comprehensive Review. *J. Clin. Med.* **2021**, *10*, 3932. [PubMed]
22. European Association for the Study of the Liver. EASL Clinical Practice Guidelines: Management of hepatocellular carcinoma. *J. Hepatol.* **2018**, *69*, 182–236.
23. Heimbach, J.K.; Kulik, L.M.; Finn, R.S.; Sirlin, C.B.; Abecassis, M.M.; Roberts, L.R.; Zhu, A.X.; Murad, M.H.; Marrero, J.A. AASLD guidelines for the treatment of hepatocellular carcinoma. *Hepatology* **2018**, *67*, 358–380.
24. Zanetto, A.; Shalaby, S.; Gambato, M.; Germani, G.; Senzolo, M.; Bizzaro, D.; Russo, F.P.; Burra, P. New Indications for Liver Transplantation. *J. Clin. Med.* **2021**, *10*, 3867. [PubMed]
25. Becchetti, C.; Gschwend, S.G.; Dufour, J.F.; Banz, V. COVID-19 in Liver Transplant Recipients: A Systematic Review. *J. Clin. Med.* **2021**, *10*, 4015.

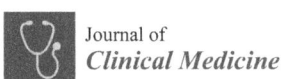

Journal of
Clinical Medicine

Review

The Management of Cholestatic Liver Diseases: Current Therapies and Emerging New Possibilities

Marta Mazzetti [1,2,*], Giulia Marconi [1], Martina Mancinelli [1], Antonio Benedetti [1], Marco Marzioni [1] and Luca Maroni [1]

[1] Clinic of Gastroenterology and Hepatology, Università Politecnica delle Marche, 60126 Ancona, Italy; giuliamarconi90@gmail.com (G.M.); martinamanci@gmail.com (M.M.); antonio.benedetti@ospedaliriuniti.marche.it (A.B.); m.marzioni@staff.univpm.it (M.M.); luca.maroni@live.it (L.M.)

[2] Department of Gastroenterology, Azienda Sanitaria Unica Regionale Marche Area Vasta 3, 62100 Macerata, Italy

* Correspondence: marta.mazzetti@virgilio.it

Abstract: Primary biliary cholangitis (PBC) and primary sclerosing cholangitis (PSC) are two chronic cholestatic liver diseases affecting bile ducts that may progress to biliary cirrhosis. In the past few years, the increasing knowledge in the pathogenesis of both diseases led to a growing number of clinical trials and possible new targets for therapy. In this review, we provide an update on the treatments in clinical use and summarize the new drugs in trials for PBC and PSC patients. Farnesoid X Receptor (FXR) agonists and Pan-Peroxisome Proliferator-Activated Receptor (PPAR) agonists are the most promising agents and have shown promising results in both PBC and PSC. Fibroblast Growth Factor 19 (FGF19) analogues also showed good results, especially in PBC, while, although PBC and PSC are autoimmune diseases, immunosuppressive drugs had disappointing effects. Since the gut microbiome could have a potential role in the pathogenesis of PSC, recent research focused on molecules that could change the microbiome, with good results. The near future of the medical management of these diseases may include new treatments or a combination of multiple drugs targeting different signaling pathways at different stages of the diseases.

Keywords: primary biliary cholangitis (PBC); primary sclerosing cholangitis (PSC); clinical trials; ursodeoxycholic acid (UDCA); Farnesoid X Receptor (FXR) agonist; Pan-Peroxisome Proliferator-Activated Receptor (PPAR) agonists

Citation: Mazzetti, M.; Marconi, G.; Mancinelli, M.; Benedetti, A.; Marzioni, M.; Maroni, L. The Management of Cholestatic Liver Diseases: Current Therapies and Emerging New Possibilities. *J. Clin. Med.* **2021**, *10*, 1763. https://doi.org/10.3390/jcm10081763

Academic Editor: Pierluigi Toniutto

Received: 21 March 2021
Accepted: 15 April 2021
Published: 18 April 2021

Publisher's Note: MDPI stays neutral with regard to jurisdictional claims in published maps and institutional affiliations.

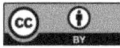

Copyright: © 2021 by the authors. Licensee MDPI, Basel, Switzerland. This article is an open access article distributed under the terms and conditions of the Creative Commons Attribution (CC BY) license (https://creativecommons.org/licenses/by/4.0/).

1. Introduction

Primary biliary cholangitis (PBC) and primary sclerosing cholangitis (PSC) are two chronic inflammatory autoimmune diseases of the bile ducts, which could culminate in biliary cirrhosis. Very few treatment options were available for decades, but in the past years many new targets and therapies were investigated, and clinical trials were performed.

The aim of this review is to provide an update on new targets and novel therapies that may change the management of these diseases in the near future.

2. Primary Biliary Cholangitis

PBC is a chronic autoimmune cholestatic liver disease that predominantly affects women. It is characterized by cholestasis, serologic reactivity to antimitochondrial antibodies (AMA) or to specific antinuclear antibodies (ANA) such as Sp100 and Gp210, and histologic evidence of chronic non-suppurative, granulomatous, lymphocytic small bile duct cholangitis. Many aspects of the aetiology and the pathogenesis of the disease are still uncertain, and the disease is often progressive, resulting in chronic cholestasis and possibly cirrhosis [1,2]. The main treatment goals include the prevention of the progression of the disease and the management of the symptoms, which may have a strong negative impact

9

on the quality of life of patients. The only two medications approved by the Food and Drug Administration (FDA) are ursodeoxycholic acid (UDCA) and obeticholic acid (OCA). However, over the past years, given the strong support of randomized clinical studies, new therapies entered into the clinical practice of many experts in the field. Moreover, others molecules are actively being investigated in different clinical trials with promising results [3]. In this section, we are going to review the principal drugs in clinical use, in clinical trial, an in a preclinical phase for PBC.

2.1. Therapies in Clinical Use

2.1.1. UDCA

UDCA, at a dosage of 13–15 mg/kg/day, is the first-line treatment for PBC [1]. It is the 7-β epimer of the chenodeoxycholic acid, a human bile acid. The complex mechanisms of action of UDCA and the evidence for its clinical use are extensively reviewed elsewhere [2,4]. Several molecular mechanisms contribute to the beneficial effect of UDCA in PBC patients. Indeed, many studies have shown that UDCA has anti-cholestatic effects due to complex post-transcriptional molecular mechanisms, a cytoprotective property, thanks to its action on endoplasmic reticulum stress, and an anti-inflammatory activity, inhibiting prostaglandin E2 [5]. UDCA administration also makes the endogenous bile acid pool more hydrophilic, and it improves therefore the biliary bicarbonate ($HCO3^-$) umbrella, which is thought to create a protective layer on the apical surface of cholangiocytes against the permeation of protonated bile acids [6]. Moreover, UDCA interferes with the pathogenesis of autoimmune diseases by decreasing the expression of Major Histocompatibility Complex (MHC) class I and class II, the eosinophil levels in blood, and the immune reaction against PAMPs [7]. The administration of UDCA in PBC patients induces a reduction in markers of cholestasis, IgM, and AMA level [8]; improves liver histology [9]; and decreases mortality, especially when started at early stage [10]. Unfortunately, one-third of the patients have an inadequate response to UDCA treatment, defined according to several scoring systems, including the Barcelona, Paris I, Paris II, Rotterdam, Toronto, Ehime, GLOBE, and UK-PBC scoring systems [1]. Recently, the UDCA Response Score (URS), calculated with pre-treatment parameters, was used to predict the UDCA response [11]. A lower probability of UDCA response was significantly associated with a higher level of ALP ($p < 0.0001$), higher levels of total bilirubin ($p = 0.0003$), lower aminotransferase concentration ($p = 0.0012$), younger age ($p < 0.0001$), longer gap from diagnosis to UDCA treatment ($p < 0.0001$), and worsening of ALP from diagnosis ($p < 0.0001$). Based on these variables, the score reached an area under the receiver operating characteristic curve of 0.83 in predicting UDCA response. Other factors that contribute to the response to treatment are male sex [12], PBC-specific ANA positivity [1], and histology [11].

2.1.2. Steroidal FXR Agonist: Obethicolic Acid (OCA)

OCA is an analogue of chenodeoxycholic acid (CDCA), with the addition of an ethyl group which gives a strong affinity for the nuclear farnesoid X receptor (FXR). FXR is the primary regulator of bile acid homeostasis, thanks to its effect on reducing production and reabsorption and increasing excretion [13]. After the good results of two phase II studies and one phase III clinical trial (POISE), in October 2016, OCA reached the EMA authorization for PBC treatment. The POISE study was a 12-month, double-blind, randomized, placebo-controlled phase III trial, evaluating 216 patients. The study included three treatment arms: OCA 10 mg ± UDCA, titration arm (OCA 5 mg ± UDCA for six months and then OCA 10 mg for the following six months), and placebo ± UDCA. The primary endpoint (i.e., ALP < 1.67 together with ALP reduction of at least 15% from baseline and normalization in total bilirubin) was reached by 46% and 47% of patients in the 5–10 mg and 10 mg OCA arms, respectively, and by 10% in the placebo group. Treatment arms also had a reduction in ALP, AST, and GGT that reached their lowest levels after three months of treatment and were maintained up to 48 months. The main adverse event was pruritus, which caused the study interruption for 7 out of 73 patients in the

OCA 10 mg group, and in 1 out of 70 in the titration arm. Concerning the lipid profile, a transient increase in LDL and a decrease in HDL, VLDL, total cholesterol, and triglycerides were detected [14,15]. The long-term efficacy and safety of OCA for PBC patients who are intolerant to UDCA or have an inadequate response to UDCA were confirmed in the three-year interim analysis of the five-year open-label extension of the pivotal phase 3 POISE trial [16]. Moreover, a sub-analysis of data from the POISE study showed that OCA treatment was associated with improvement or stabilization of histological features of the disease (ductular injury, fibrosis, and collagen deposition), but final analyses of fibrosis-related endpoints are ongoing [17]. OCA monotherapy (10 mg and 50 mg) was also studied in a double-blind, placebo-controlled phase 2 study in patients with PBC. After three months, a significant decrease in ALP was observed in both of the groups, and a similar effect was detected through six years of open-label extension treatment [18]. Thus, OCA is recommended by international guidelines as a first-line therapy in patients who are intolerant to UDCA, and as a second-line therapy in addition to UDCA in patients with an incomplete response to UDCA. Of note, special attention should be paid in cirrhotic patients. In fact, severe liver injury or death was reported in patients treated with incorrectly high doses, and the FDA has issued a Black Box Warning for OCA. Guidelines recommend starting OCA at a dose of 5 mg weekly (with a maximum dose of 10 mg twice weekly) in Child Pugh B or C cirrhotic patients, and to use caution in Child Pugh A patients [1,19,20].

2.1.3. PPARs Agonist: Bezafibrate

Bezafibrate is a pan-peroxisome proliferator-activated receptor (PPAR) agonist and, in combination with UDCA, was demonstrated to have a potent activity in PBC due to its specific anticholestatic properties. PPARs are nuclear receptors regulating the transcription of genes involved in metabolic pathways and inflammation. They exist in three isotypes (PPAR-α, PPAR-γ, and PPAR-β/δ), with different tissue distributions and actions. PPARα are mainly expressed in hepatocytes, where they stimulate multidrug resistance protein 3 (MDR3) expression, which protects cholangiocytes against bile salt due to its effect on phosphatidylcholine secretion [21]. Moreover, PPARα has an anti-inflammatory action that is based on trans-repression of AP1 and NF-kB signaling, transcription factors responsible for the expression of many genes involved in inflammation, oncogenesis, and apoptosis [2]. PPARβ/δ, specifically expressed in hepatocytes, cholangiocytes, Kupffer cells, and hepatic stellate cells, plays a role in the progression of PBC due to its anti-inflammatory effects. PPARδ is also involved in the transport and the absorption of bile components [22]. PPAR-γ, expressed in Kupffer cells, has anti-inflammatory activity, and its agonist is proved to reduce portal inflammation in murine models of PBC [23]. Bezafibrate was evaluated in the BEZURSO trial, a two-month, double-blind, randomized, placebo-controlled phase 3 trial, in which the combination of UDCA and bezafibrate 400 mg was compared with UDCA and placebo in 100 patients who had an inadequate response to UDCA according to the Paris 2 criteria. The primary endpoint of the study was a complete biochemical normalization at 24 months. Interesting, the primary endpoint was achieved by 37% of patients treated with bezafibrate and 0% of patients in the control group. Moreover, 67% of the patients treated with bezafibrate reported a normalization of ALP, compared to 2% in the placebo group. Itch improved in almost one-third of patients. Histologic data were too limited to determine whether bezafibrate had a role in the reduction of liver fibrosis and hepatic inflammation; however, a significant decrease in liver stiffness and Enhanced Liver Fibrosis score was observed. With the exception of the well-known side effects of fibrates (myalgias and increases in creatinine and transaminases), no statistical differences regarding adverse events between the two groups were observed. As a precaution, bezafibrate should be administered with caution in patients at risk for chronic kidney disease (e.g., diabetes, hypertension, or established renal disease) [24]. Moreover, another study on PBC patients with a suboptimal response to UDCA proved that a long-term treatment with UDCA and bezafibrate has an excellent effect on pruritus. As a matter of fact, after a median of

38 months, all but one patient reported a partial or complete itching relief, and a recurrence or worsening of pruritus was observed after bezafibrate discontinuation [25].

Fenofibrate is another PPARα-agonist, and it was also studied in PBC patients. A retrospective study on patients treated with UDCA and fenofibrate, compared with patients treated only with UDCA, proved that the fenofibrate-treated group had a significant improvement in the biochemical parameters, in particular ALP and ALT [26]. The same effect on ALP was demonstrated in another retrospective study on PBC patients with a suboptimal response to UDCA treated with fenofibrate and UDCA [27], but more studies and randomized controlled trials are needed to understand its role in PBC.

2.1.4. Corticosteroid: Budesonide

Budesonide is a potent synthetic corticosteroid with a high first-pass metabolism within the liver, resulting in few systemic side effects compared to other systemic steroids. It is an agonist of the nuclear glucocorticoid receptor (GR) and pregnane X receptor (PXR). Budesonide and UDCA have a synergic activity in increasing the expression of the biliary chloride/bicarbonate anion exchanger 2 (AE2) with the result of an increase in biliary secretion of bicarbonate and stabilization of the biliary bicarbonate umbrella [3]. Previous studies showed that budesonide improves liver histology and biochemistry in PBC patients with interface hepatitis on biopsy [28,29]. In contrast, in a recent three-year phase-III, double-blind, randomized trial comparing budesonide vs. placebo, patients treated with UDCA showed that budesonide combined with UDCA was not associated with an improvement in liver histology in patients with PBC and an inadequate response to UDCA. It is important to mention that the study was underpowered for the evaluation of the liver histology due to challenges in patient recruitment. Improvements in biochemical markers of disease activity were demonstrated in secondary analyses [30]. Budesonide should be avoided in cirrhotic patients because of the increased risk of portal vein thrombosis and uncontrolled systemic shunting of the drug [31].

2.2. Therapies Evaluated in Clinical Trials

The main aspects of the clinical trials are described in Table 1.

Table 1. Principal characteristics of the study of the drugs in clinical trials.

	Study	Phase	Pt Number	Dose	Study Duration	Primary Endpoint	Primary Endpoint Met	Note
Non-Bile Acids FXR agonists (*drugs*)								
Cilofexor	[32]	2	71	30 mg, 100 mg	12 weeks	Safety and tolerability of Cilofexor	yes	
Tropifexor	[33]	2	61	30 μg, 60 μg, 90 μg	12 weeks	Change in GGT in 4 weeks	yes	at interim analysis
EDP-305	NCT03394924	2	68	Dose 1 dose 2	12 weeks	20% reduction in ALP or normalization of ALP in 12 weeks	n/a	ongoing

Table 1. *Cont.*

	Study	Phase	Pt Number	Dose	Study Duration	Primary Endpoint	Primary Endpoint Met	Note
PPAR agonists (*drugs*)								
Seladelpar	[34]	2	70	50 mg, 200 mg	12 weeks	Change in ALP		Early stopped (grade 3 increases in ALT)
	[35]	2		5 mg, 10 mg	12 weeks	Change in ALP	yes	
	NCT02955602	2	119	2 mg, 5 mg, 10 mg	8 weeks with 44 weeks extension	Change in ALP	n/a	ongoing
	NCT03602560 (EN-HANCE)	3	240 *	5–10 mg, 10 mg	52 weeks	Change in ALP and bilirubin		suspended (interface hepatits)
Elafibranor	[36]	2	45	80 mg, 120 mg	12 weeks	Change in ALP	yes	
Fibroblast growth factor 19 (FGF19) analogues (*drugs*)								
NGM282	[37]	2	45	0.3 mg, 3 mg	28 days	Change in ALP	yes	
Antifibrotic agent (*drugs*)								
Setanaxib	[38]	2	111	400 mg od/bd	24 weeks	Change in GGT	yes	at interim analysis
Immunomodulatory Strategies (*drugs*)								
Rituximab	[39]	Open label	6	1 g (2 doses)	52 weeks	Reduction in ALP, IgM and AMA after 36 week		
	[40]	Open label	14	1 g (2 doses)	6 months	Normalization or ALP < 25% from baseline	no	
	[41]	2	57	1 g (2 doses)	12 months	Fatigue (PBC 40)	no	
Ustekimumab	[42]	Open label	20	90 mg	28 weeks	ALP < 40% from baseline	no	
Abataceb	[43]	Open label	16	125 mg	24 weeks	ALP normalization or <40% from baseline	no	
Baricitinib	NCT03742973	2	2	2 mg, 4 mg	12 weeks	Change in ALP	no	Enrollment futility
FFP104	NCT02193360	1/2	24 (estimated)	1 mg/kg, 2.5 mg/kg, 2 mg/kg ev	12 weeks	Safety and tolerability	n/a	Recruitment status unknown
E6011	NCT03092765	2	29	High or low dose	64 weeks	ALP change at week 12	n/a	Terminated
Etrasimod	NCT03155932	Open label	2		24 weeks	ALP change	n/a	ongoing
Other treatment								
S-adenosyl-L-methionine	[44]	Open label	24	1.2 g	6 months	PBC 40 improvement	yes	significant decrease of ALP in non-cirrhotic patients

* estimated.

2.2.1. Non-Bile Acids FXR Agonists

Many FXR non-steroid agonists were investigated in PBC.

Cilofexor, a synthetic nonsteroidal FXR ligand, is involved in the transcriptional regulation of genes that play a role in bile acid metabolism. Cilofexor was tested in a phase 2 placebo-controlled, 12-week study on PBC patients. Cilofexor 100 led to a decrease in ALP (median reduction −13.8%; $p = 0.005$ vs. placebo), in GGT (−47.7%; $p < 0.001$), in ALT (−17.8%, $p = 0.08$), and in C-reactive protein (CRP; −33.6%, $p = 0.03$). Unfortunately, grade 2–3 pruritus occurred in 39% of the patients treated with Cilofexor 100 mg, compared with 10% in Cilofexor 30 mg and in 8% of patients treated with placebo. Pruritus led also to treatment discontinuation in 7% of patients on Cilofexor 100 mg [32].

Tropifexor (LJN452) is a non-bile acid FXR agonist investigated in a double-blind, randomized, placebo-controlled, phase 2 study ("A Multi-part, Double Blind Study to Assess Safety, Tolerability and Efficacy of Tropifexor (LJN452) in PBC Patients", NCT02516605) that evaluated the safety and the efficacy of different doses of Tropifexor (30 μg, 60 μg, and 90 μg) in patients with an inadequate response to UDCA [33]. As opposed to OCA, Tropifexor should not have major effects on the lipid profile, being a non-steroidal molecule. To elude the confounding effect of ALP gene induction mediated by FXR, the endpoint of this trial was set on the reduction in GGT levels. After four weeks, interim analysis showed a dose-dependent reduction in GGT, ALP, and hepatocellular damage (ALT). Therefore, this study indicates the potential benefit of Tropifexor in PBC, and further studies are warranted [45].

EDP-305 is another FXR agonist that was evaluated in PBC because of its antifibrotic effect in animal models [46]. A phase 2 double-blind, placebo-controlled trial assessing the safety, pharmacokinetics, and efficacy in patients with PBC and inadequate response or intolerance to UDCA was just completed ("A Study to Assess the Safety, Tolerability, Pharmacokinetics and Efficacy of EDP-305 in Subjects With Primary Biliary Cholangitis", NCT03394924). In the intent-to-treat analysis recently announced, EDP-305 did not meet the primary endpoint as defined by at least a 20% reduction in ALP, but key secondary endpoints (changes in ALT, AST, and GGT compared with placebo) at week 12 were reached in both the EDP-305 1 mg arm and the 2.5 mg arm.

2.2.2. PPAR Agonists

Seladelpar is a new selective agonist of the PPARδ receptor, which has an anti-inflammatory and choleretic activity. The first phase 2 clinical trial that investigated the effect in PBC patients nonresponsive to UDCA was prematurely terminated because of the occurrence of a reversible grade 3 increase in transaminase levels in three patients [34]. A new phase 2 study evaluating a lower dose of Seladelpar (5 mg and 10 mg) was recently performed. The 12-week interim results, first published at the AASLD Liver Meeting in 2017, showed a drop in ALP in 45% and 82% of patients in the 5 mg group and 10 mg group, respectively, and a normalization of ALP in 12% of the 5 mg group and 45% of the 10 mg group, respectively [35]. Given the promising results of the interim analysis, another clinical trial evaluating the efficacy and the safety of Seladelpar 2 mg, 5 mg, and 10 mg is ongoing (NCT02955602). Finally, at the end of 2018, the ENHANCE trial started. It was a 52-week, double-blind, placebo-controlled, randomized phase 3 study that included subjects with PBC and an inadequate response to UDCA or intolerance to UDCA ("ENHANCE: Seladelpar in Subjects With Primary Biliary Cholangitis (PBC) and an Inadequate Response to or an Intolerance to Ursodeoxycholic Acid (UDCA)", NCT03602560) [45]. Unfortunately, the open-label extension phase of this study was suspended after the onset of a similar trial evaluating the role of Seladelpar in NASH that found the occurrence of interface hepatitis in histological specimens. However, an independent panel of expert hepatologists and pathologists deemed that study-stopping was not warranted, since liver injury was within the expected changes seen in NASH patients and could not be attributed to Seladelpar. Recruitment has therefore restarted for Seadelpar in PBC patients after being put on hold. The phase 3 RESPONSE trial (NCT04620733) is currently recruiting patients.

Elafibranor, a dual PPAR-α/δ agonist, also studied in non-alcoholic steatohepatitis (NASH) [47], was recently tested in a multicenter, randomized, double-blind, placebo-controlled phase 2 study clinical trial recruiting patients with PBC non-responders to UDCA. Data were discussed at the International Liver Congress in Vienna in April 2019 [36]. Forty-five patients were randomized into three arms: Elafibranor 80 mg, Elafibranor 120 mg, and placebo. After 12 weeks of treatment, a reduction in ALP from baseline was observed in 48% patients in the 80 mg group and in 41% in the 120 mg arm; an increase of 3% was detected with placebo. Moreover, 67% patients in the 80 mg group ($p = 0.001$) and 79% of patients in the 120 mg group ($p < 0.001$) reached the secondary endpoint (serum ALP < 1.67 ULN, ALP decrease > 15%, total bilirubin < ULN) (NCT03124108). Thus, in July 2019, the USA FDA and the European Medicines Agency approved Orphan Drug Designation to Elafibranor for the treatment of PBC [48].

2.2.3. Fibroblast Growth Factor 19 (FGF19) Analogues

FGF19 acts as a hormone on a cell surface receptor complex in hepatocytes, decreasing bile acid synthesis, gluconeogenesis, and lipogenesis. FGF19 expression is induced by bile-acid-mediated activation of FXR in the gut [49], and it reaches the liver through portal circulation. In the liver, FGF19 suppresses bile acid synthesis due to the inhibition of cholesterol 7-α-hydroxylase (CYP7A1) and sterol 12-α-hydroxylase (CYP8B1). Moreover, FXR decreases hepatic fibrogenesis by reducing collagen and by increasing matrix metalloprotease activity in hepatic stellate cells [50].

NGM282 (Aldafermin), an engineered analogue of FGF19, was tested in a 28-day, double-blind, placebo-controlled phase 2 trial. Forty-five PBC patients with an inadequate response to UDCA were treated with subcutaneous daily doses of NGM282 at 0.3 mg (n = 14), 3 mg (n = 16), or placebo (n = 15). ALP level had a significant drop in the treatment group, as well as transaminase levels and markers of cholestasis, hepatocellular injury, and inflammation (IgM levels). The reduction in complement component 4 (C4) levels suggests that NGM282 acts with a direct inhibition in the de-novo bile acid synthesis through the classical pathway. The main adverse effect was diarrhea. No effect on itch was detected [37]. In contrast to FGF19, no increase in liver cancer risk was observed in animal models treated with NGM282 [51]. Longer studies are needed to evaluate the long-term efficacy and safety of this molecule.

2.2.4. Antifibrotic Agent

Setanaxib (GKT137831) is an inhibitor of Nicotinamide Adenine Dinucleotide Phosphate (NADPH) oxidases isoforms 1 and 4. NADPH oxidase enzymes, generating reactive species of oxygen, play a central role in inflammation and stellate cell-mediated fibrogenesis [52]. It was demonstrated in animal models of acute biliary injury and steatohepatitis that GKT137831 reduces hepatocyte apoptosis and liver fibrosis [53]. Thus, a multicenter, randomized, double-blind, placebo-controlled phase 2 study evaluating the safety and the efficacy of GKT137831 OD or BID in 111 patients with PBC and incomplete response to UDCA was performed (NCT03226067). Interim analysis showed a reduction in GGT and ALP level in six weeks, without a significant concomitant adverse event. A decrease in GGT of 7%, 12%, and 23% were observed in the placebo, 400 mg OD, and 400 mg BID groups, respectively ($p < 0.01$ for 400 mg BID vs. placebo). A greater GGT reduction was reached in patients with more advanced disease (GGT $\geq$ 2.5 X ULN at baseline). Changes in ALP were statistically significant in the 400 mg BID versus placebo [38].

2.2.5. Immunomodulatory Strategies

Since PBC is an autoimmune condition characterized by anti-mitochondrial autoantibodies (AMA) and high levels of immunoglobulin M (IgM), many immunosuppressive drugs were studied in PBC, including corticosteroid [54], azathioprine [55], cyclosporine [56], methotrexate [57], and mycophenolate mofetil [58]. However, results were consistently unsatisfactory. Recently, other molecules were studied in PBC.

Rituximab, an anti-CD20 antibody currently used in lymphomas and autoimmune syndromes, was evaluated in PBC due to its promising results in murine models of autoimmune cholangitis [58]. Three clinical trials in PBC patients with an incomplete response to UDCA were reported. In an open label study, Rituximab (two doses of 1000 mg) induced a decrease in AMA and IgM levels, with only a marginal reduction of ALP after 36 weeks [39]. Unfortunately, a similar study including 14 PBC patients showed a significant but only transitory reduction in ALP [40]. Finally, Rituximab was demonstrated not to have an impact on fatigue, assessed by PBC-40 [41].

Ustekinumab is an anti-interleukin (IL)-12/23 monoclonal antibody commonly used in several autoimmune syndromes and inflammatory bowel diseases (IBD). IL-12 and IL-23-mediated Th1/Th17 signaling pathways play a role in the etiopathogenesis of PBC [59]. Unfortunately, a multicenter open label trial did not reach the primary endpoint of reduction in ALP of 40% from the baseline. However, at week 24, a statistically significant decrease of 12.1% in ALP from baseline was observed [42].

Abatacept is a Cytotoxic T-Lymphocyte Antigen 4 IgG antibody used in rheumatoid and psoriatic arthritis. An open-label, 24-week trial was performed in PBC patients, but no significant changes in biochemical enzymes were observed [43].

The efficacy of Baricitinib (LY3009104), a reversible inhibitor of Janus kinase 1 (JAK1) and JAK2 currently used in rheumatoid arthritis, is currently being evaluated in an ongoing, placebo controlled phase 2 trial (NCT03742973) [45].

Other types of molecules are undergoing clinical evaluation in phase 1 and phase 2 trials: FFP104 blocks the CD40/CD40L interaction between CD4+ T helper lymphocytes and B cells that are involved in the pathogenesis of PBC (NCT02193360) [60]; E6011 is an anti-chemokine-adhesion molecule CX3CL1 (fractalkine) antibody, which is elevated in the serum of PBC patients (NCT03092765); Etrasimod is a selective sphingosine-1-phosphate (S1P) receptor (S1PR) modulator targeting S1P receptor subtypes 1, 4, and 5, leading to an inhibition of activated lymphocytes from migrating to sites of inflammation (NCT03155932) [3].

2.2.6. Other Treatment

S-adenosyl-L-methionine, added to UDCA in non-cirrhotic PBC patients, was demonstrated to have a positive effect on markers of cholestasis and quality of life, probably due to its hepatoprotective effects [44]. In this open label on 24 PBC patients, there was a significant decrease of ALP, GGT, and total cholesterol over a period of six months. A significant improvement of fatigue and pruritus on the PBC-40 questionnaire was also observed.

2.3. Therapies Evaluated in Pre-Clinical Studies

24-norursodeoxycholic acid (norUDCA) differs from UDCA due to the resistance in conjugation with taurine or glycine. NorUDCA increases the cholehepatic shunt of bile salts, leading to a supra-physiological secretion of bicarbonate. NorUDCA showed promising results in the treatment of PSC [61], but its efficacy in PBC has yet to be clarified. Up to now, improvements in fibrosis and inflammation were demonstrated in preclinical studies on animal model with cholestatic liver diseases [2].

Na+ -Taurocholate Cotransporting Polypeptide (NTCP) is a hepatocellular uptake transporter of bile salts, and its inhibition by myrcludex B results in hepatoprotective effects, increasing the biliary phospholipid/bile salt ratio. In 3.5-diethoxycarbonyl-1.4-dihydrocollidine-fed mice, a murine model of cholestasis, and in Atp8b1-G308V mice, used for chronic cholestasis, bile salt levels increased in treated animals from 604 ± 277 to 1746 ± 719 μm and from 432 ± 280 to 762 ± 288 μm, respectively, while phospholipid output was maintained, resulting in a higher phospholipid/bile salt ratio. Thus, it may be beneficial in some forms of cholestasis, but further studies need to be performed [62].

3. Primary Sclerosing Cholangitis

Primary sclerosing cholangitis (PSC) is a chronic bile duct disease with a prevalence of 1–16 per 100,000. PSC is more common in men (comprising 60–70% of patients) and is reported more frequently in Northern European countries and in North America. Moreover, 70% of the patients have ulcerative colitis [63]. The diagnosis is based on a combination of clinical, laboratory, imaging, and histological factors. Endoscopic retrograde cholangiopancreatography (ERCP) plays a very limited role in the diagnosis of PSC, while it may be used for the treatment of dominant stenosis [64]. It is well-known that patients affected by PSC have a higher risk of cholangiocarcinoma and gallbladder cancer. Up to now, no pharmacological treatment is universally approved for PSC. The lack of a clear pathogenesis and the absence of consistent endpoints have contributed to the difficulties in unravelling novel molecular targets and in designing effective clinical trials for PSC treatment [45]. The principal promising treatments and ongoing trials will be summarized in this section.

3.1. Therapies in Clinical Use
UDCA

The use of UDCA in PSC patients remains controversial to date. Previous small and uncontrolled studies of short duration consistently reported an improvement in liver tests in PSC treated with UDCA [65,66]. The first randomized controlled trial of UDCA (13 to 15 mg/kg) in PSC patients appeared in 1992. Beuers et al. showed a significant improvement of biochemical parameters, such as bilirubin, ALP, GGT, and transaminases, in six PSC patients treated for one year as compared to placebo [67]. A number of subsequent studies evaluated the effect of UDCA at different dosages in PSC. Despite the amelioration of biochemical parameters that appears to be relatively constant in all studies, definite proof for an improvement in "hard endpoints" such as survival, liver transplantation, or progression to CCA is still lacking. In a small cohort of 26 PSC patients, Mitchell et al. reported beneficial effects of UDCA (20 mg/kg) not only on liver tests but also on the cholagiographic appearance of the biliary tree evaluated by ERCP and liver fibrosis [68]. A subsequent randomized controlled trial in 219 PSC patients treated with UDCA (17 to 23 mg/kg) or placebo failed to show a significant improvement in the combined endpoint "death or liver transplantation", despite a trend to a reduction in both (31% and 34% reduction, respectively) [69]. Moreover, high doses of UDCA in the range of 28–30 mg/kg were shown to be associated with an increased risk of disease progression to cirrhosis, development of varices, CCA, liver transplantation, or death [70]. Unfortunately, three meta-analyses also failed to show an effect of UDCA on mortality or liver transplantation [71–73]. To date, the most recent guidelines by the British Society of Gastroenterology recommend not to treat newly diagnosed PSC patients with UDCA routinely [74].

3.2. Therapies Evaluated in Clinical Trials

The principal characteristics of the clinical trials are described in Table 2.

Table 2. Principal characteristics of the study of the drugs in clinical trials.

	Study	Phase	Pt Number	Dose	Study Duration	Primary Endpoint	Primary Endpoint Met	Note
24-norursodeoxycholic acid (norUDCA)	[61]	2	161	500 mg, 1 g, 1.5 gr	16 weeks	Change in ALP	yes	
	NCT03872921	3	300 *	250 mg 6 cps/d	2 years	Change in ALP and histology	n/a	ongoing
FXR agonist (drugs)								
OCA	[75]	2	77	1.5–3 mg 5–10 mg	24 weeks	Change in ALP	yes	5–10 mg

Table 2. *Cont.*

	Study	Phase	Pt Number	Dose	Study Duration	Primary Endpoint	Primary Endpoint Met	Note
Cilofexor	[76]	2	52	100 mg 30 mg	12 weeks	Safety and liver enzyme improve-ment	yes	
NGM282	[77]	2	62	1 mg 3 mg	12 weeks	Change in ALP	no	
ATRA	[78]	Pilot study	15	45 mg/m/d	12 weeks	ALP < 30% from baseline	no	Decrease in ALT and C4
	NCT03359174	2	2	10 mg bd	24 weeks	Change in ALP	n/a	ongoing
PPAR agonists								
Bezafibrates	[79]	2	11	200 mg BID	12 weeks	improvements in liver function test	yes	
Bezafibrates	[79]	2	11	200 mg BID	12 weeks	improvements in liver function test	yes	
Antifibrotic therapy (drugs)								
Simtuzumab	[80]	2	234	75 mg, 125 mg	96 weeks	Hepaticcollagencontento		
Immunomodulator (drugs)								
Timolumab	NCT02239211	2	23	8 mg/kg	11 weeks	ALP < 25% from baseline	n/a	Awaiting results
Cenicriviroc	NCT02653625	Open label	24	150 mg	24 weeks	Change in ALP	yes	
Vedolizumab	[81]	Retrospective	102		412 days (median)		no	ALP < 20% from baseline
Vidofludimus	NCT03722576	2	14	30 mg	6 months	Change in ALP	n/a	Awaiting results
Modulation of gut microbioma (drugs)								
Vancomycin	NCT03710122	2/3	102 *		24 months	Change in ALP	n/a	ongoing
Rifaximin	[82]	Open label	16	550 mg bd	12 weeks	Change in ALP	no	
Minocycline	[83]	Pilot study	16	100 mg bd	1 year	Change in biochemistry	yes	
FMT	[84]	Open label	10		24 weeks	safety	yes	
Other treatments (drugs)								
Sulfasalazine	NCT03561584	2	42	500 mg bd	14 weeks	Change in ALP	n/a	ongoing
Curcumin	[85]	Open label	258	750 mg bd	12 weeks	ALP < 1.5 ULN or <40% from baseline	no	
HTD1801	NCT03333928	2	59	500 mg 1 gr	18 weeks	Change in ALP	n/a	Awaiting results

Table 2. *Cont.*

	Study	Phase	Pt Number	Dose	Study Duration	Primary Endpoint	Primary Endpoint Met	Note
DUR-928	NCT03394781	2	5	10 mg 50 mg	28 days	Change in ALP	n/a	ongoing
Docosahexaenoic acid	[86]	Open label	23	800 mg bd	12 months	Change in ALP and safety	yes	
Hymecromone	NCT02780752	1	18 *	1.2 gr 2.4 gr 3.6 gr	4 days	Change in spu	n/a	ongoing
Orbcel-C	NCT02997878	2	56 *	0.5, 1.0, 2.5 million cells/kg	56 days	Safety, change in ALP e ALT	n/a	ongoing

* estimated.

3.2.1. 24-Norursodeoxycholic Acid (norUDCA)

24-norursodeoxycholic acid (norUDCA) has a molecular structure similar to UDCA, except for the lack of a methylene group, resulting in a resistance to conjugation. NorUDCA is therefore passively absorbed from cholangiocytes and goes through cholehepatic shunt, which leads to the stimulation of a bicarbonate-rich choleresis. Moreover, norUDCA has anti-lipotoxic, anti-proliferative, anti-fibrotic, and anti-inflammatory effects, and, in vitro, it is less toxic than UDCA for hepatocytes and cholangiocytes due to its hydrophilicity [2]. A phase 2 clinical trial on 161 PSC patients without concomitant UDCA therapy, evaluating the efficacy of three doses of oral norUDCA, showed a significant dose-dependent reduction in ALP values after 12 weeks, without significant adverse events. The authors showed a significant reduction in ALP levels of 12.3%, 17.3%, and 26.0% in patients treated with 500 mg, 1000 mg, and 1500 mg per day of norUDCA, respectively; placebo-treated patients had a minor increase in ALP levels (1.2%) [61]. Despite some concerns of possible worsening of the disease due to the choleretic effects of norUDCA (especially in PSC patients with dominant strictures), these effects need to be clarified in longer studies; the association of UDCA and norUDCA has the potential to offer additive beneficial effects for PSC patients [87]. A phase 3 double-blind, randomized clinical trial is actively recruiting patients across several worldwide centers (NCT03872921).

3.2.2. FXR Agonists

FXR agonists are evaluated in PSC because of their inhibition in bile acid synthesis in the liver, as previous explained [45].

OCA was tested in PSC patients in the AESOP trial (a randomized, double-blind, placebo-controlled phase II study). Seventy-seven PSC patients were recruited, and they were treated for 24 weeks with titrating doses of 1.5–3 mg/day and 5–10 mg/day OCA, or placebo, after 12 weeks. At the end of the study, serum ALP was significantly reduced with OCA 5–10 mg compared with the placebo arm (least-square mean difference of −83.4 U/L; $p = 0.043$). Interestingly, the effective dose of OCA is already in use for PBC therapy. The effect of OCA 5–10 mg was independent of administration of UDCA, despite a greater reduction in ALP that was registered in patients without UDCA at baseline (25–30% ALP reduction in patients without UDCA at baseline vs. 14–16% ALP reduction in patients with UDCA at baseline). The main side effect was dose-dependent pruritus, which occurred in 67% of patients in the OCA 5–10 mg group, in 60% of patients in the OCA 1.5–3 mg group, and in 45% of patients in the placebo arm. Discontinuation due to pruritus occurred only in one patient in the OCA 1.5–3.0 mg group and in three patients in the OCA 5–10 mg group [75]. A phase 3 trial is actively recruiting patients (NCT02177136).

Cilofexor (GS-9674), a non-steroidal FXR agonist, was tested in a phase 2, randomized, double-blind, placebo-controlled trial of 52 non-cirrhotic PSC patients with ALP levels greater than 1.67 ULN. Patients treated with Cilofexor 100 mg had a significant drop in ALP, gamma-GT, ALT, and primary bile acids (ALP mean reduction of -13.8%, $p = 0.005$; gamma-GT mean reduction of 47.7%, $p < 0.001$; ALT mean reduction of -17.8%, $p = 0.08$; primary bile acids reduction of -30.5%, $p = 0.0008$). The main limitations of this trial were the inclusion of only large-duct PSC cases without cirrhosis and the low prevalence of IBD [76].

NGM282, a FGF19 analogue, was recently studied in a phase 2, randomized, double-blind, placebo-controlled trial in PSC patients with ALP levels greater than $1.5 \times$ ULN. Despite that no significant changes in ALP from baseline were observed, fibrosis biomarkers (Enhanced Liver Fibrosis test score and Pro-C3) were significantly improved in the treatment group [77]. This trial has stimulated discussion about the most appropriated target in PSC [88]. There are no established endpoints in PSC. A recent consensus of the International Primary Sclerosing Cholangitis Study Group, reviewing available literature, concluded that the only few candidates as surrogate endpoints in PSC may be ALP, transient elastography, histology, or the combination of ALP and histology and bilirubin; however, no one exceeds level 3 validation [89].

All-trans retinoic acid (ATRA), currently used in acne and in acute promyelocytic leukemia, represses bile acid synthesis through the FXR/RXR nuclear receptor complex pathway [90]. The efficacy of the combination of UDCA (15–23 mg/kg/day) and ATRA (45 mg/m^2/day) was tested in 15 PSC patients. Despite ATRA, admiration did not reach the primary endpoint of the study (30% reduction in serum ALP), and a decrease in ALT and C4 levels were observed [78]. An open-label phase 2 trial evaluating efficacy and the safety of a lower dose of ATRA is currently ongoing (NCT03359174).

3.2.3. PPAR Agonists

There is a rising number of studies on the efficacy of fibrates in PSC. However, the majority of available data comes from observational or retrospective analyses [3]. A recent retrospective French-Spanish study reported a 40% reduction in ALP levels, together with amelioration of pruritus, after fenofibrate 200 mg/day or bezafibrate 400 mg/day treatment (median duration of therapy of about 1.5 years) in 20 PSC patients [91]. Interestingly, the authors reported a rebound in ALP levels after discontinuation of the PPAR agonist based on occurrence of biliary stones, tolerability, or worsening of liver tests. It has to be mentioned, however, that the liver stiffness evaluated by transient elastography significantly increased during the study. A small prospective study evaluated the efficacy of bezafibrate (200 mg bid) in 11 PSC patients. After 12 weeks of treatment, ALP and ALT levels significantly improved in 7 out of 11 (64%) patients and subsequently increased after treatment discontinuation [79]. Further studies on fibrates for PSC are warranted.

3.2.4. Antifibrotic Therapy

Despite fibrosis being central in the pathogenesis of the disease, very few antifibrotic drugs have been studied. Lysyl oxidase like-2 (LOXL2) is an enzyme that catalyzes the crosslinking of collagen and elastin fibers, thereby strengthening the extracellular matrix structure. Previous studies showed that LOXL2 levels in the serum and liver of PSC patients are correlated with disease severity [92]. Moreover, the administration of a LOXL2 inhibitor in rodents was shown to reduce the accumulation of hepatic and biliary fibrosis and also accelerate its reversal [93,94]. Unfortunately, no improvement in liver fibrosis was observed in a placebo-controlled, phase 2b trial testing Simtuzumab, a LOXL2 inhibitor. In the trial, a total of 234 patients with compensated PSC were randomized on a 1:1:1 basis to receive placebo, weekly subcutaneous injections of Simtuzumab 75 mg, or weekly subcutaneous injections of Simtuzumab 125 mg for 96 weeks. The study failed to demonstrate any effect of Simtuzumab on hepatic collagen content (measured by morphometry on liver biopsy) and fibrosis stage (measured by the Ishak fibrosis stage) [80].

3.2.5. Immunomodulators

Although PSC is an immune-mediated disease, traditional immunosuppressive approaches so far failed to demonstrate a clinical benefit in PSC [95]. Timolumab (BTT1023), a human monoclonal anti-VAP-1 antibody, was shown to prevent fibrosis in murine models of liver injury [96]. A phase 2 clinical trial (BUTEO trial) evaluating the effect of Timolumab in PSC over a 78-day treatment (primary endpoint: reduction of ALP levels by >25% from baseline) is still ongoing (NCT02239211) [97]. Cenicriviroc, a CCR2/CCR5 antagonist, was tested in a phase 2 trial (PERSEUS trial), and it was proven to cause a modest reduction in ALP (median 18%) after 24 weeks among 24 patients [98]. Moreover, it was shown to have anti-inflammatory and antifibrotic effects in NASH animal models and in Abcb4 (Mdr2−/−) mice [99].

Vedolizumab is a monoclonal antibody directed against the α4β7 integrin, which is used in the treatment of inflammatory bowel disease. MADCAM-1 is the ligand for α4β7 integrin and is normally expressed in the gut. Since MADCAM-1 is also found in the liver, administration of vedolizumab is thought to reduce MADCAM-1-induced leucocyte migration between the gut and the liver [100]. Despite these promising premises, in a retrospective analysis, Vedolizumab treatment did not show any improvement in liver biochemistry in patients affected by IBD and PSC who received at least three doses of vedolizumab. About 20% of patients experienced a reduction of at least 20% in ALP levels; however, this outcome was independently associated only with the presence of cirrhosis [81]. Similar results were reported in a previous retrospective study in 34 patients with PSC and IBD (16 patients affected by Crohn's disease and 18 patients by ulcerative colitis) treated with vedolizumab [101].

Vidofludimus is an inhibitor of the dihydroorotate dehydrogenase that blocks the replication of activated T- and B-cells and interferes with the JAK/signal transducer [45]. A phase 2, open-label clinical trial evaluating the safety and the efficacy of vidofludimus in patients with PSC will start in 2020 (NCT03722576).

3.2.6. Modulation of the Gut Microbiome

Recent research focused on the gut microbiome as a potential element in the pathogenesis of PSC. One of the hypothesis is that gut microbiome activates innate immunity within the liver, resulting in inflammation and fibrosis in the bile duct [102]. Moreover, studies on the microbiome and PSC demonstrated that the microbiome of PSC patients is different from healthy controls and IBD-patients [103]. Thus, changing the composition of the gut microbiome might reduce inflammation and fibrosis in the bile ducts.

Vancomycin is a glycopeptide antibiotic that also has an immunomodulatory effect due to the decrease in T cell cytokine production [104]. Vancomycin was compared to metronidazole [105] and to placebo [106] in two randomized trials in PSC patients with or without IBD, and a significant reduction in ALP levels and the Mayo score was reported. A phase 2, multicenter clinical trial aiming to recruit 102 adult participants with PSC and evaluating ALP levels at 6, 12, and 18 months is still ongoing (NCT03710122).

Other interesting antibiotics are rifaximin and minocycline. Rifaximin had no effect in decreasing cholestatic markers and the Mayo score in 16 PSC patients [82]. In contrast, minocycline was shown to cause an improvement in ALP levels and the Mayo score in 16 patients [83].

Fecal Microbiome Transplantation (FMT) is a promising treatment for PSC patients. In one small pilot study, patients with PSC underwent FMT, and three of them experienced a ≥50% decrease in ALP levels. Its effect may be correlated with the bacterial diversity and donor engraftment [84].

3.2.7. Other Treatments

Anti-inflammatory drugs such as sulfasalazine and curcumin were tested in PSC patients. A multicenter, randomized, double-blinded, placebo-controlled trial to assess the benefit and the safety of sulfasalazine in the treatment of PSC just ended, and results are not available (NCT03561584). No significant improvements in cholestasis or symptoms were seen in patients treated with Curcumin [85].

Various minor drugs with different mechanisms of action could have a role in the treatment of PSC, and they were evaluated in different clinical trials. HTD1801 was studied in two phase 2 ongoing trials due to its action on lipid metabolism (NCT03333928, NCT03678480). DUR-928 is an endogenous epigenetic regulator that was studied in a phase 2 study on PSC patients due to its anti-inflammatory properties and its role in lipid metabolism and cell survival (NCT03394781) [3]. Docosahexaenoicacid supplementation, increasing PPAR signaling, was associated with a drop in ALP levels in patients with PSC, in a 12-month, open-label, pilot study on 23 PSC patients [86]. Another ongoing phase 1/2 trial is evaluating the potential effect of Hymecromone, a hyaluronic acid synthesis inhibitor (NCT02780752). Additionally, selected mesenchymal stromal cells (Orbcel-C) are in an ongoing phase 2 trial on PSC patients (NCT02997878) [3].

4. Current Therapeutic Management with Patients Newly Diagnosed with PBC and PSC

Overall, the current codified treatment for patients with PBC consists of UDCA, OCA, and bezafibrate. We provide a flowchart for the standard management of patients with a new diagnosis of PBC (Figure 1). Unfortunately, an analogue algorithm could not be performed for the management of PSC. As a matter of fact, as previously explained, there is not a codified treatment of PSC.

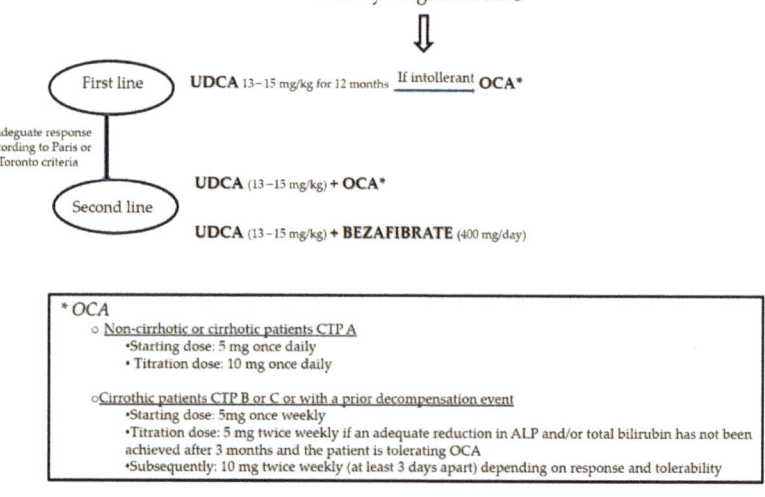

Figure 1. Current algorithm of the treatment in PBC.

5. Conclusions

In this review, we provided an update on the drugs in clinical use and an overview of the new molecules in evaluation for the treatment of PBC and PSC patients. Recently, a deeper understanding of the pathophysiology of these diseases unveiled new molecular targets and, consequently, offered new chances for treatment. Given the complex nature of PBC and PSC, it appears unlikely that a single drug will be able to address all patients for each disease correctly. Instead, the near future of the medical management of chronic cholestatic liver diseases will most probably rely on a combination of multiple drugs targeting different signaling pathways at different stages of the disease. It will be essential to design clinical trials to address these issues specifically and to guide clinical management. A better knowledge of the molecular basis of the diseases and a more detailed disease stratification based on patient characteristics and disease behavior remain therefore the cornerstones to devise new effective treatments for PBC and PSC patients.

Author Contributions: M.M. (Marta Mazzetti) writing—original draft preparation, conceptualisation, methodology; G.M. data curation, writing—review and editing; M.M. (Martina Mancinelli) data curation, writing—review and editing; A.B. supervision, validation; M.M. (Marco Marzioni) supervision, validation; L.M. conceptualisation, validation, writing—review and editing. All authors have read and agreed to the published version of the manuscript.

Funding: This research received no external funding.

Institutional Review Board Statement: Not applicable.

Informed Consent Statement: Not applicable.

Data Availability Statement: No new data were created or analyzed in this study. Data sharing is not applicable to this article.

Conflicts of Interest: The authors declare no conflict of interest.

References

1. European Association for the Study of the Liver. Electronic address eee, European Association for the Study of the L: EASL Clinical Practice Guidelines: The diagnosis and management of patients with primary biliary cholangitis. *J. Hepatol.* **2017**, *67*, 145–172. [CrossRef]
2. Beuers, U.; Trauner, M.; Jansen, P.; Poupon, R. New paradigms in the treatment of hepatic cholestasis: From UDCA to FXR, PXR and beyond. *J. Hepatol.* **2015**, *62* (Suppl. 1), S25–S37. [CrossRef]
3. Wagner, M.; Fickert, P. Drug Therapies for Chronic Cholestatic Liver Diseases. *Annu. Rev. Pharmacol. Toxicol.* **2020**, *60*, 503–527. [CrossRef] [PubMed]
4. Beuers, U. Drug insight: Mechanisms and sites of action of ursodeoxycholic acid in cholestasis. *Nat. Clin. Pract. Gastroenterol. Hepatol.* **2006**, *3*, 318–328. [CrossRef] [PubMed]
5. Paumgartner, G.; Beuers, U. Ursodeoxycholic acid in cholestatic liver disease: Mechanisms of action and therapeutic use revisited. *Hepatology* **2002**, *36*, 525–531. [CrossRef] [PubMed]
6. Beuers, U.; Maroni, L.; Elferink, R.O. The biliary HCO(3)(-) umbrella: Experimental evidence revisited. *Curr. Opin. Gastroenterol.* **2012**, *28*, 253–257. [CrossRef] [PubMed]
7. Floreani, A.; Mangini, C. Primary biliary cholangitis: Old and novel therapy. *Eur. J. Intern. Med.* **2018**, *47*, 1–5. [CrossRef] [PubMed]
8. Ter Borg, P.C.; Schalm, S.W.; Hansen, B.E.; van Buuren, H.R.; Dutch, P.B.C.S.G. Prognosis of ursodeoxycholic Acid-treated patients with primary biliary cirrhosis. Results of a 10-yr cohort study involving 297 patients. *Am. J. Gastroenterol.* **2006**, *101*, 2044–2050. [CrossRef]
9. Corpechot, C.; Carrat, F.; Bonnand, A.M.; Poupon, R.E.; Poupon, R. The effect of ursodeoxycholic acid therapy on liver fibrosis progression in primary biliary cirrhosis. *Hepatology* **2000**, *32*, 1196–1199. [CrossRef]
10. Harms, M.H.; van Buuren, H.R.; Corpechot, C.; Thorburn, D.; Janssen, H.L.A.; Lindor, K.D.; Hirschfield, G.M.; Pares, A.; Floreani, A.; Mayo, M.J.; et al. Ursodeoxycholic acid therapy and liver transplant-free survival in patients with primary biliary cholangitis. *J. Hepatol.* **2019**, *71*, 357–365. [CrossRef]
11. Carbone, M.; Nardi, A.; Flack, S.; Carpino, G.; Varvaropoulou, N.; Gavrila, C.; Spicer, A.; Badrock, J.; Bernuzzi, F.; Cardinale, V.; et al. Pretreatment prediction of response to ursodeoxycholic acid in primary biliary cholangitis: Development and validation of the UDCA Response Score. *Lancet Gastroenterol. Hepatol.* **2018**, *3*, 626–634. [CrossRef]
12. Carbone, M.; Mells, G.F.; Pells, G.; Dawwas, M.F.; Newton, J.L.; Heneghan, M.A.; Neuberger, J.M.; Day, D.B.; Ducker, S.J.; Consortium, U.P.; et al. Sex and age are determinants of the clinical phenotype of primary biliary cirrhosis and response to ursodeoxycholic acid. *Gastroenterology* **2013**, *144*, 560–569. [CrossRef] [PubMed]
13. Invernizzi, P.; Floreani, A.; Carbone, M.; Marzioni, M.; Craxi, A.; Muratori, L.; Vespasiani Gentilucci, U.; Gardini, I.; Gasbarrini, A.; Kruger, P.; et al. Primary Biliary Cholangitis: Advances in management and treatment of the disease. *Dig. Liver Dis.* **2017**, *49*, 841–846. [CrossRef] [PubMed]
14. Hirschfield, G.M.; Mason, A.; Luketic, V.; Lindor, K.; Gordon, S.C.; Mayo, M.; Kowdley, K.V.; Vincent, C.; Bodhenheimer, H.C., Jr.; Pares, A.; et al. Efficacy of obeticholic acid in patients with primary biliary cirrhosis and inadequate response to ursodeoxycholic acid. *Gastroenterology* **2015**, *148*, 751–761.e758. [CrossRef]
15. Nevens, F.; Andreone, P.; Mazzella, G.; Strasser, S.I.; Bowlus, C.; Invernizzi, P.; Drenth, J.P.; Pockros, P.J.; Regula, J.; Beuers, U.; et al. A Placebo-Controlled Trial of Obeticholic Acid in Primary Biliary Cholangitis. *N. Engl. J. Med.* **2016**, *375*, 631–643. [CrossRef]
16. Trauner, M.; Nevens, F.; Shiffman, M.L.; Drenth, J.P.H.; Bowlus, C.L.; Vargas, V.; Andreone, P.; Hirschfield, G.M.; Pencek, R.; Malecha, E.S.; et al. Long-term efficacy and safety of obeticholic acid for patients with primary biliary cholangitis: 3-year results of an international open-label extension study. *Lancet Gastroenterol. Hepatol.* **2019**, *4*, 445–453. [CrossRef]

17. Bowlus, C.L.; Pockros, P.J.; Kremer, A.E.; Pares, A.; Forman, L.M.; Drenth, J.P.H.; Ryder, S.D.; Terracciano, L.; Jin, Y.; Liberman, A.; et al. Long-Term Obeticholic Acid Therapy Improves Histological Endpoints in Patients with Primary Biliary Cholangitis. *Clin. Gastroenterol. Hepatol.* **2020**, *18*, 1170–1178.e1176. [CrossRef]

18. Kowdley, K.V.; Luketic, V.; Chapman, R.; Hirschfield, G.M.; Poupon, R.; Schramm, C.; Vincent, C.; Rust, C.; Parés, A.; Mason, A.; et al. A randomized trial of obeticholic acid monotherapy in patients with primary biliary cholangitis. *Hepatology* **2018**, *67*, 1890–1902. [CrossRef]

19. Hirschfield, G.M.; Dyson, J.K.; Alexander, G.J.M.; Chapman, M.H.; Collier, J.; Hübscher, S.; Patanwala, I.; Pereira, S.P.; Thain, C.; Thorburn, D.; et al. The British Society of Gastroenterology/UK-PBC primary biliary cholangitis treatment and management guidelines. *Gut* **2018**, *67*, 1568–1594. [CrossRef]

20. Lindor, K.D.; Bowlus, C.L.; Boyer, J.; Levy, C.; Mayo, M. Primary Biliary Cholangitis: 2018 Practice Guidance from the American Association for the Study of Liver Diseases. *Hepatology* **2019**, *69*, 394–419.

21. Kok, T.; Bloks, V.W.; Wolters, H.; Havinga, R.; Jansen, P.L.; Staels, B.; Kuipers, F. Peroxisome proliferator-activated receptor alpha (PPARalpha)-mediated regulation of multidrug resistance 2 (Mdr2) expression and function in mice. *Biochem. J.* **2003**, *369 Pt 3*, 539–547. [CrossRef]

22. Mukundan, L.; Odegaard, J.I.; Morel, C.R.; Heredia, J.E.; Mwangi, J.W.; Ricardo-Gonzalez, R.R.; Goh, Y.P.; Eagle, A.R.; Dunn, S.E.; Awakuni, J.U.; et al. PPAR-delta senses and orchestrates clearance of apoptotic cells to promote tolerance. *Nat. Med.* **2009**, *15*, 1266–1272. [CrossRef]

23. Nozaki, Y.; Harada, K.; Sanzen, T.; Nakanuma, Y. PPARgamma ligand attenuates portal inflammation in the MRL-lpr mouse: A new strategy to restrain cholangiopathy in primary biliary cirrhosis. *Med. Mol. Morphol.* **2013**, *46*, 153–159. [CrossRef] [PubMed]

24. Corpechot, C.; Chazouillères, O.; Rousseau, A.; Le Gruyer, A.; Habersetzer, F.; Mathurin, P.; Goria, O.; Potier, P.; Minello, A.; Silvain, C.; et al. A Placebo-Controlled Trial of Bezafibrate in Primary Biliary Cholangitis. *N. Engl. J. Med.* **2018**, *378*, 2171–2181. [CrossRef] [PubMed]

25. Reig, A.; Sese, P.; Pares, A. Effects of Bezafibrate on Outcome and Pruritus in Primary Biliary Cholangitis with Suboptimal Ursodeoxycholic Acid Response. *Am. J. Gastroenterol.* **2018**, *113*, 49–55. [CrossRef]

26. Cheung, A.C.; Lapointe-Shaw, L.; Kowgier, M.; Meza-Cardona, J.; Hirschfield, G.M.; Janssen, H.L.; Feld, J.J. Combined ursodeoxycholic acid (UDCA) and fenofibrate in primary biliary cholangitis patients with incomplete UDCA response may improve outcomes. *Aliment. Pharm. Ther.* **2016**, *43*, 283–293. [CrossRef]

27. Duan, W.; Ou, X.; Wang, X.; Wang, Y.; Zhao, X.; Wang, Q.; Wu, X.; Zhang, W.; Ma, H.; You, H.; et al. Efficacy and safety of fenofibrate add-on therapy for patients with primary biliary cholangitis and a suboptimal response to UDCA. *Rev. Esp. Enferm. Dig.* **2018**, *110*, 557–563. [CrossRef] [PubMed]

28. Rautiainen, H.; Karkkainen, P.; Karvonen, A.L.; Nurmi, H.; Pikkarainen, P.; Nuutinen, H.; Farkkila, M. Budesonide combined with UDCA to improve liver histology in primary biliary cirrhosis: A three-year randomized trial. *Hepatology* **2005**, *41*, 747–752. [CrossRef]

29. Leuschner, M.; Maier, K.P.; Schlichting, J.; Strahl, S.; Herrmann, G.; Dahm, H.H.; Ackermann, H.; Happ, J.; Leuschner, U. Oral budesonide and ursodeoxycholic acid for treatment of primary biliary cirrhosis: Results of a prospective double-blind trial. *Gastroenterology* **1999**, *117*, 918–925. [CrossRef]

30. Hirschfield, G.M.; Beuers, U.; Kupcinskas, L.; Ott, P.; Bergquist, A.; Farkkila, M.; Manns, M.P.; Pares, A.; Spengler, U.; Stiess, M.; et al. A placebo-controlled randomised trial of budesonide for PBC following an insufficient response to UDCA. *J. Hepatol.* **2021**, *74*, 321–329. [CrossRef]

31. Hempfling, W.; Grunhage, F.; Dilger, K.; Reichel, C.; Beuers, U.; Sauerbruch, T. Pharmacokinetics and pharmacodynamic action of budesonide in early- and late-stage primary biliary cirrhosis. *Hepatology* **2003**, *38*, 196–202. [CrossRef]

32. Kowdley, K.V.; Minuk, G.Y.; Pagadala, M.R.; Gulamhusein, A.; Swain, M.G.; Neff, G.W.; Zogg, D.; Bowlus, C.L.; Agarwal, K.; Yoshida, E.M. The nonsteroidal farnesoid x receptor (FXR) agonist cilofexor improves liver biochemistry in patients with primary biliary cholangitis (PBC): A phase 2, randomized, placebo-controlled trial. In *Hepatology*; Wiley: Hoboken, NJ, USA, 2019; pp. 31A–32A.

33. Schramm, C.; Hirschfield, G.; Mason, A.; Wedemeyer, H.; Klickstein, L.; Neelakantham, S.; Koo, P.; Sanni, J.; Badman, M.; Jones, D. Early assessment of safety and efficacy of tropifexor, a potent non bile-acid FXR agonist, in patients with primary biliary cholangitis: An interim analysis of an ongoing phase 2 study. *J. Hepatol.* **2018**, *68*, S103. [CrossRef]

34. Jones, D.; Boudes, P.F.; Swain, M.G.; Bowlus, C.L.; Galambos, M.R.; Bacon, B.R.; Doerffel, Y.; Gitlin, N.; Gordon, S.C.; Odin, J.A.; et al. Seladelpar (MBX-8025), a selective PPAR-delta agonist, in patients with primary biliary cholangitis with an inadequate response to ursodeoxycholic acid: A double-blind, randomised, placebo-controlled, phase 2, proof-of-concept study. *Lancet Gastroenterol. Hepatol.* **2017**, *2*, 716–726. [CrossRef]

35. Treatment Efficacy and Safety of Low Dose Seladelpar, a Selective PPAR-δ Agonist, in Patients with Primary Biliary CholanGitis: Twelve-Week Interim Analysis of an International, Randomized, Dose Ranging, Phase 2 Study. Available online: https://aasldpubs.onlinelibrary.wiley.com/doi/abs/10.1002/hep.29634 (accessed on 21 January 2021).

36. Jörn, P.D.S.; Pares, A.; Kowdley, K.V.; Heneghan, M.; Caldwell, S.; Pratt, D.; Bonder, A.; Hirschfield, G.M.; Bchir, M.; Cynthia, L. LBO-02-Elafibranor, a peroxisome proliferator-activted receptor alpha and delta agonist demonstrates favourable efficacy and safety in patients with primary biliary cholangitis and inadequate response to ursodeoxycholic acid treatment. *J. Hepatol.* **2019**, *70*, e128. [CrossRef]

37. Mayo, M.J.; Wigg, A.J.; Leggett, B.A.; Arnold, H.; Thompson, A.J.; Weltman, M.; Carey, E.J.; Muir, A.J.; Ling, L.; Rossi, S.J.; et al. NGM282 for Treatment of Patients with Primary Biliary Cholangitis: A Multicenter, Randomized, Double-Blind, Placebo-Controlled Trial. *Hepatol. Commun.* **2018**, *2*, 1037–1050. [CrossRef] [PubMed]
38. Dalekos, G.; Invernizzi, P.; Nevens, F.; Hans, V.V.; Zigmond, E.; Andrade, R.J.; Ben Ari, Z.; Heneghan, M.; Huang, J.; Harrison, S. Efficacy of GKT831 in patients with primary biliary cholangitis and inadequate response to ursodeoxycholic acid: Interim efficacy results of a phase 2 clinical trial. *J. Hepatol.* **2019**, *70*, E1–E2. [CrossRef]
39. Tsuda, M.; Moritoki, Y.; Lian, Z.X.; Zhang, W.; Yoshida, K.; Wakabayashi, K.; Yang, G.X.; Nakatani, T.; Vierling, J.; Lindor, K.; et al. Biochemical and immunologic effects of rituximab in patients with primary biliary cirrhosis and an incomplete response to ursodeoxycholic acid. *Hepatology* **2012**, *55*, 512–521. [CrossRef]
40. Myers, R.P.; Swain, M.G.; Lee, S.S.; Shaheen, A.A.; Burak, K.W. B-cell depletion with rituximab in patients with primary biliary cirrhosis refractory to ursodeoxycholic acid. *Am. J. Gastroenterol.* **2013**, *108*, 933–941. [CrossRef] [PubMed]
41. Khanna, A.; Jopson, L.; Howel, D.; Bryant, A.; Blamire, A.; Newton, J.L.; Jones, D.E. Rituximab Is Ineffective for Treatment of Fatigue in Primary Biliary Cholangitis: A Phase 2 Randomized Controlled Trial. *Hepatology* **2019**, *70*, 1646–1657. [CrossRef] [PubMed]
42. Hirschfield, G.M.; Gershwin, M.E.; Strauss, R.; Mayo, M.J.; Levy, C.; Zou, B.; Johanns, J.; Nnane, I.P.; Dasgupta, B.; Li, K.; et al. Ustekinumab for patients with primary biliary cholangitis who have an inadequate response to ursodeoxycholic acid: A proof-of-concept study. *Hepatology* **2016**, *64*, 189–199. [CrossRef] [PubMed]
43. Bowlus, C.L.; Yang, G.X.; Liu, C.H.; Johnson, C.R.; Dhaliwal, S.S.; Frank, D.; Levy, C.; Peters, M.G.; Vierling, J.M.; Gershwin, M.E. Therapeutic trials of biologics in primary biliary cholangitis: An open label study of abatacept and review of the literature. *J. Autoimmun.* **2019**, *101*, 26–34. [CrossRef] [PubMed]
44. Wunsch, E.; Raszeja-Wyszomirska, J.; Barbier, O.; Milkiewicz, M.; Krawczyk, M.; Milkiewicz, P. Effect of S-adenosyl-L-methionine on liver biochemistry and quality of life in patients with primary biliary cholangitis treated with ursodeoxycholic acid. A prospective, open label pilot study. *J. Gastrointestin. Liver Dis.* **2018**, *27*, 273–279. [CrossRef] [PubMed]
45. Gerussi, A.; D'Amato, D.; Cristoferi, L.; O'Donnell, S.E.; Carbone, M.; Invernizzi, P. Multiple therapeutic targets in rare cholestatic liver diseases: Time to redefine treatment strategies. *Ann. Hepatol.* **2020**, *19*, 5–16. [CrossRef]
46. An, P.; Wei, G.; Huang, P.; Li, W.; Qi, X.; Lin, Y.; Vaid, K.A.; Wang, J.; Zhang, S.; Li, Y.; et al. A novel non-bile acid FXR agonist EDP-305 potently suppresses liver injury and fibrosis without worsening of ductular reaction. *Liver Int.* **2020**, *40*, 1655–1669. [CrossRef]
47. Ratziu, V.; Harrison, S.A.; Francque, S.; Bedossa, P.; Lehert, P.; Serfaty, L.; Romero-Gomez, M.; Boursier, J.; Abdelmalek, M.; Caldwell, S.; et al. Elafibranor, an Agonist of the Peroxisome Proliferator-Activated Receptor-alpha and -delta, Induces Resolution of Nonalcoholic Steatohepatitis Without Fibrosis Worsening. *Gastroenterology* **2016**, *150*, 1147–1159.e1145. [CrossRef]
48. Galoosian, A.; Hanlon, C.; Zhang, J.; Holt, E.W.; Yimam, K.K. Clinical Updates in Primary Biliary Cholangitis: Trends, Epidemiology, Diagnostics, and New Therapeutic Approaches. *J. Clin. Transl. Hepatol.* **2020**, *8*, 49–60. [CrossRef]
49. Kliewer, S.A.; Mangelsdorf, D.J. Bile Acids as Hormones: The FXR-FGF15/19 Pathway. *Dig. Dis.* **2015**, *33*, 327–331. [CrossRef]
50. Schumacher, J.D.; Kong, B.; Wu, J.; Rizzolo, D.; Armstrong, L.E.; Chow, M.D.; Goedken, M.; Lee, Y.H.; Guo, G.L. Direct and Indirect Effects of Fibroblast Growth Factor (FGF) 15 and FGF19 on Liver Fibrosis Development. *Hepatology* **2020**, *71*, 670–685. [CrossRef]
51. Zhou, M.; Learned, R.M.; Rossi, S.J.; DePaoli, A.M.; Tian, H.; Ling, L. Engineered fibroblast growth factor 19 reduces liver injury and resolves sclerosing cholangitis in Mdr2-deficient mice. *Hepatology* **2016**, *63*, 914–929. [CrossRef]
52. Lambeth, J.D. NOX enzymes and the biology of reactive oxygen. *Nat. Rev. Immunol.* **2004**, *4*, 181–189. [CrossRef] [PubMed]
53. Aoyama, T.; Paik, Y.H.; Watanabe, S.; Laleu, B.; Gaggini, F.; Fioraso-Cartier, L.; Molango, S.; Heitz, F.; Merlot, C.; Szyndralewiez, C.; et al. Nicotinamide adenine dinucleotide phosphate oxidase in experimental liver fibrosis: GKT137831 as a novel potential therapeutic agent. *Hepatology* **2012**, *56*, 2316–2327. [CrossRef]
54. Wolfhagen, F.H.; van Buuren, H.R.; Schalm, S.W. Combined treatment with ursodeoxycholic acid and prednisone in primary biliary cirrhosis. *Neth. J. Med.* **1994**, *44*, 84–90.
55. Wolfhagen, F.H.; van Hoogstraten, H.J.; van Buuren, H.R.; van Berge-Henegouwen, G.P.; ten Kate, F.J.; Hop, W.C.; van der Hoek, E.W.; Kerbert, M.J.; van Lijf, H.H.; den Ouden, J.W.; et al. Triple therapy with ursodeoxycholic acid, prednisone and azathioprine in primary biliary cirrhosis: A 1-year randomized, placebo-controlled study. *J. Hepatol.* **1998**, *29*, 736–742. [CrossRef]
56. Wiesner, R.H.; Ludwig, J.; Lindor, K.D.; Jorgensen, R.A.; Baldus, W.P.; Homburger, H.A.; Dickson, E.R. A controlled trial of cyclosporine in the treatment of primary biliary cirrhosis. *N. Engl. J. Med.* **1990**, *322*, 1419–1424. [CrossRef] [PubMed]
57. Combes, B.; Emerson, S.S.; Flye, N.L.; Munoz, S.J.; Luketic, V.A.; Mayo, M.J.; McCashland, T.M.; Zetterman, R.K.; Peters, M.G.; Di Bisceglie, A.M.; et al. Methotrexate (MTX) plus ursodeoxycholic acid (UDCA) in the treatment of primary biliary cirrhosis. *Hepatology* **2005**, *42*, 1184–1193. [CrossRef] [PubMed]
58. Treiber, G.; Malfertheiner, P. Mycophenolate mofetil for the treatment of primary biliary cirrhosis in patients with an incomplete response to ursodeoxycholic acid. *J. Clin. Gastroenterol.* **2005**, *39*, 837–838; author reply 838. [CrossRef]
59. Yang, C.Y.; Ma, X.; Tsuneyama, K.; Huang, S.; Takahashi, T.; Chalasani, N.P.; Bowlus, C.L.; Yang, G.X.; Leung, P.S.; Ansari, A.A.; et al. IL-12/Th1 and IL-23/Th17 biliary microenvironment in primary biliary cirrhosis: Implications for therapy. *Hepatology* **2014**, *59*, 1944–1953. [CrossRef] [PubMed]

60. Tanaka, H.; Yang, G.X.; Iwakoshi, N.; Knechtle, S.J.; Kawata, K.; Tsuneyama, K.; Leung, P.; Coppel, R.L.; Ansari, A.A.; Joh, T.; et al. Anti-CD40 ligand monoclonal antibody delays the progression of murine autoimmune cholangitis. *Clin. Exp. Immunol.* **2013**, *174*, 364–371. [CrossRef]

61. Fickert, P.; Hirschfield, G.M.; Denk, G.; Marschall, H.U.; Altorjay, I.; Farkkila, M.; Schramm, C.; Spengler, U.; Chapman, R.; Bergquist, A.; et al. norUrsodeoxycholic acid improves cholestasis in primary sclerosing cholangitis. *J. Hepatol.* **2017**, *67*, 549–558. [CrossRef] [PubMed]

62. Slijepcevic, D.; Roscam Abbing, R.L.P.; Fuchs, C.D.; Haazen, L.C.M.; Beuers, U.; Trauner, M.; Oude Elferink, R.P.J.; van de Graaf, S.F.J. Na(+) -taurocholate cotransporting polypeptide inhibition has hepatoprotective effects in cholestasis in mice. *Hepatology* **2018**, *68*, 1057–1069. [CrossRef]

63. Tabibian, J.H.; Ali, A.H.; Lindor, K.D. Primary Sclerosing Cholangitis, Part 1: Epidemiology, Etiopathogenesis, Clinical Features, and Treatment. *Gastroenterol. Hepatol.* **2018**, *14*, 293–304.

64. European Society of Gastrointestinal Endoscopy; European Association for the Study of the Liver. Role of endoscopy in primary sclerosing cholangitis: European Society of Gastrointestinal Endoscopy (ESGE) and European Association for the Study of the Liver (EASL) Clinical Guideline. *J. Hepatol.* **2017**, *66*, 1265–1281. [CrossRef] [PubMed]

65. Chazouilleres, O.; Poupon, R.; Capron, J.P.; Metman, E.H.; Dhumeaux, D.; Amouretti, M.; Couzigou, P.; Labayle, D.; Trinchet, J.C. Ursodeoxycholic acid for primary sclerosing cholangitis. *J. Hepatol.* **1990**, *11*, 120–123. [CrossRef]

66. O'Brien, C.B.; Senior, J.R.; Arora-Mirchandani, R.; Batta, A.K.; Salen, G. Ursodeoxycholic acid for the treatment of primary sclerosing cholangitis: A 30-month pilot study. *Hepatology* **1991**, *14*, 838–847. [CrossRef] [PubMed]

67. Beuers, U.; Spengler, U.; Kruis, W.; Aydemir, U.; Wiebecke, B.; Heldwein, W.; Weinzierl, M.; Pape, G.R.; Sauerbruch, T.; Paumgartner, G. Ursodeoxycholic acid for treatment of primary sclerosing cholangitis: A placebo-controlled trial. *Hepatology* **1992**, *16*, 707–714. [CrossRef] [PubMed]

68. Mitchell, S.A.; Bansi, D.S.; Hunt, N.; Von Bergmann, K.; Fleming, K.A.; Chapman, R.W. A preliminary trial of high-dose ursodeoxycholic acid in primary sclerosing cholangitis. *Gastroenterology* **2001**, *121*, 900–907. [CrossRef]

69. Olsson, R.; Boberg, K.M.; de Muckadell, O.S.; Lindgren, S.; Hultcrantz, R.; Folvik, G.; Bell, H.; Gangsoy-Kristiansen, M.; Matre, J.; Rydning, A.; et al. High-dose ursodeoxycholic acid in primary sclerosing cholangitis: A 5-year multicenter, randomized, controlled study. *Gastroenterology* **2005**, *129*, 1464–1472. [CrossRef]

70. Lindor, K.D.; Kowdley, K.V.; Luketic, V.A.; Harrison, M.E.; McCashland, T.; Befeler, A.S.; Harnois, D.; Jorgensen, R.; Petz, J.; Keach, J.; et al. High-dose ursodeoxycholic acid for the treatment of primary sclerosing cholangitis. *Hepatology* **2009**, *50*, 808–814. [CrossRef]

71. Shi, J.; Li, Z.; Zeng, X.; Lin, Y.; Xie, W.F. Ursodeoxycholic acid in primary sclerosing cholangitis: Meta-analysis of randomized controlled trials. *Hepatol. Res.* **2009**, *39*, 865–873. [CrossRef]

72. Poropat, G.; Giljaca, V.; Stimac, D.; Gluud, C. Bile acids for primary sclerosing cholangitis. *Cochrane Database Syst. Rev.* **2011**, CD003626. [CrossRef]

73. Triantos, C.K.; Koukias, N.M.; Nikolopoulou, V.N.; Burroughs, A.K. Meta-analysis: Ursodeoxycholic acid for primary sclerosing cholangitis. *Aliment. Pharm. Ther.* **2011**, *34*, 901–910. [CrossRef]

74. Chapman, M.H.; Thorburn, D.; Hirschfield, G.M.; Webster, G.G.J.; Rushbrook, S.M.; Alexander, G.; Collier, J.; Dyson, J.K.; Jones, D.E.; Patanwala, I.; et al. British Society of Gastroenterology and UK-PSC guidelines for the diagnosis and management of primary sclerosing cholangitis. *Gut* **2019**, *68*, 1356–1378. [CrossRef] [PubMed]

75. Kowdley, K.V.; Vuppalanchi, R.; Levy, C.; Floreani, A.; Andreone, P.; LaRusso, N.F.; Shrestha, R.; Trotter, J.; Goldberg, D.; Rushbrook, S.; et al. A randomized, placebo-controlled, phase II study of obeticholic acid for primary sclerosing cholangitis. *J. Hepatol.* **2020**, *73*, 94–101. [CrossRef] [PubMed]

76. Trauner, M.; Gulamhusein, A.; Hameed, B.; Caldwell, S.; Shiffman, M.L.; Landis, C.; Eksteen, B.; Agarwal, K.; Muir, A.; Rushbrook, S.; et al. The Nonsteroidal Farnesoid X Receptor Agonist Cilofexor (GS-9674) Improves Markers of Cholestasis and Liver Injury in Patients with Primary Sclerosing Cholangitis. *Hepatology* **2019**, *70*, 788–801. [CrossRef] [PubMed]

77. Hirschfield, G.M.; Chazouilleres, O.; Drenth, J.P.; Thorburn, D.; Harrison, S.A.; Landis, C.S.; Mayo, M.J.; Muir, A.J.; Trotter, J.F.; Leeming, D.J.; et al. Effect of NGM282, an FGF19 analogue, in primary sclerosing cholangitis: A multicenter, randomized, double-blind, placebo-controlled phase II trial. *J. Hepatol.* **2019**, *70*, 483–493. [CrossRef] [PubMed]

78. Assis, D.N.; Abdelghany, O.; Cai, S.Y.; Gossard, A.A.; Eaton, J.E.; Keach, J.C.; Deng, Y.; Setchell, K.D.; Ciarleglio, M.; Lindor, K.D.; et al. Combination Therapy of All-Trans Retinoic Acid with Ursodeoxycholic Acid in Patients with Primary Sclerosing Cholangitis: A Human Pilot Study. *J. Clin. Gastroenterol.* **2017**, *51*, e11–e16. [CrossRef]

79. Mizuno, S.; Hirano, K.; Isayama, H.; Watanabe, T.; Yamamoto, N.; Nakai, Y.; Sasahira, N.; Tada, M.; Omata, M.; Koike, K. Prospective study of bezafibrate for the treatment of primary sclerosing cholangitis. *J. Hepatobiliary Pancreat. Sci.* **2015**, *22*, 766–770. [CrossRef]

80. Muir, A.J.; Levy, C.; Janssen, H.L.A.; Montano-Loza, A.J.; Shiffman, M.L.; Caldwell, S.; Luketic, V.; Ding, D.; Jia, C.; McColgan, B.J.; et al. Simtuzumab for Primary Sclerosing Cholangitis: Phase 2 Study Results with Insights on the Natural History of the Disease. *Hepatology* **2019**, *69*, 684–698. [CrossRef]

81. Lynch, K.D.; Chapman, R.W.; Keshav, S.; Montano-Loza, A.J.; Mason, A.L.; Kremer, A.E.; Vetter, M.; de Krijger, M.; Ponsioen, C.Y.; Trivedi, P.; et al. Effects of Vedolizumab in Patients with Primary Sclerosing Cholangitis and Inflammatory Bowel Diseases. *Clin. Gastroenterol. Hepatol.* **2020**, *18*, 179–187. [CrossRef]

82. Tabibian, J.H.; Gossard, A.; El-Youssef, M.; Eaton, J.E.; Petz, J.; Jorgensen, R.; Enders, F.B.; Tabibian, A.; Lindor, K.D. Prospective Clinical Trial of Rifaximin Therapy for Patients with Primary Sclerosing Cholangitis. *Am. J. Ther.* **2017**, *24*, e56–e63. [CrossRef]

83. Silveira, M.G.; Torok, N.J.; Gossard, A.A.; Keach, J.C.; Jorgensen, R.A.; Petz, J.L.; Lindor, K.D. Minocycline in the treatment of patients with primary sclerosing cholangitis: Results of a pilot study. *Am. J. Gastroenterol.* **2009**, *104*, 83–88. [CrossRef]

84. Allegretti, J.R.; Kassam, Z.; Carrellas, M.; Mullish, B.H.; Marchesi, J.R.; Pechlivanis, A.; Smith, M.; Gerardin, Y.; Timberlake, S.; Pratt, D.S.; et al. Fecal Microbiota Transplantation in Patients with Primary Sclerosing Cholangitis: A Pilot Clinical Trial. *Am. J. Gastroenterol.* **2019**, *114*, 1071–1079. [CrossRef] [PubMed]

85. Eaton, J.E.; Nelson, K.M.; Gossard, A.A.; Carey, E.J.; Tabibian, J.H.; Lindor, K.D.; LaRusso, N.F. Efficacy and safety of curcumin in primary sclerosing cholangitis: An open label pilot study. *Scand. J. Gastroenterol.* **2019**, *54*, 633–639. [CrossRef]

86. Martin, C.R.; Blanco, P.G.; Keach, J.C.; Petz, J.L.; Zaman, M.M.; Bhaskar, K.R.; Cluette-Brown, J.E.; Gautam, S.; Sheth, S.; Afdhal, N.H.; et al. The safety and efficacy of oral docosahexaenoic acid supplementation for the treatment of primary sclerosing cholangitis—A pilot study. *Aliment. Pharm. Ther.* **2012**, *35*, 255–265. [CrossRef] [PubMed]

87. Chazouilleres, O. 24-Norursodeoxycholic acid in patients with primary sclerosing cholangitis: A new "urso saga" on the horizon? *J. Hepatol.* **2017**, *67*, 446–447. [CrossRef] [PubMed]

88. Tabibian, J.H.; Lindor, K.D. NGM282, an FGF19 analogue, in primary sclerosing cholangitis: A nebulous matter. *J. Hepatol.* **2019**, *70*, 348–350. [CrossRef] [PubMed]

89. Ponsioen, C.Y.; Chapman, R.W.; Chazouilleres, O.; Hirschfield, G.M.; Karlsen, T.H.; Lohse, A.W.; Pinzani, M.; Schrumpf, E.; Trauner, M.; Gores, G.J. Surrogate endpoints for clinical trials in primary sclerosing cholangitis: Review and results from an International PSC Study Group consensus process. *Hepatology* **2016**, *63*, 1357–1367. [CrossRef]

90. Cai, S.Y.; He, H.; Nguyen, T.; Mennone, A.; Boyer, J.L. Retinoic acid represses CYP7A1 expression in human hepatocytes and HepG2 cells by FXR/RXR-dependent and independent mechanisms. *J. Lipid Res.* **2010**, *51*, 2265–2274. [CrossRef]

91. Lemoinne, S.; Pares, A.; Reig, A.; Ben Belkacem, K.; Kemgang Fankem, A.D.; Gaouar, F.; Poupon, R.; Housset, C.; Corpechot, C.; Chazouilleres, O. Primary sclerosing cholangitis response to the combination of fibrates with ursodeoxycholic acid: French-Spanish experience. *Clin. Res. Hepatol. Gastroenterol.* **2018**, *42*, 521–528. [CrossRef]

92. Muir, A.; Goodman, Z.; Bowlus, C.; Caldwell, S.; Invernizzi, P.; Luketic, V.; Minuk, G.; Hirschfield, G.; Myers, R.; Ding, D. Serum lysyl oxidase-like-2 (SLOXL2) levels correlate with disease severity in patients with primary sclerosing cholangitis. *J. Hepatol.* **2016**, *64*, S428. [CrossRef]

93. Ikenaga, N.; Peng, Z.W.; Vaid, K.A.; Liu, S.B.; Yoshida, S.; Sverdlov, D.Y.; Mikels-Vigdal, A.; Smith, V.; Schuppan, D.; Popov, Y.V. Selective targeting of lysyl oxidase-like 2 (LOXL2) suppresses hepatic fibrosis progression and accelerates its reversal. *Gut* **2017**, *66*, 1697–1708. [CrossRef] [PubMed]

94. Barry-Hamilton, V.; Spangler, R.; Marshall, D.; McCauley, S.; Rodriguez, H.M.; Oyasu, M.; Mikels, A.; Vaysberg, M.; Ghermazien, H.; Wai, C.; et al. Allosteric inhibition of lysyl oxidase-like-2 impedes the development of a pathologic microenvironment. *Nat. Med.* **2010**, *16*, 1009–1017. [CrossRef] [PubMed]

95. Karlsen, T.H.; Folseraas, T.; Thorburn, D.; Vesterhus, M. Primary sclerosing cholangitis—A comprehensive review. *J. Hepatol.* **2017**, *67*, 1298–1323. [CrossRef]

96. Weston, C.J.; Shepherd, E.L.; Claridge, L.C.; Rantakari, P.; Curbishley, S.M.; Tomlinson, J.W.; Hubscher, S.G.; Reynolds, G.M.; Aalto, K.; Anstee, Q.M.; et al. Vascular adhesion protein-1 promotes liver inflammation and drives hepatic fibrosis. *J. Clin. Investig.* **2015**, *125*, 501–520. [CrossRef] [PubMed]

97. Arndtz, K.; Corrigan, M.; Rowe, A.; Kirkham, A.; Barton, D.; Fox, R.P.; Llewellyn, L.; Athwal, A.; Wilkhu, M.; Chen, Y.Y.; et al. Investigating the safety and activity of the use of BTT1023 (Timolumab), in the treatment of patients with primary sclerosing cholangitis (BUTEO): A single-arm, two-stage, open-label, multi-centre, phase II clinical trial protocol. *BMJ Open* **2017**, *7*, e015081. [CrossRef] [PubMed]

98. Eksteen, B.; Bowlus, C.L.; Montano-Loza, A.J.; Lefebvre, E.; Fischer, L.; Vig, P.; Martins, E.B.; Ahmad, J.; Yimam, K.K.; Pockros, P.J.; et al. Efficacy and Safety of Cenicriviroc in Patients with Primary Sclerosing Cholangitis: PERSEUS Study. *Hepatol. Commun.* **2021**, *5*, 478–490. [CrossRef] [PubMed]

99. Guicciardi, M.E.; Trussoni, C.E.; Krishnan, A.; Bronk, S.F.; Lorenzo Pisarello, M.J.; O'Hara, S.P.; Splinter, P.L.; Gao, Y.; Vig, P.; Revzin, A.; et al. Macrophages contribute to the pathogenesis of sclerosing cholangitis in mice. *J. Hepatol.* **2018**, *69*, 676–686. [CrossRef] [PubMed]

100. Wiest, R.; Albillos, A.; Trauner, M.; Bajaj, J.S.; Jalan, R. Targeting the gut-liver axis in liver disease. *J. Hepatol.* **2017**, *67*, 1084–1103. [CrossRef]

101. Christensen, B.; Micic, D.; Gibson, P.R.; Yarur, A.; Bellaguarda, E.; Corsello, P.; Gaetano, J.N.; Kinnucan, J.; Rao, V.L.; Reddy, S.; et al. Vedolizumab in patients with concurrent primary sclerosing cholangitis and inflammatory bowel disease does not improve liver biochemistry but is safe and effective for the bowel disease. *Aliment. Pharm. Ther.* **2018**, *47*, 753–762. [CrossRef]

102. Dupont, H.L.; Jiang, Z.D.; Dupont, A.W.; Utay, N.S. The Intestinal Microbiome in Human Health and Disease. *Trans. Am. Clin. Climatol. Assoc.* **2020**, *131*, 178–197.

103. Kummen, M.; Holm, K.; Anmarkrud, J.A.; Nygard, S.; Vesterhus, M.; Hoivik, M.L.; Troseid, M.; Marschall, H.U.; Schrumpf, E.; Moum, B.; et al. The gut microbial profile in patients with primary sclerosing cholangitis is distinct from patients with ulcerative colitis without biliary disease and healthy controls. *Gut* **2017**, *66*, 611–619. [CrossRef] [PubMed]

104. Maurice, J.B.; Thorburn, D. Precision medicine in primary sclerosing cholangitis. *J. Dig. Dis.* **2019**, *20*, 346–356. [CrossRef] [PubMed]
105. Tabibian, J.H.; Weeding, E.; Jorgensen, R.A.; Petz, J.L.; Keach, J.C.; Talwalkar, J.A.; Lindor, K.D. Randomised clinical trial: Vancomycin or metronidazole in patients with primary sclerosing cholangitis—A pilot study. *Aliment. Pharm. Ther.* **2013**, *37*, 604–612. [CrossRef] [PubMed]
106. Rahimpour, S.; Nasiri-Toosi, M.; Khalili, H.; Ebrahimi-Daryani, N.; Nouri-Taromlou, M.K.; Azizi, Z. A Triple Blinded, Randomized, Placebo-Controlled Clinical Trial to Evaluate the Efficacy and Safety of Oral Vancomycin in Primary Sclerosing Cholangitis: A Pilot Study. *J. Gastrointestin. Liver Dis.* **2016**, *25*, 457–464. [CrossRef]

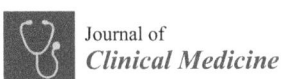

Journal of
Clinical Medicine

Article

Real-World Clinical Management of Patients with Primary Biliary Cholangitis—A Retrospective Multicenter Study from Germany

Anne-Christin Beatrice Wilde [1,*,†], Charlotte Lieb [1,†], Elise Leicht [1], Lena Maria Greverath [1], Lara Marleen Steinhagen [1], Nina Wald de Chamorro [1], Jörg Petersen [2], Wolf Peter Hofmann [3], Holger Hinrichsen [4], Renate Heyne [5], Thomas Berg [6], Uwe Naumann [7], Jeannette Schwenzer [8], Johannes Vermehren [9], Andreas Geier [10], Frank Tacke [1] and Tobias Müller [1]

1   Department of Hepatology and Gastroenterology, Charité Universitätsmedizin Berlin, 13353 Berlin, Germany; charlotte.lieb@charite.de (C.L.); elise.leicht@charite.de (E.L.); lena-maria.greverath@charite.de (L.M.G.); Lara.Steinhagen@outlook.de (L.M.S.); nina.wald-de-chamorro@charite.de (N.W.d.C.); frank.tacke@charite.de (F.T.); tobias.mueller@charite.de (T.M.)
2   IFI Institute for Interdisciplinary Medicine, Asklepios Klinik St. Georg, 20099 Hamburg, Germany; petersen@ifi-medizin.de
3   Center of Gastroenterology Am Bayerischen Platz, 10825 Berlin, Germany; wolfpeter.hofmann@icloud.com
4   GHZ-Center of Gastroenterology and Hepatology, 24105 Kiel, Germany; holger.hinrichsen@gastroenterologie-kiel.eu
5   Liver Center Checkpoint, 10961 Berlin, Germany; heyne@leberzentrum-checkpoint.de
6   Division of Hepatology, Department of Medicine II, Leipzig University, Medical Center, 04103 Leipzig, Germany; thomas.berg@medizin.uni-leipzig.de
7   UBN/PRAXIS, 14059 Berlin, Germany; info@ubn-praxis.de
8   Center of Gastroenterology Biesdorf, 12683 Berlin, Germany; schwenzer@bauchzentrum-biesdorf.de
9   Department of Hepatology and Gastroenterology, University Hospital Frankfurt Am Main, 60590 Frankfurt am Main, Germany; johannes.vermehren@kgu.de
10 Internal Medicine, University Hospital Wuerzburg, 97080 Wuerzburg, Germany; geier_a2@ukw.de
*   Correspondence: anne-christin.wilde@charite.de
†   These authors contributed equally.

Citation: Wilde, A.-C.B.; Lieb, C.; Leicht, E.; Greverath, L.M.; Steinhagen, L.M.; Wald de Chamorro, N.; Petersen, J.; Hofmann, W.P.; Hinrichsen, H.; Heyne, R.; et al. Real-World Clinical Management of Patients with Primary Biliary Cholangitis—A Retrospective Multicenter Study from Germany. *J. Clin. Med.* **2021**, *10*, 1061. https://doi.org/10.3390/jcm10051061

Academic Editor: Pierluigi Toniutto

Received: 14 February 2021
Accepted: 1 March 2021
Published: 4 March 2021

Publisher's Note: MDPI stays neutral with regard to jurisdictional claims in published maps and institutional affiliations.

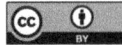
Abstract: Background: Clinical practice guidelines for patients with primary biliary cholangitis (PBC) have been recently revised and implemented for well-established response criteria to standard first-line ursodeoxycholic acid (UDCA) therapy at 12 months after treatment initiation for the early identification of high-risk patients with inadequate treatment responses who may require treatment modification. However, there are only very limited data concerning the real-world clinical management of patients with PBC in Germany. Objective: The aim of this retrospective multicenter study was to evaluate response rates to standard first-line UDCA therapy and subsequent Second-line treatment regimens in a large cohort of well-characterized patients with PBC from 10 independent hepatological referral centers in Germany prior to the introduction of obeticholic acid as a licensed second-line treatment option. Methods: Diagnostic confirmation of PBC, standard first-line UDCA treatment regimens and response rates at 12 months according to Paris-I, Paris-II, and Barcelona criteria, the follow-up cut-off alkaline phosphatase (ALP) $\leq 1.67 \times$ upper limit of normal (ULN) and the normalization of bilirubin (bilirubin $\leq 1 \times$ ULN) were retrospectively examined between June 1986 and March 2017. The management and hitherto applied second-line treatment regimens in patients with an inadequate response to UDCA and subsequent response rates at 12 months were also evaluated. Results: Overall, 480 PBC patients were included in this study. The median UDCA dosage was 13.2 mg UDCA/kg bodyweight (BW)/d. Adequate UDCA treatment response rates according to Paris-I, Paris-II, and Barcelona criteria were observed in 91, 71.3, and 61.3% of patients, respectively. In 83.8% of patients, ALP $\leq 1.67 \times$ ULN were achieved. A total of 116 patients (24.2%) showed an inadequate response to UDCA according to at least one criterion. The diverse second-line treatment regimens applied led to significantly higher response rates according to Paris-II (35 vs. 60%, $p = 0.005$), Barcelona (13 vs. 34%, $p = 0.0005$), ALP $\leq 1.67 \times$ ULN and bilirubin $\leq 1 \times$ ULN (52.1 vs. 75%, $p = 0.002$). The addition of bezafibrates appeared to induce the

J. Clin. Med. **2021**, *10*, 1061. https://doi.org/10.3390/jcm10051061   https://www.mdpi.com/journal/jcm

J. Clin. Med. **2021**, *10*, 1061

strongest beneficial effect in this cohort (Paris II: 24 vs. 74%, $p = 0.004$; Barcelona: 50 vs. 84%, $p = 0.046$; ALP $< 1.67 \times$ ULN and bilirubin $\leq 1 \times$ ULN: 33 vs. 86%, $p = 0.001$). Conclusion: Our large retrospective multicenter study confirms high response rates following UDCA first-line standard treatment in patients with PBC and highlights the need for close monitoring and early treatment modification in high-risk patients with an insufficient response to UDCA since early treatment modification significantly increases subsequent response rates of these patients.

Keywords: primary biliary cholangitis; autoantibodies; ursodeoxycholic acid; treatment response; second line therapy

1. Introduction

Primary biliary cholangitis (PBC) is a rare chronic inflammatory biliary disease characterized by the progressive destruction of intrahepatic bile ducts, leading to cholestasis and subsequent liver damage. Although immune-mediated processes are widely considered as a major underlying cause, the exact etiology of biliary inflammation still remains to be fully elucidated but likely comprises additional factors such as environmental stimuli and epigenetic factors [1]. If untreated, PBC may lead to end-stage liver cirrhosis and eventually liver failure. Orthotopic liver transplantation is the only definitive therapy for PBC patients with end-stage liver disease. Early treatment with weight-based ursodeoxycholic acid (UDCA) has been proven to extend transplant-free survival and is therefore recommended at a dosage of 13 to 15 mg UDCA/kg bodyweight (BW)/d as a standard first-line therapy by national and international PBC clinical practice guidelines [2–4]. These guidelines also implemented the evaluation of specific response criteria at 12 months after the initiation of UDCA treatment for the early detection of high-risk patients with inadequate treatment responses who need treatment modification. The most commonly applied Paris-I, Paris-II, and Barcelona criteria have been widely accepted for treatment monitoring including laboratory parameters such as bilirubin and alkaline phosphatase (ALP). Recently, ALP levels $\leq 1.67 \times$ upper limit of normal (ULN) or ALP normalization and the normalization of bilirubin values (bilirubin $\leq 1 \times$ ULN) have been proven to yield prognostic relevance [5,6]. The risk of PBC disease progression to severe liver disease in patients with PBC may also be estimated using the UK-PBC risk score, which is based on continuous variables that have been specifically developed to identify patients at an increased risk for progression to death or liver transplantation after 5, 10, and 15 years [7,8].

In December 2016, obeticholic acid was licensed as a second-line treatment option in combination with UDCA for patients with an inadequate UDCA response or monotherapy for patients with an intolerance to UDCA and is therefore recommended by current PBC clinical practice guidelines. Bezafibrates have also been shown to increase response rates in patients with an inadequate response to first-line UDCA therapy [9] and have therefore been depicted as a potential off-label second-line treatment option in combination with UDCA in the current guidelines.

There are only very limited data concerning the real-world clinical management of patients with PBC in Germany [10]. Moreover, a recent German population-based study reported the rising prevalence of PBC and deficits in their subsequent clinical management [11]. We therefore aimed to evaluate real-world diagnostic approaches, standard first-line UDCA treatment regimens and respective response rates at 12 months applying Paris-I, Paris-II, and Barcelona criteria, ALP levels $\leq 1.67 \times$ ULN, and bilirubin $\leq 1 \times$ ULN in a large cohort of well-characterized patients with PBC in a retrospective multicenter study from 10 independent hepatological referral centers in Germany. The real-world management of patients with an inadequate response to standard first-line UDCA treatment including the hitherto applied individual second-line treatment regimens prior to the introduction of obeticholic acid and the subsequent response rates at 12 months were also evaluated.

2. Methods

2.1. Diagnostic Criteria

The records of patients suspected to have PBC between June 1986 and March 2017 were evaluated in a large retrospective multicenter study from 10 independent German hepatological referral centers, comprising four tertiary-care university hospitals in Berlin, Frankfurt am Main, Würzburg, and Leipzig and six hepatological centers in Berlin, Hamburg, and Kiel. The study was approved by the local Ethics Committees of the Universities of Berlin, Frankfurt, Leipzig, and Würzburg and written informed consent was obtained from all participants. The diagnosis of PBC was accepted if the patients fulfilled at least two of the following criteria (1) chronic cholestasis for more than six months; (2) the presence of anti-mitochondrial antibody (AMA) titer > 1:40 or other specific autoantibodies, including sp100 or gp210, if AMA-negative (3) the histological conformation of lymphocytic destructive cholangitis and destruction of interlobular bile ducts. Patients with concomitant features of autoimmune hepatitis (AIH) as defined by the current PBC treatment guidelines (according to liver biopsy or high simplified score according to Hennes et al. or patients who fulfilled the Paris criteria for AIH-PBC-Overlap) [3,4,12] showed lower response rates to UDCA in a previous study [13]; therefore, these patients were excluded to eliminate this bias. Furthermore, patients with concomitant features of primary sclerosing cholangitis, biliary obstruction, drug-induced cholestatic liver disease, severe non-alcoholic fatty liver disease, hemochromatosis, Wilson's disease, alpha1-antitrypsin deficiency, alcohol abuse, chronic hepatitis B, or hepatitis C were excluded from the study by extended laboratory testing and imaging including abdominal ultrasound and magnetic resonance cholangiopancreatography. All patients underwent thorough clinical exams supplemented by laboratory tests at baseline and follow-up visits every three to four months in an outpatient setting. The clinical course of disease including the development of liver cirrhosis was evaluated.

2.2. Baseline Characteristics

Baseline characteristics comprised sex, age at onset of therapy, weight, serum levels of alaninaminotransferase (ALT), aspartataminotransferase (AST), alkaline phosphatase (ALP), γ-glutamyltransferase (γGT), bilirubin, albumin, prothrombin time, platelet count, immunoglobulin A (IgA), G (IgG), M (IgM), anti-mitochondrial antibodies (AMA), anti-smooth muscle antibodies (SMA), anti-nuclear antibodies (ANA), anti-sp100, anti-gp210, and, if available, a histological evaluation of PBC.

2.3. Evaluation of Standard First-Line UDCA Treatment Regimens and Response Rates at 12 Months

Standard first-line UDCA treatment regimens in mg UDCA/kg bodyweight per day (mg UDCA/kg BW/d) were evaluated. At 12 months, the ALP, AST, and bilirubin levels were assessed to evaluate Paris-I, Paris-II, and Barcelona criteria, ALP levels $\leq 1.67 \times$ ULN, and bilirubin $\leq 1 \times$ ULN to define an adequate respectively inadequate UDCA response.

2.4. Management of Patients with an Inadequate Response to First-Line UDCA Treatment

The management of patients with an inadequate response to first-line UDCA treatment including the evaluation of hitherto applied second-line treatment regimens was evaluated. Subsequent response rates at 12 months after treatment modification were assessed by applying Paris-I, Paris-II, and Barcelona criteria, ALP cut-off levels $\leq 1.67 \times$ ULN, and bilirubin $\leq 1 \times$ ULN.

2.5. Statistical Analysis

Analyses were performed by IBM SPSS Statistic Version 24 for Windows (IBM, Armonk, NY, USA) and Prism 6.0 (GraphPad Software, La Jolla, CA, USA). Comparison between groups were made by using the Kruskal–Wallis test, Mann–Whitney test, and Fischer's exact test. Data are presented as the median and interquartile range (IQR). The Kaplan–Meier survival curve with the Mantel–Cox test was examined to assess the relationship between the response to therapy according to Paris-II and the development of liver cirrhosis and the log-rank test for statistical assessment. This study was performed in accordance with the ethical guidelines of the 1975 Declaration of Helsinki and was approved by the local Ethics Committee (EA2/035/07; 03-2015).

3. Results

3.1. Study Population

As depicted in Figure 1, a total of 763 records from patients suspected with PBC was identified through an extended database search. Among them, 283 patients were excluded from this study, mainly due to subsequent incomplete data sets (150 patients), liver transplantation (124 patients) or lack of subsequent UDCA treatment (nine patients). Patients with apparent autoimmune hepatitis overlap were also excluded. Therefore, 480 patients with PBC were enrolled for first-line therapy analysis. A total of 116 patients showed an inadequate response to UDCA according to at least one criterion and were therefore included for second-line therapy analysis.

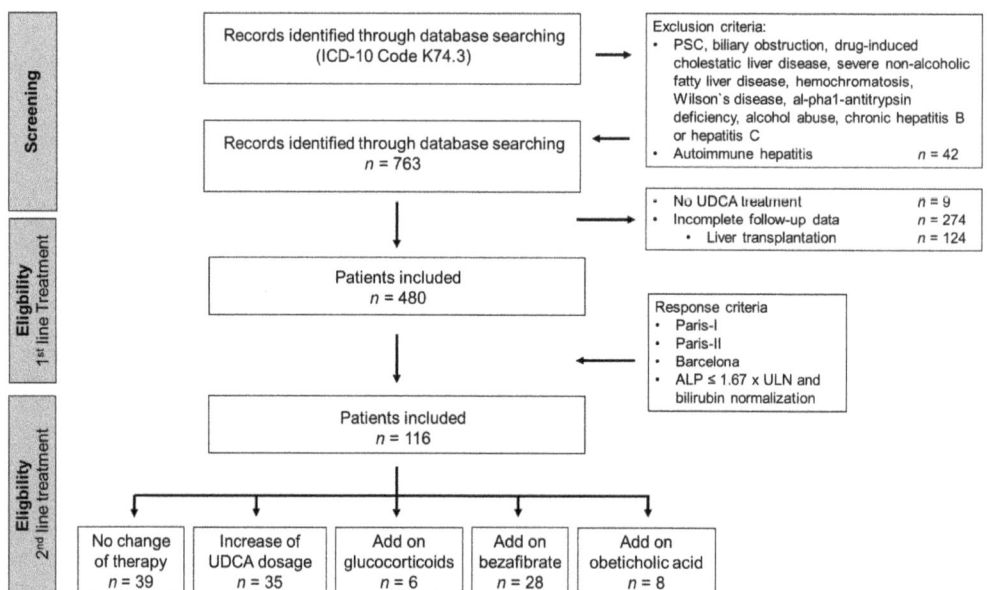

Figure 1. Study flow diagram. In total, 763 patients with confirmed PBC from 10 independent hepatological referral centers were screened for study eligibility and real-world first-line UDCA treatment regimens and subsequent response rates at 12 months after the initiation of treatment were evaluated in 480 patients. Patients with an inadequate response to at least one of the response criteria (*n* = 116) were evaluated for hitherto available second-line treatment regimens and subsequent response rates at 12 months after treatment modification.

3.2. Baseline Characteristics

The overall study population of 480 patients with PBC comprised 431 females (89.8%) and 49 (10.2%) males (Table S1). The median age at UDCA treatment initiation was 57 years (Q1–Q3: 48 to 64 years). In 83.5% (401/480) of the patients, the diagnosis of PBC was established based on cholestatic biochemical patterns and PBC-specific autoantibodies. In total, 399 (86.9%) patients out of 459 were AMA-positive. Autoantibodies against sp100 were determined in 112 patients, of which 28 (25%) had a positive result. A liver biopsy was carried out in 26.5% (127/480) and varied largely between the different centers (17.1 to 50%).

3.3. Standard First-Line UDCA Treatment Regimens and Response Rates at 12 Months

In the overall cohort, the median UDCA dosage was 13.2 mg UDCA/kg BW/d and ranged between a minimum of 5 mg UDCA/kg BW/d and a maximum of 28.3 mg UDCA/kg BW/d (IQR: 3.9 (Q1–Q3: 11.1 to 15 mg UDCA/kg BW/d)).

As depicted in Table 1, at 12 months after the initiation of UDCA treatment, Paris-I criteria for adequate treatment response were met in 91% (253/278) of patients. Applying Paris-II, and Barcelona criteria, an adequate UDCA treatment response was achieved in 71.3% (201/282) and 61.3% (273/439) of patients, respectively. In total, 83% (365/440) of the patients showed ALP levels $\leq 1.67 \times$ ULN, 95.5% (383/401) and achieved the normalization of bilirubin, and 81% (325/402) showed ALP $\leq 1.67 \times$ ULN and bilirubin normalization. In 64 patients, full clinical follow-up data were available, allowing for the assessment of the UK-PBC risk score. In these patients, an inadequate response to UDCA at 12 months after treatment initiation according to Paris-I and Paris-II criteria was associated with a significantly higher UK-PBC risk score compared to patients with an adequate UDCA response ($p < 0.001$; Table S2). The risk of experiencing an event (increase in bilirubin value above 100 μmol/L, liver transplantation, or death) within 15 years varied from 9.80 (± 8.17; Paris-II) and 18.28% (± 10.98; Paris-I) among non-responders. However, when using the Barcelona criteria, patients who did not adequately respond to UDCA were not at a significantly higher risk after 15 years as compared to patients with an adequate response (8.06 vs. 7.06%; $p = 0.423$). Moreover, we evaluated the proportion of patients who developed liver cirrhosis in relation to the one-year response rate under UDCA. Overall, significantly more patients with an inadequate one-year response to UDCA according to Paris-I and Paris-II developed liver cirrhosis (Figure S1).

Table 1. First line UDCA treatment response at 12 months.

Response Criteria at 12 Months of Standard UDCA Therapy	Total
Paris-I ALP < 3 × ULN + AST < 2 × ULN + bilirubin normalization	91.0% (253/278)
Paris-II ALP < 1.5 × ULN + AST < 1.5 × ULN + bilirubin normalization	71.3% (201/282)
Barcelona ALP ≤ 1 × ULN or reduction of ALP > 40%	61.3% (273/439)
ALP ≤ 1.67 × ULN	83.0% (365/440)
Bilirubin ≤ 1 × ULN	95.5% (383/401)
AP ≤ 1.67 × ULN + bilirubin normalization	80.8% (325/402)

UDCA: ursodeoxycholic acid; ALP: alkaline phosphatase; ULN: upper limit of normal; AST: aspartataminotransferase.

3.4. Management of Patients with Inadequate UDCA Treatment Response

As depicted in Figure 1, a total of 116 patients showed an inadequate response to the standard first-line UDCA treatment at 12 months after treatment initiation according to at least one criterion. Within this group of patients, 34% (39/116) of patients did not undergo any change of treatment and 66% (77/116) underwent treatment modification: 30% (35/116) obtained an increased UDCA dosage, 24% (28/116) obtained fibrates as an add-on therapy to UDCA, 5% (6/116) obtained glucocorticoids as an add-on therapy to UDCA and 7% (4/63) obtained obeticholic acid as an add-on therapy to UDCA.

At 12 months after the initiation of second-line therapy, Paris-I and Paris-II criteria were available in 58 patients, Barcelona criteria in 90 patients and ALP levels $\leq 1.67 \times$ ULN and bilirubin normalization in 83 patients (Table 2). Overall, the diverse second-line treatment regimens applied led to significantly higher response rates according to Paris-II (35% vs. 60%, $p = 0.005$), Barcelona (13% vs. 34%, $p = 0.0005$), ALP $\leq 1.67 \times$ ULN and bilirubin normalization (52.1 vs. 75%, $p = 0.002$).

Table 2. Second line treatment response in patients with inadequate UDCA response.

Response Criteria at 12 Months of UDCA Therapy	Before Initiation of 2nd Line Therapy and After at Least 12 of Therapy with UDCA	12 Months After Initiation of 2nd Line Therapy	*p*
Paris-I ALP < 3 × ULN + AST < 2 × ULN + Bilirubin ≤ 1mg/dL	76.8% (53/69)	84.5% (49/58)	0.371
Paris-II ALP < 1.5 × ULN + AST < 1.5 × ULN + Bilirubin ≤ 1mg/dL	34.9% (24/69)	60.3% (35/58)	**0.005**
Barcelona ALP ≤ 1 × ULN or reduction of ALP > 40%	12.9% (13/101)	34.4% (31/90)	**0.0005**
ALP ≤ 1.67 × ULN + Bilirubin ≤ 1 × ULN	52.1% (50/96)	74.7% (62/83)	**0.002**

Bold values indicates a statistical significance ($p < 0.05$).

As depicted in Figure 2 (Table S3), the UDCA dosage intensification and the addition of glucocorticoids did not increase response rates in patients with an inadequate UDCA response, whereas the addition of fibrates significantly enhanced response rates according to Paris-II ($p = 0.004$) and Barcelona criteria ($p = 0.046$) and ALP levels ≤ 1.67 × ULN and bilirubin normalization ($p = 0.001$) at 12 months after the initiation of treatment modification. In the small group of patients obtaining additional obeticholic acid since approval in December 2016, there was a trend towards higher response rates with respect to ALP levels ≤ 1.67 × ULN and bilirubin normalization.

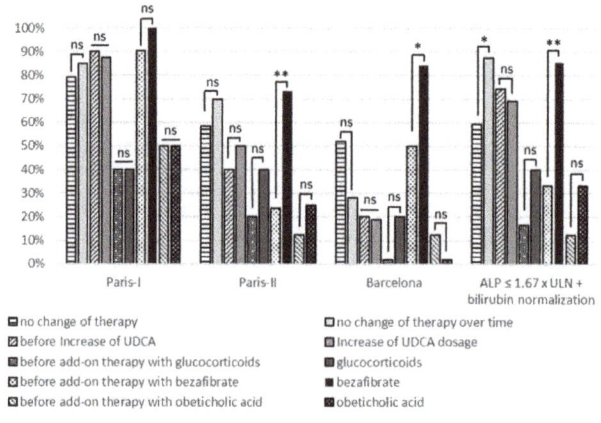

Figure 2. Management of patients with inadequate response to standard UDCA first-line treatment. The real-world management of 116 patients with inadequate response to standard first-line UDCA treatment according to at least one criterion is depicted, including patients without treatment modification ($n = 39$), increase of UDCA dosage ($n = 35$), addition of glucocorticoids ($n = 6$), bezafibrates ($n = 28$) or obeticholic acid ($n = 4$). Treatment response rates according to Paris-I, Paris-II, and Barcelona criteria and ALP levels ≤ 1.67 × ULN and bilirubin ≤ 1 × ULN at 12 months after treatment modification, respectively; continuation of UDCA-monotherapy was analyzed. * $p < 0.05$, ** $p < 0.01$, not significant (ns) = $p ≥ 0.05$.

3.5. Evaluation of Liver Biochemistry

As depicted in Figure 3, intensified UDCA treatment and/or the addition of glucocorticoids did not improve liver biochemistry, whereas the addition of fibrates significantly reduced ALP ($p < 0.001$) and gamma-glutamyl transferase (gGT) levels ($p = 0.023$). Additional treatment with obeticholic acid also showed a reduction of gGT levels ($p = 0.043$). Bilirubin levels, which normalized in the vast majority of patients during first-line therapy, showed no further decrease irrespective of the second-line therapy applied.

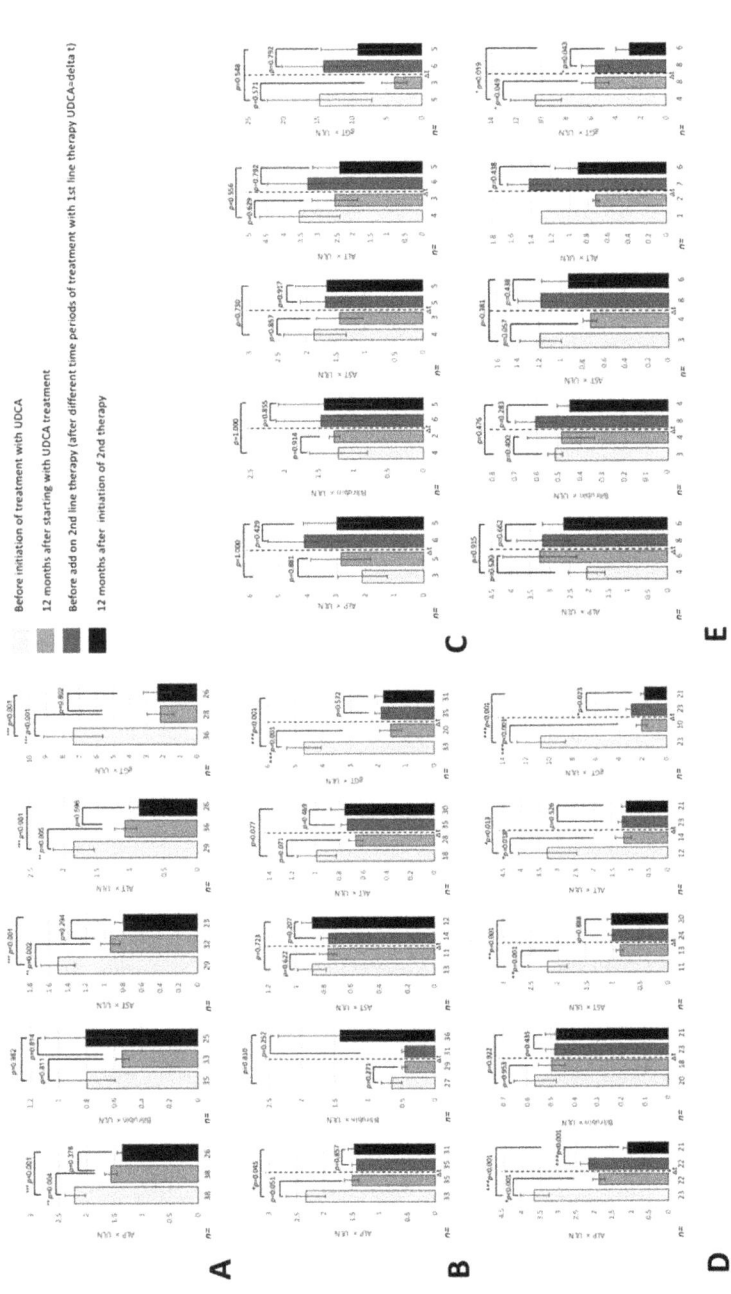

Figure 3. Evaluation of liver biochemistry. The course of liver biochemistry in patients with inadequate response to standard first-line UDCA treatment according to the subsequent individual management (**A**): no treatment modification (*n* = 39), (**B**): increase of UDCA dosage (*n* = 35), (**C**): addition of glucocorticoids (*n* = 6), (**D**): bezafibrates (*n* = 28) or (**E**): obeticholic acid (*n* = 4) is shown. The first bar represents the baseline values for alkaline phosphatase [ALP], bilirubin, aspartate aminotransferase [AST], alanine aminotransferase [ALT] and gamma-glutamyl transferase [gGT]. The second bar represents the laboratory results at 12 months after the initiation of standard first-line UDCA treatment. The third bar represents baseline values before the start of second-line treatment after different time periods under UDCA treatment. The fourth bar depicts the effect on liver biochemistry at 12 months after treatment modification. * $p < 0.05$, ** $p < 0.01$, *** $p < 0.001$, ns = $p \geq$ 0.05.

4. Discussion

Primary biliary cholangitis may be associated with considerable morbidity despite recent advances in the management of this disease [2]. Thus, there is an unmet clinical need to improve the management of PBC, in particular in patients with an inadequate response to standard first-line treatment with weight-based UDCA. In this retrospective multicenter study, so-far the largest, we provide insight into the real-world clinical management of patients with PBC with respect to the recently revised national and international clinical practice guidelines. In this study from 10 independent hepatological centers in Germany, the diagnosis of PBC was established by serological parameters in 83.5% of all patients, i.e., chronic cholestasis and specific autoantibodies, whereas in 26.5% of all patients, an additional histological examination were carried out. Detailed analysis of the treatment regimens applied by the different centers revealed a median UDCA dosage of 13.2 mg/kg BW/d as the standard first-line therapy in the study cohort, achieving adequate treatment response rates in 60 to 90% of patients at 12 months after the initiation of therapy depending on the response criteria applied. Therefore, up to 40% of patients showed an inadequate UDCA response at 12 months after the standard UDCA first-line therapy. Of note, in almost one third of these patients in this high-risk group, there was no obvious treatment modification, whereas in the majority of cases the UDCA dosage was increased. Other treatment modifications included the off-label addition of fibrates or, less frequently, the addition of budesonide. Since 2017, the patients were also treated with obeticholic acid as the only licensed second-line therapy. Therefore, the number of patients receiving obeticholic acid was very limited. Taken together, the diverse second-line treatment regimens applied led to significantly higher response rates according to Paris-II and Barcelona criteria, and ALP $\leq 1.67 \times$ ULN and bilirubin normalization. The addition of fibrates appeared to induce the strongest beneficial effect in this cohort.

Several limitations of the present study need to be acknowledged. Due to the retrospective character of this study, a systematic evaluation of all biochemical parameters in every study participant was not available, leading to inconsistent patient numbers depending on the different response criteria in the overall cohort. Additionally, patients who underwent liver transplantation were excluded due to incomplete data. Another limitation of the study is that the data available on further follow-up in patients without treatment modification are limited and therefore do not allow to draw a solid conclusion. Moreover, a certain selection bias cannot be excluded since all study participants were recruited from four tertiary care centers and six hepatological referral centers, leading to a potential selection of difficult-to-diagnose cases, which likely explains the rather low proportion of patients with PBC-specific autoantibodies in the present cohort. However, a recent population-based study with non-selected PBC patients revealed no obvious difference to earlier hospital-based studies [14].

However, we would like to strengthen the fact that this is, so far, the largest retrospective multicenter study addressing the real-world management of patients with PBC in Germany, comprising patients from 10 different hepatological referral centers. The baseline characteristics of the present PBC cohort were consistent with previous PBC study populations, showing a clear predominance of female patients with a female-to-male ratio of 9:1. An increasing proportion of male patients, as postulated in a recent epidemiological study [15] and a recent German retrospective study [11], was not observed in the present cohort. The median age at treatment initiation was 57 years, which was in line with the age peak described in the literature between the fifth and seventh decade of life. Of note, depending on the individual participating center, between 5 and 16% of all PBC patients were AMA-negative, whereas previous studies described only 5 to 10% AMA-negative patients [16–18]. However, in a recent Polish study [19], the proportion of AMA-negative patients was 18.9%, suggesting that the proportion of AMA-negative patients in special populations might be higher than previously reported. In our first-line study, 399 of 459 patients were AMA-positive whereas only 112 cases were tested for the presence of specific autoantibodies against protein sp100 with a positive result in 25% of patients, which might be due to the fact that these antibodies are not readily available in daily routine use. However, our observation was in line with the very heterogeneous results of previous meta-analyses from 2014, describing antibodies against sp100 in 7 to 60% of all patients [20].

With respect to the applied first-line UDCA therapy, the median dosage of 13.2 mg UDCA/kg BW/d was close to the lower limit of the recommended dosage of 13 to 15 mg UDCA/kg BW/d. Adequate UDCA response rates in 91% of patients at 12 months after treatment initiation according to Paris-I criteria was higher compared to previous studies of other countries. In a Dutch study from 2009, the overall response rate according to Paris-I criteria was 66% [21]; in a French study from 2011, it was 76% [22]; and in a large multicenter British study from 2013, it was 79% [23]. This discrepancy might be explained by the large proportion of patients with early PBC stages in the present cohort defined by normal bilirubin levels prior to the start of UDCA treatment. Interestingly, a recent German prospective study from 2019 showed a similarly high response rate according to Paris-I criteria [10]. This study also described a high number of patients in an early stage of PBC. Therefore, Paris-II criteria might be more adequate to examine the response rate in the present cohort. In a recently published study, Murillo-Perez et al. highlighted that not only a reduction of ALP level, but both bilirubin normalization and an ALP level below $1 \times$ ULN significantly contributes to a more accurate risk stratification and improved survival [6]. Therefore, not only one criterion but several criteria (the Barcelona criterion together with Paris-II criterion and ALP level $\leq 1.67 \times$ ULN with bilirubin normalization) should be used for each patient; furthermore, a complete normalization of ALP and bilirubin level should possibly be targeted in the future to determine the lowest risk for a disease progression and, if needed, to intensify the therapy.

In line with this hypothesis, applying Paris-II and Barcelona criteria, adequate response rates of 71 (Paris-II) and 61% (Barcelona) at 12 months after treatment initiation were consistent with previous observations [22,24].

Our findings demonstrate higher treatment response rates at 12 months after treatment modification under real-world conditions. Of note, comparison of different treatment regimens in patients with an inadequate therapy response showed particularly higher response rates among patients receiving additional fibrates. These results are in line with previous studies showing higher response rates for fibrates as an add-on therapy to UDCA [9,25,26]. In the other large cohort of the study—patients without any change of treatment regime—there was no significant improvement in treatment response according to Paris-I, Paris-II, and Barcelona criteria. However, there was a significant increase in patients achieving ALP levels $\leq 1.67 \times$ ULN and bilirubin normalization. These results are in line with a recent study from Germany by Sebode et al., who also showed that the guideline recommended treatment regime of patients with PBC was partly not applied [11]. Follow-up data for treatment modification with obeticholic acid were missing due to the short period of this recently licensed therapy. However, we already observed a clear trend towards a better therapy response rate regarding the ALP-level $\leq 1.67 \times$ ULN and bilirubin normalization and a significant reduction of gGT after the addition of obeticholic acid to UDCA. However, our data are in line with the findings by Nevens et al. who showed an improved response rate according to ALP levels below $1.67 \times$ ULN and bilirubin normalization under obeticholic acid [27].

In conclusion, this large real-world multicenter study confirms high response rates following UDCA first-line standard treatment in patients with PBC and highlights the need for close monitoring and early treatment modification in high-risk patients with an insufficient response to UDCA since early treatment modification significantly increases the subsequent response rates of these patients. A large prospective observation study has already been initiated and will provide further long-term outcomes.

Supplementary Materials: The following are available online at https://www.mdpi.com/2077-038 3/10/5/1061/s1. Figure S1: Development of liver cirrhosis in relation to 12 months UDCA treatment response, Table S1: Baseline characteristics, Table S2: UK-PBC-Risk-Score in relation to 12 months UDCA treatment response, Table S3: Treatment response before and after 12 months of second line therapy in detail.

Author Contributions: Conceptualization, T.M. and A.-C.B.W.; methodology, T.M. and A.-C.B.W.; formal analysis, A.-C.B.W., C.L. and E.L.; investigation, A.-C.B.W., C.L., E.L., L.M.G., L.M.S., N.W.d.C., J.P., W.P.H., H.H., R.H., T.B., U.N., J.S., J.V. and A.G.; writing-original draft preparation, A.-C.B.W.; writing-review and editing, T.M., F.T.; visualization, A.-C.B.W.; supervision, T.M.; project administration, T.M.; funding acquisition, T.M. All authors have read and agreed to the published version of the manuscript.

Funding: This study was supported by the German Research Foundation Grants MU 2864/1-3 and MU 2864/3-1 and by unrestricted research grants from Intercept Pharmaceuticals and Falk Pharma GmbH. The supporting parties had no influence on the study design, data collection and analyses, writing of the manuscript or on the decision to submit the manuscript for publication.

Institutional Review Board Statement: The study was approved by the local Ethics Committees of the Universities of Berlin, Frankfurt, Leipzig and Würzburg and written informed consent was obtained from all participants. This study was performed in accordance with the ethical guidelines of the 1975 Declaration of Helsinki and was approved by the local Ethics Committee (EA2/035/07; 03-2015).

Informed Consent Statement: Informed consent was obtained from all subjects involved in the study.

Data Availability Statement: The data presented in this study are available on request.

Conflicts of Interest: The authors declare no conflict of interest. The funders had no role in the design of the study; in the collection, analyses, or interpretation of data; in the writing of the manuscript, or in the decision to publish the results.

References

1. Carey, E.J.; Ali, A.H.; Lindor, K.D. Primary biliary cirrhosis. *Lancet* **2015**, *386*, 1565–1575. [CrossRef]
2. Lindor, K.D.; Bowlus, C.L.; Boyer, J.; Levy, C.; Mayo, M. Primary Biliary Cholangitis: 2018 Practice Guidance from the American Association for the Study of Liver Diseases. *J. Hepatol.* **2018**, *69*, 394–419. [CrossRef]
3. Hirschfield, G.M.; Beuers, U.; Corpechot, C.; Invernizzi, P.; Jones, D.; Marzioni, M. EASL Clinical Practice Guidelines: The diagnosis and management of patients with primary biliary cholangitis. *J. Hepatol.* **2017**, *67*, 145–172. [CrossRef]
4. Strassburg, C.P.; Beckebaum, S.; Geier, A.; Gotthardt, D.; Klein, R.; Melter, M.; Schott, E.; Spengler, U.; Tacke, F.; Trauner, M.; et al. S2k Leitlinie Autoimmune Lebererkrankungen. *Zeitschrift für Gastroenterologie* **2017**, *55*, 1135–1226. [CrossRef]
5. Lammert, C.; Juran, B.D.; Schlicht, E.; Chan, L.L.; Atkinson, E.J.; de Andrade, M.; Lazaridis, K.N. Biochemical response to ursodeoxycholic acid predicts survival in a North American cohort of primary biliary cirrhosis patients. *J. Gastroenterol.* **2014**, *49*, 1414–1420. [CrossRef]
6. Perez, C.F.; Harms, M.H.; Lindor, K.D.; Van Buuren, H.R.; Hirschfield, G.M.; Corpechot, C.; Van Der Meer, A.J.; Feld, J.J.; Gulamhusein, A.; Lammers, W.J.; et al. Goals of treatment for improved survival in primary biliary cholangitis: Treatment target should be bilirubin within the normal range and normalization of alkaline phosphatase. *Am. J. Gastroenterol.* **2020**, *115*, 1066–1074. [CrossRef] [PubMed]
7. Carbone, M.; Sharp, S.J.; Flack, S.; Paximadas, D.; Spiess, K.; Adgey, C.; Griffiths, L.; Lim, R.; Trembling, P.; Williamson, K.; et al. The UK-PBC risk scores: Derivation and validation of a scoring system for long-term prediction of end-stage liver disease in primary biliary cholangitis. *Hepatology* **2016**, *63*, 930–950. [CrossRef] [PubMed]
8. Efe, C.; Tas, K. Validation of Risk Scoring Systems in Ursodeoxycholic Acid-Treated Patients with Primary Biliary Cholangitis. *J. Gastroenterol.* **2019**, *114*, 1101–1108. [CrossRef] [PubMed]
9. Corpechot, C.; Chazouillères, O.; Rousseau, A.; Le Gruyer, A.; Habersetzer, F.; Mathurin, P.; Goria, O.; Potier, P.; Minello, A.; Silvain, C.; et al. A Placebo-Controlled Trial of Bezafibrate in Primary Biliary Cholangitis. *N. Engl. J. Med.* **2018**, *378*, 2171–2181. [CrossRef]
10. Kaps, L.; Grambihler, A.; Yemane, B.; Nagel, M.; Labenz, C.; Ploch, P.; Michel, M.; Galle, P.R.; Wörns, M.A.; Schattenberg, J.M. Symptom Burden and Treatment Response in Patients with Primary Biliary Cholangitis (PBC). *Dig. Dis. Sci.* **2019**, 1–8. [CrossRef]
11. Sebode, M.; Kloppenburg, A.; Aigner, A.; Lohse, A.W.; Schramm, C.; Linder, R. Population-based study of autoimmune hepatitis and primary biliary cholangitis in Germany: Rising prevalences based on ICD codes, yet defits in medical treatment. *Zeitschrift für Gastroenterologie* **2020**, *58*, 431–438.

12. Hennes, E.M.; Zeniya, M.; Czaja, A.J.; Parés, A.; Dalekos, G.N.; Krawitt, E.L.; Bittencourt, P.L.; Porta, G.; Boberg, K.M.; Hofer, H.; et al. Simplified criteria for the diagnosis of autoimmune hepatitis. *Hepatology* **2008**, *48*, 169–176. [CrossRef]
13. Wen, M.; Men, R.; Fan, X.; Shen, Y.; Ni, P.; Hu, Z.; Yang, L. Worse Response to Ursodeoxycholic Acid in Primary Biliary Cholangitis Patients with Autoimmune Hepatitis Features. *Dig. Dis.* **2020**. [CrossRef] [PubMed]
14. Örnolfsson, K.T.; Lund, S.H.; Olafsson, S.; Bergmann, O.M.; Björnsson, E.S. Biochemical response to ursodeoxycholic acid among PBC patients: A nationwide population-based study. *Scand. J. Gastroenterol.* **2019**, *54*, 609–616. [CrossRef]
15. Lleo, A.; Jepsen, P.; Morenghi, E.; Carbone, M.; Moroni, L.; Battezzati, P.M.; Podda, M.; Mackay, I.R.; Gershwin, M.E.; Invernizzi, P. Evolving Trends in Female to Male Incidence and Male Mortality of Primary Biliary Cholangitis. *Sci. Rep.* **2016**, *6*, 25906. [CrossRef]
16. Lindor, K.D.; Gershwin, M.E.; Poupon, R.; Kaplan, M.; Bergasa, N.V.; Heathcote, E.J. Primary biliary cirrhosis. *Hepatology* **2009**, *50*, 291–308. [CrossRef] [PubMed]
17. Liu, B.; Shi, X.H.; Zhang, F.C.; Zhang, W.; Gao, L.X. Antimitochondrial antibody-negative primary biliary cirrhosis: A subset of primary biliary cirrhosis. *Liver Int.* **2008**, *28*, 233–239. [CrossRef] [PubMed]
18. Hirschfield, G.M.; Heathcote, E.J. Antimitochondrial antibody-negative primary biliary cirrhosis. *Clin. Liver Dis.* **2008**, *12*, 323–331. [CrossRef]
19. Raszeja-Wyszomirska, J.; Wunsch, E.; Krawczyk, M.; Rigopoulou, E.I.; Kostrzewa, K.; Norman, G.L.; Bogdanos, D.P.; Milkiewicz, P. Assessment of health related quality of life in polish patients with primary biliary cirrhosis. *Clin. Res. Hepatol. Gastroenterol.* **2016**, *40*, 471–479. [CrossRef] [PubMed]
20. Hu, S.-L.; Zhao, F.-R.; Hu, Q.; Chen, W.-X. Meta-analysis assessment of GP210 and SP100 for the diagnosis of primary biliary cirrhosis. *PLoS ONE* **2014**, *9*, e101916. [CrossRef] [PubMed]
21. Kuiper, E.M.; Hansen, B.E.; de Vries, R.A.; den Ouden–Muller, J.W.; Van Ditzhuijsen, T.J.; Haagsma, E.B.; Houben, M.H.; Witteman, B.J.; van Erpecum, K.J.; van Buuren, H.R.; et al. Improved Prognosis of Patients With Primary Biliary Cirrhosis That Have a Biochemical Response to Ursodeoxycholic Acid. *Gastroenterology* **2009**, *136*, 1281–1287. [CrossRef] [PubMed]
22. Corpechot, C.; Chazouillères, O.; Poupon, R. Early primary biliary cirrhosis: Biochemical response to treatment and prediction of long-term outcome. *J. Hepatol.* **2011**, *55*, 1361–1367. [CrossRef]
23. Carbone, M.; Mells, G.F.; Pells, G.; Dawwas, M.F.; Newton, J.L.; Heneghan, M.A.; Neuberger, J.M.; Day, D.B.; Ducker, S.J.; Sandford, R.N.; et al. Sex and age are determinants of the clinical phenotype of primary biliary cirrhosis and response to ursodeoxycholic acid. *Gastroenterology* **2013**, *144*, 560–569.e7. [CrossRef] [PubMed]
24. Parés, A.; Caballería, L.; Rodés, J. Excellent Long-Term Survival in Patients With Primary Biliary Cirrhosis and Biochemical Response to Ursodeoxycholic Acid. *Gastroenterology* **2006**, *130*, 715–720. [CrossRef]
25. Itakura, J.; Izumi, N.; Nishimura, Y.; Inoue, K.; Ueda, K.; Nakanishi, H.; Tsuchiya, K.; Hamano, K.; Asahina, Y.; Kurosaki, M.; et al. Prospective randomized crossover trial of combination therapy with bezafibrate and UDCA for primary biliary cirrhosis. *Hepatol. Res.* **2008**, *38*, 557–564. [CrossRef] [PubMed]
26. Iwasaki, S.; Ohira, H.; Nishiguchi, S.; Zeniya, M.; Kaneko, S.; Onji, M.; Ishibashi, H.; Sakaida, I.; Kuriyama, S.; Ichida, T.; et al. The eficacy of ursodeoxycholic acid and bezafibrate combination therapy for primary biliary cirrhosis: Aprospectiv, multicenter study. *Hepatol. Res.* **2008**, *38*, 557–564. [CrossRef] [PubMed]
27. Nevens, F.; Andreone, P.; Mazzella, G.; Strasser, S.I.; Bowlus, C.; Invernizzi, P.; Drenth, J.P.; Pockros, P.J.; Regula, J.; Beuers, U.; et al. A placebo-controlled trial of obeticholic acid in primary biliary cholangitis. *N. Engl. J. Med.* **2016**, *375*, 631–643. [CrossRef] [PubMed]

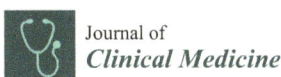

Journal of
Clinical Medicine

Review

Prevention of Cirrhosis Complications: Looking for Potential Disease Modifying Agents

Giacomo Zaccherini [1]**, Manuel Tufoni** [2]**, Mauro Bernardi** [1] **and Paolo Caraceni** [1,2,3,]*

1   Department of Medical and Surgical Sciences, University of Bologna, 40138 Bologna, Italy; giacomo.zaccherini@unibo.it (G.Z.); mauro.bernardi@unibo.it (M.B.)
2   IRCCS AOU di Bologna—Policlinico di S. Orsola, 40138 Bologna, Italy; manuel.tufoni@aosp.bo.it
3   Center for Biomedical Applied Research, University of Bologna, 40138 Bologna, Italy
*   Correspondence: paolo.caraceni@unibo.it

Abstract: The current therapeutic strategies for the management of patients with cirrhosis rely on the prevention or treatment of specific complications. The removal of the causative agents (i.e., viruses or alcohol) prevents decompensation in the vast majority of patients with compensated cirrhosis. In contrast, even when etiological treatment has been effective, a significant proportion of patients with decompensated cirrhosis remains at risk of further disease progression. Therefore, therapies targeting specific key points in the complex pathophysiological cascade of decompensated cirrhosis could represent a new approach for the management of these severely ill patients. Some of the interventions currently employed for treating or preventing specific complications of cirrhosis or used in other diseases (i.e., poorly absorbable oral antibiotics, statins, albumin) have been proposed as potential disease-modifying agents in cirrhosis (DMAC) since clinical studies have shown their capacity of improving survival. Additional multicenter, large randomized clinical trials are awaited to confirm these promising results. Finally, new drugs able to antagonize key pathophysiological mechanisms are under pre-clinical development or at the initial stages of clinical assessment.

Keywords: decompensated cirrhosis; portal hypertension; ascites; non-selective beta-blockers; TIPS; rifaximin; human albumin; statins

Citation: Zaccherini, G.; Tufoni, M.; Bernardi, M.; Caraceni, P. Prevention of Cirrhosis Complications: Looking for Potential Disease Modifying Agents. *J. Clin. Med.* **2021**, *10*, 4590. https://doi.org/10.3390/jcm10194590

Academic Editors: Pierluigi Toniutto and Hiroki Nishikawa

Received: 25 July 2021
Accepted: 4 October 2021
Published: 5 October 2021

Publisher's Note: MDPI stays neutral with regard to jurisdictional claims in published maps and institutional affiliations.

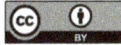
1. Introduction

In the natural history of liver cirrhosis, the onset of a major complication of the disease represents a crucial clinical event. Indeed, the occurrence of ascites, portal hypertensive gastrointestinal bleeding, hepatic encephalopathy, and deep jaundice, alone or in combination, hallmarks the transition from the compensated to the decompensated phase of cirrhosis. About 5–7% of patients with compensated cirrhosis cross this border every year, thus entering a clinical history punctuated by further complications, frequent hospitalizations, worsening of quality of life and shortening of life expectancy [1].

In this context, the current therapeutic strategies aim to treat or control each complication individually [2]. However, even though their efficacy has been proven in randomized clinical trials (RCTs), such approaches do not significantly affect the course of the disease, thus making it difficult to bring out a clear survival benefit for patients [3,4]. Treatments proven to prevent the progression of the disease are not currently available. However, some potential candidates are under investigation and subject to debate in the scientific community [5,6].

The only interventions showing a clear influence on the natural history of cirrhosis so far are etiological treatments targeted to the elimination of the cause of the disease (i.e., antivirals for hepatitis B and C or prolonged abstinence for alcohol use disorders). In the decompensated stage, even though a slowdown of the disease progression or even a reversion to the compensated state can occur, progression can be seen in up to one-third of cases [4,7,8]. Thus, alternative approaches are warranted.

41

Recent investigations contributed to uncover hitherto unknown pathophysiological mechanisms of decompensated cirrhosis [9]. It is now clear that the systemic spread of bacterial products from the gut due to abnormal translocation and substances from the liver where inflammation and cell death occur activates immune cells. The consequent release of pro-inflammatory cytokines and chemokines gives rise to sustained systemic inflammation and oxidative stress. These events lead to cardiocirculatory dysfunction responsible for reducing effective volemia and diffuse microvascular damage. These mechanisms provide the pathophysiological substrate for multi-organ dysfunction and, ultimately failure [10].

From this knowledge, novel therapeutic perspectives emerged relying on mechanistic approaches. Their goal is to counteract key pathophysiological events: portal hypertension, bacterial translocation, circulatory dysfunction, systemic inflammation, oxidative stress, and immunological dysfunction. This kind of mechanism is exploited by disease-modifying agents (DMA) who have proven to exert beneficial effects on the course of a disease. These interventions are well established in several fields of medicine, especially in rheumatologic and neurologic disorders. Whether this approach is transferable to cirrhosis (DMAC) has recently emerged as the subject of debate [6]. In any case, some basic principles are unavoidable. Indeed, once a strong rationale for the use of a potential DMAC is established and its efficacy at the pre-clinical level achieved, solid evidence of clinical benefit has to be pursued, preferably through multicenter phase III randomized clinical trials (RCTs) having patient survival as the primary endpoint [11,12]. Given the high clinical heterogeneity of decompensated cirrhosis and its rapidly evolving clinical course [1,13,14], two other characteristics should be clearly identified: the target population receiving the highest benefit from the treatment, and temporary or permanent "stopping rules" in case of loss of efficacy or potential harm.

This review will critically analyze the available evidence supporting that interventions able to counteract key pathophysiological mechanisms can play a role as DMAC in decompensated cirrhosis.

2. Etiological Treatments

Whenever possible, removing or neutralizing the cause of the persisting liver insult is the ideal goal to be attempted in all patients with chronic liver disease. Indeed, successful etiological treatments can halt or at least slow down the progression of cirrhosis [5,15].

This is particularly true in the compensated stage of the disease, when the removal of the causative agent generally prevents decompensation, reduces the risk of hepatocellular carcinoma (HCC) and prolongs survival. Thus, etiological treatments undoubtedly represent the first choice in this setting [15]. Etiological treatments remain of primary importance in decompensated cirrhosis, but the extent of their effects is variable. Indeed, the successful elimination of the causative agent can temper the turbulent course of decompensated cirrhosis, or even induce the regression of the disease to a significant extent. However, a portion of patients do not obtain a relevant clinical improvement, remaining at risk of further decompensation, poor quality of life, and reduced life expectancy [5,7,16].

Patients with HBV-related cirrhosis should be treated with specific anti-viral drugs as evidence shows that clinical improvement occurs in most cases [16–18]. Once the decompensated stage has been reached, improvement in the severity of cirrhosis and survival rate occurs in about half to two-thirds of cases [19]. There is solid evidence that clinical improvement generally occurs once viral clearance is obtained in patients with HCV-related cirrhosis [20,21]. However, long-term effects on the occurrence of complications and survival remain less defined. First, not all patients benefit to the same extent. Patients with severe portal hypertension and advanced disease, as defined by a model for end-stage liver disease (MELD) score exceeding a certain threshold (between 15 and 20), seem to be less susceptible to sustained clinical improvement [7,21,22]. Second, most patients with decompensated cirrhosis followed for a median period of 4 years after viral clearance did not significantly improve their liver function and MELD score remaining at risk for severe complications, death and need of liver transplantation [8]. Another important issue is related to patients waitlisted for liver transplantation that achieve a modest reduction in the MELD score after HCV viral clearance without improving their clinical conditions to a substantial extent. As a result, they remain at risk of complications and death, yet their priority on the waiting list is negatively affected. Thus, an appropriate evaluation of the timing of antiviral therapy is needed [23,24].

Alcohol withdrawal and abstinence from alcohol are crucial to improving the clinical course and outcomes in patients with chronic alcoholic liver disease, regardless of their disease state [2]. In patients with compensated cirrhosis, such an approach can prevent disease progression and decompensation [15], while in decompensated patients it can at least prevent further deterioration and stabilize the clinical course in most cases [25,26].

No clearly effective and approved drugs are available for patients with non-alcoholic fatty liver disease (NAFLD), so the treatment cornerstone relies on correcting or attenuating the cofactors of the metabolic syndrome, such as optimizing glycemic control in diabetic patients and or lowering body weight in case of obesity. However, great caution is needed in recommending unsupervised weight loss in patients with cirrhosis, since sarcopenia is a highly prevalent and impactful comorbidity [27,28] that can be worsened by incautious weight loss. However, a monitored weight loss associated with lifestyle interventions (like tailored dietary counseling and adapted physical activity) can obtain improvement in portal hypertension and general conditions [29], thus rendering patients more suitable for liver transplantation.

Finally, sporadic data are only available on the effects of etiological treatments in patients with cirrhosis of less frequent etiologies. Indeed, the beneficial effects of removing causative factors in these settings have yet to be demonstrated. The sole exception is autoimmune cirrhosis, whose response to immunosuppressive therapy is followed by an improvement in long-term outcomes [30]. However, an appropriate balance between effective immune suppression and risk for infection can be difficult to achieve in this context.

Summarizing the available evidence, etiological treatments are often effective in slowing down the course of cirrhosis and are of primary importance in the management of patients. However, they present limitations in the decompensated stage of the disease [2,5]. Indeed, once cirrhosis has reached a self-perpetuating "point of no return", even the removal of the causative agent cannot arrest the disease progression so that the patient long-term prognosis is not influenced. Therefore, the effective management of patients with advanced cirrhosis also requires the adoption of strategies able to counteract the key pathophysiological mechanisms.

3. Pathophysiological Treatments

Besides new approaches still under development, interventions directed at counteracting pathophysiological mechanisms include treatments currently used to manage specific complications of cirrhosis. However, to employ them as DMAC, they should be handled in the context of novel strategies. This section will review the available treatments, both already tested and under investigation, able to antagonize one or more key events in the complex pathophysiological network of decompensated cirrhosis (Figure 1).

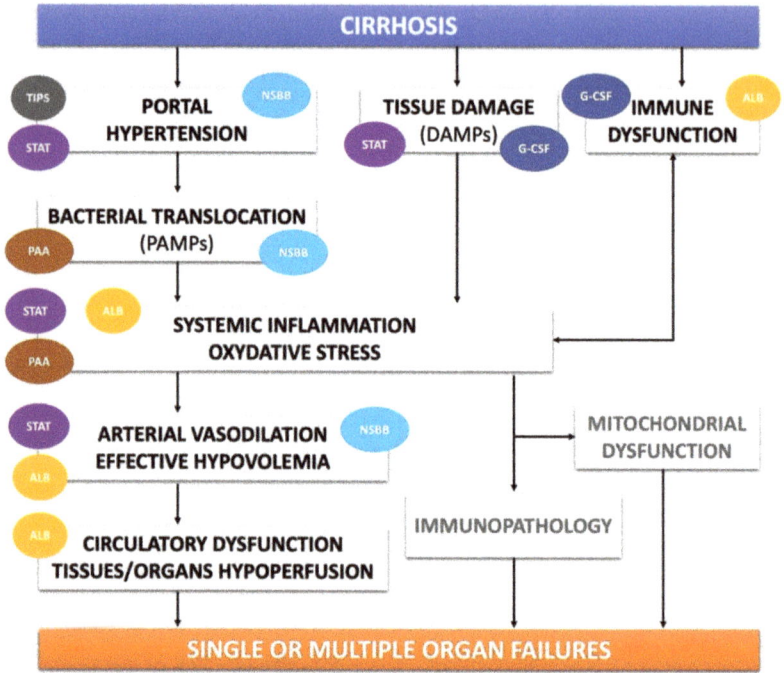

Figure 1. Targets of action of available treatments antagonizing key pathophysiological events in decompensated cirrhosis. See text for details. TIPS: trans-jugular intra-hepatic porto-systemic shunt; STAT: statins; NSBB: non-selective beta-blockers; G-CSF: granulocyte colony stimulating factors; PAA: poorly absorbable antibiotics.

3.1. Non-Selective β-Blockers

Non-selective β-blockers (NSBBs) were introduced in the management of patients with cirrhosis about 40 years ago when their lowering effect on portal pressure was demonstrated. At present, NSBBs still are the only drugs recommended for long-term treatment of portal hypertension [2,31,32].

Propranolol was the first NSBB employed. Its effect on portal pressure is mainly related to the reduction in cardiac output and the unopposed α-adrenergic tone in the splanchnic arterial bed. As a result, portal pressure declines because of a reduced splanchnic blood inflow [33]. About 20 years ago, carvedilol was also introduced in the management of portal hypertension [34]. This NSBB is provided with intrinsic anti-α1-adrenergic activity, contributing to lower portal pressure by decreasing intrahepatic vascular resistance. This characteristic, however, may induce a greater reduction in systemic blood pressure [35]. NSBBs also exert non-hemodynamic effects, as they decrease intestinal permeability, bacterial translocation, and systemic inflammation [36]. Whether these effects are relevant in mediating their effect in humans is still unclear.

The RCTs that evaluated the effect of NSBBs in cirrhosis had the prevention of the first or recurrent variceal bleeding as primary endpoints. Even though most of these trials excluded patients in the advanced stages of cirrhosis, several also included patients with decompensated disease. Interestingly, metanalyses showed that bleeding prevention was more pronounced in decompensated than in compensated patients [37,38].

Unfortunately, data to ascertain if NSBBs administration to patients with decompensated cirrhosis prevents other complications beyond variceal bleeding are insufficient. A first systematic search did not find sufficient evidence supporting a NSBBs effect on other complications of cirrhosis. This negative result was possibly due to the underreporting of non-bleeding complications [39]. Indeed, a more recent meta-analysis pooling data from 15 studies showed that patients lowering portal pressure gradient below 12 mmHg or more than 20% from baseline exhibited lower bleeding rates, lower incidence of complications, and a greater improvement in survival than non-responders [40]. This suggests that NSBBs may substantially modify the course of the disease.

Two recent clinical trials reinforced this concept. The PREDESCI trial showed that NS-BBs administration to patients with compensated cirrhosis delays decompensation, mainly preventing ascites formation [41]. Another study [42] assessed the effects of carvedilol, carefully titrated based on blood pressure and heart rate, in patients with acute-on-chronic liver failure diagnosed according to the definition of the Asian-Pacific Association for the Study of the Liver [43]. In this placebo-controlled trial, carvedilol reduced the incidence of bacterial infections and acute kidney injury and lowered mortality.

Soon after the first reports on the use of propranolol in patients with cirrhosis, a word of caution rose on its use in patients with ascites as they may risk for developing hepatorenal syndrome (HRS) [44]. Safety signals on either survival or kidney function did not emerge from the numerous RCTs comparing NSBBs with placebo in patients with cirrhosis. However, most studies did not enroll patients with refractory ascites. Further emphasis on this matter derived from observational studies reporting worse outcomes in patients with refractory ascites [45] or spontaneous bacterial peritonitis (SBP) [46]. The concept of a "therapeutic window" beyond which NSBBs may become detrimental was proposed [47], and several subsequent studies were dedicated to this matter. Unfortunately, conflicting results were provided [48].

Different effects of NSBBs on intrarenal hemodynamics of patients with responsive or refractory ascites may explain their potential adverse effects in the latter. Indeed, as opposed to patients with diuretic responsive ascites, NSBBs lower renal perfusion pressure below the critical threshold for autoregulation (65 mmHg) in 55% of the patients with refractory ascites. This phenomenon is likely due to an excessive reduction of cardiac output due to systolic dysfunction [49]. Thus, the question arises as to how identifying patients who may receive harm from NSBBs treatment. Possibly, arterial pressure is the simplest biomarker to establish when the therapeutic window for NSBBs closes. A prospective observational study reported that mean arterial pressure levels <65 mmHg defines the threshold below which NSBBs do not improve transplant-free survival of patients with ascites, particularly in those with SBP and ACLF [50]. Similar results were observed using the threshold of 90 mmHg of systolic blood pressure, which is recommended in current guidelines as a threshold for dose reduction or discontinuation of NSBBs [2,31,32].

In summary, the current indication for NSBBs administration to patients with cirrhosis remains the prevention of variceal bleeding or rebleeding. Nonetheless, when an effective lowering in portal pressure is achieved, more general effects can be observed on the incidence of complications and patients' survival, suggesting the potential role of NSBBs as DMAC. However, besides the prophylactic action on portal hypertensive bleeding or re-bleeding, NSBBs effects vary in different stages of the disease. On the one hand, prevention of decompensation (mainly ascites) can be seen in compensated cirrhosis; on the other, renal dysfunction and HRS can occur in patients with very advanced cirrhosis. Therefore, further studies are eagerly needed to identify target subgroups of patients who may benefit most from long-term NSBBs administration.

3.2. Transjugular Intrahepatic Porto-Systemic Shunt

As already reported, portal hypertension plays a crucial causative role in most complications of cirrhosis. Therefore, interventions targeted to decrease portal pressure, such as transjugular intrahepatic porto-systemic shunt (TIPS), can potentially modify the long-term clinical course of patients with cirrhosis [51]. To date, the main clinical settings for the use of TIPS are the management of variceal bleeding and the control of refractory ascites. However, the main contentious points remain the identification of target patients and appropriate timing for TIPS placement.

The role of "pre-emptive" TIPS as a potential DMAC emerged from 3 RCTs in patients with cirrhosis and variceal hemorrhage [52–54] (Table 1). They showed that TIPS placement within 24 or 72 h is effective in controlling bleeding, preventing rebleeding, and improving survival in patients at high risk of uncontrolled bleeding and bleeding-related mortality (HVPG > 20 mmHg, Child C [10–13 points] or B with active bleeding). Moreover, 2 recent large multicenter observational studies highlighted that "pre-emptive" TIPS also improves survival in patients with acute variceal bleeding and ACLF [55,56]. In patients with persistent bleeding or severe rebleeding within five days, "rescue/salvage" TIPS is used when other therapeutic alternatives are not available, but, despite a high rate of bleeding control, a clear benefit on survival has not been established [31,32]. Similarly, although there is consensus for TIPS insertion as secondary prophylaxis of bleeding in patients who failed to respond to endoscopic banding plus non-selective beta-blockers (NSBBs), a benefit on survival has not been consistently observed likely because of the high heterogeneity of the patients included in the studies [31,32].

Table 1. RCTs assessing pre-emptive TIPS vs. endoscopic treatment in acute variceal bleeding.

Reference	Study Population (Randomized Patients)	Exclusion Criteria	Survival-Related Endpoints of the Study	Effect on Survival
Monescillo A., et al. (Hepatology, 2004)	52 patients with cirrhosis admitted for AVB and HVPG ≥20 mmHg	Age <18/>75 years HCC PVT Previous TIPS HIV infection Chronic heart or renal failure	Primary endpoint: Prospective assessment of treatment failure as well as short- and long-term survival	Mortality reduced by TIPS: In hospital: 11% vs. 31%, $p = 0.02$; ARR 20% 1-year: 38% vs. 65%, $p = 0.01$; ARR 27% Bleeding-related: 19% vs. 38%, $p < 0.05$
Garcia-Pagan JC, et al. (N. Engl. J. Med., 2010)	63 patients with cirrhosis admitted for AVB (CTP B with active bleeding at endoscopyor CTP C ≤13 points)	Age <18/>75 years HCC outside Milan criteria Occlusive PVT Previous TIPS Failure of NSBB plus EVL, Bleeding from GV/ectopic varices Creatinine >3 mg/dL Chronic heart failure	Secondary endpoint: 6-weeks and 1-year mortality	Mortality reduced by TIPS: 6-week: 3% vs. 33%; ARR 30% 1-year: 14% vs. 39%, ARR 25% ($p = 0.001$)
Lv Y., et al. (Lancet Gastroenterol. Hepatol., 2019)	132 patients with cirrhosis admitted for AVB (CTP B patients with and without active bleeding at endoscopy or CTP C ≤13 points)	As above + Recurrent HE (without precipitating factors)	Primary endpoint: Transplant-free survival	Survival improved by TIPS: 6-weeks: 99 vs. 84%; $p = 0.02$ 1-year: 86% vs. 73%; $p = 0.046$ 2-years: 79% vs. 64%; $p = 0.04$

ARR: absolute risk reduction; AVB: acute variceal bleeding; CTP: Child–Turcotte–Pugh; EVL: endoscopic variceal ligation; HCC: hepatocellular carcinoma; HE: hepatic encephalopathy; HVPG: hepatic vein pressure gradient; IGV: isolated gastric varices; NSBB: non-selective beta-blockers; PVT: portal vein thrombosis; RCT: randomized clinical trial.

When TIPS insertion is related to the treatment of ascites, the available evidence for its capacity of modifying the course of the disease is less clearly defined. So far, seven RCTs compared the effect of TIPS versus large-volume paracentesis plus albumin, the standard of care for patients with refractory ascites [57–63] (Table 2). TIPS showed a superior efficacy in controlling ascites in all trials, although only shunts performed with covered stents positively affected survival [63]. A similar effect on survival occurred in patients with less advanced disease [62] or "recurrent/recidivant" ascites not fulfilling criteria for refractory ascites [58,61,63]. Furthermore, the high incidence of adverse events, such as hepatic encephalopathy, liver failure, and cardiac dysfunction, requires great caution in TIPS use in these patients [51], thus strengthening the need for a thoughtful selection of target patients. Promising results for expanding the application of TIPS could come from the use of smaller diameter stents (6–8 mm instead of 10 mm), which showed similar efficacy, but a lower incidence of adverse events, likely by preventing excessive shunting [64,65].

Table 2. RCTs assessing TIPS vs. LVP + Albumin in recurrent/refractory ascites.

Reference	Study Population (Randomized Patients)	Exclusion Criteria	Survival Related Endpoints of the Study	Effects on Survival
Lebrec D., et al. (J. Hepatol., 1996)	25 patients with cirrhosis and refractory ascites (no response after 5 days of in-hospital maximal diuretic therapy or ≥2 episodes of tense ascites in the previous 4 months)	Age >70 years, HE ≥grade 2 PVT Biliary obstruction Creatinine >1.7 mg/dL HCC Active bacterial infection Severe extra-hepatic disease Pulmonary hypertension	Not specified	LVP + Albumin vs. TIPS: 2-year overall survival: 60% vs. 29% ($p = 0.03$)
Rossle M., et al. (N. Engl. J. Med., 2000)	60 patients with cirrhosis and refractory ascites or recurrent ascites (ICA criteria)	HE ≥grade 2 PVT Bilirubin >5 mg/dL, Creatinine >3mg/dL Advanced HCC Hepatic hydrothorax Failure of paracentesis(defined as persistence of ascites after paracentesis or need for large-volume paracentesis more than once per week)	Primary endpoint: Transplant-free survival	LVP + Albumin vs. TIPS: 1-year: 69% vs. 58% 2-year: 58% vs. 32% ($p = 0.11$)
Ginès P., et al. (Gastroenterology, 2002)	70 patients with cirrhosis and refractory ascites (ICA criteria)	Age <18/>75 years PVT HE ≥grade 2 Bilirubin >10 mg/dL, Creatinine >3 mg/dL INR >2.5 Platelet <40.000/mm^3 Chronic Heart Failure HCC Organic renal failure	Primary endpoint: Transplant-free survival	LVP + Albumin vs. TIPS: 1-year: 41% vs. 35% 2-year: 26% vs. 30% ($p = 0.51$)
Sanyal A.J., et al. (Gastroenterology, 2003)	109 patients with cirrhosis and refractory ascites (ICA criteria) plus creatinine <1.5 mg/dL	HE ≥grade 2 PVT Bilirubin >5 mg/dL INR >2 HCC Bacterial infection Alcoholic hepatitis Chronic heart failure Pulmonary hypertension Organic kidney disease Recent gastrointestinal bleeding Severe extra-hepatic disease	Primary endpoint: Overall and transplant-free survival	LVP + Albumin vs. TIPS: Overall: 41.3 vs. 38.2 months; $p = 0.84$ Transplant-free: 19.6 vs. 12.4 months; $p = 0.77$
Salerno F., et al. (Hepatology, 2004)	66 patients with cirrhosis and refractory ascites (ICA criteria) or "recidivant" ascites (recurrence of at least 3 episodes of tense ascites within a 12-month period despite prescription of low sodium diet and adequate diuretic doses)	Age >72 years HE ≥grade 2 PVT CTP score >11 Bilirubin >6 mg/dL Creatinine >3 mg/dL Advanced HCC Bacterial infection Chronic heart failure Recent gastrointestinal bleeding	Primary endpoint: Transplant-free survival	LVP + Albumin vs. TIPS: 1-year: 52% vs. 77% 2-year: 29% vs. 59% ($p = 0.021$)
Narahara Y., et al. (J. Gastroenterol., 2011)	60 patients with cirrhosis and refractory ascites (ICA criteria) plus: CTP score <11 Bilirubin <3 mg/dL Creatinine <1.9 mg/dL	Age >70 years Episodes of HE PV cavernoma HCC Other malignancy Active infection Active severe cardiac or pulmonary disease Organic kidney disease >6 LVPs in the previous 3 months Waitlisted for LT or expected to receive LT within the next 6 months Recurrent overt HE	Primary endpoint: Overall survival	LVP + Albumin vs. TIPS: 1-year: 49% vs. 80% 2-year: 35% vs. 64% ($p < 0.005$)
Bureau C., et al. (Gastroenterology, 2017)	62 patients (>18/<70 year) with cirrhosis and recurrent tense ascites (requiring ≥2 LVP in the previous 3 weeks) PFTE-covered stents	PVT CTP score >12 Bilirubin >5.8 mg/dL Creatinine >2.8 mg/dL HCC Chronic heart failure Pulmonary hypertension	Primary endpoint: Transplant-free survival	LVP + Albumin vs. TIPS: 1-year: 93% vs. 52%; $p = 0.003$

CTP: Child–Turcotte–Pugh; HCC: hepatocellular carcinoma; ICA: International Club of Ascites; INR: international normalized ratio; HE: hepatic encephalopathy; HRS: hepatorenal syndrome; LT: liver transplantation; PFTE: polytetrafluoroethylene; PHT: portal hypertension; PVT: portal vein thrombosis.

The reduction in portal pressure induced by TIPS insertion is associated with beneficial effects on renal function in patients with cirrhosis and ascites, including an increase in sodium and water excretion and reduced activity of vasoconstrictor and antinatriuretic systems [2,51]. This could represent a valid rationale for the use of TIPS also in patients with HRS. The results of the available trials [66–68], although limited by a non-controlled design and small sample sizes, support this therapeutical approach, especially for non-transplantable patients. Furthermore, the practical applicability is usually limited by the concomitant severe degree of liver failure [2].

In summary, by acting against a key pathophysiological mechanism as portal hypertension, TIPS has a great potential to serve as DMAC. However, two factors limit its widespread use to this end. On the one hand, available studies evaluated the effects of TIPS in patients who develop either portal hypertensive bleeding or difficult-to-treat ascites. Its impact in patients with clinically significant portal hypertension but without these complications has never been assessed. On the other, the occurrence of severe TIPS-related complications often prevents its insertion in patients with refractory ascites. The use of a small-diameter covered stent may help in overcoming these limitations.

3.3. Poorly Absorbable Antibiotics

Acting on the intestinal microbiota to limit the abnormal translocation of bacteria and bacterial products is another treatment strategy of relevant importance in patients with cirrhosis. The use of antibiotics would appear an obvious choice, whose main limitation derives from the induction of bacterial resistance. Most available studies assessed the effects of non- or poorly-adsorbable antibiotics to limit their activities in the intestinal environment.

3.3.1. Quinolones

The enhanced susceptibility to bacterial infections by patients with cirrhosis has long been known. The high prevalence of episodes sustained by Gram-negative microorganisms of intestinal origin led to recognize the relevance of the abnormal bacterial translocation from the gut [69–71].

The proof-of-concept of the efficacy of antibiotic prophylaxis derives from an RCT comparing 12 months of treatment with norfloxacin versus placebo for 12 months to prevent SBP recurrence [72]. Norfloxacin remarkably reduced the recurrences due to Gram-negative bacteria, without side effects. Subsequent studies showed that either norfloxacin or ciprofloxacin significantly prevented SBP occurrence in high-risk patients with low protein concentration in ascites, liver failure, and/or gastrointestinal bleeding. The benefit deriving from either norfloxacin or ciprofloxacin in either primary or secondary prophylaxis of SBP was confirmed by most meta-analyses [73,74]. Interestingly, norfloxacin reduced circulating bacterial products associated with improved systemic inflammatory markers and circulatory dysfunction [75].

These results potentially demonstrate a pathophysiological effect beyond SBP prevention. However, a benefit on survival and the occurrence of complications of cirrhosis still needs to be convincingly established. A pivotal study in decompensated patients with a low protein content in ascitic fluid (<1.5 g/dL) and severe cirrhosis (Child–Pugh ≥9 with serum bilirubin ≥3 mg/dL) or impaired renal function (serum creatinine ≥1.2 mg/dL, blood urea nitrogen ≥25 mg/dL or serum sodium ≤130 mEq/L), showed that norfloxacin prophylaxis not only reduced the incidence of SBP but also lessened one-year risk for HRS and improved one-year survival compared with placebo [76]. However, both survival and incidence of HRS were secondary endpoints, and the study sample size was inadequate. More recently, a large multicenter RCT did not demonstrate a survival advantage in Child C patients receiving norfloxacin prophylaxis, although a post-hoc analysis unveiled a reduction in six-month mortality confined to the subgroup with low ascites protein concentration [77]. Finally, concerns about the safety of quinolones being a risk factor for the development of infections due to drug-resistant bacteria have been raised over the years [71], although more recent reports did not confirm these findings [77,78].

In conclusion, several important questions regarding the use of quinolones in decompensated cirrhosis remain unanswered, so that their administration as a DMAC cannot be currently proposed.

3.3.2. Rifaximin

There has been growing interest in the possible efficacy of rifaximin in preventing infections and other complications of portal hypertension in cirrhosis. Rifaximin is a minimally absorbed antibiotic with activity against Gram-negative and Gram-positive bacteria [79]. Moreover, it can improve the gut epithelial layer homeostasis, decrease inflammatory pathways, impair bacterial adhesion to enterocytes, and modulate the gut microbiome, thus positively affecting the entire gut liver-axis [80–82].

Currently, the only recognized indication for rifaximin use in patients with cirrhosis is the prevention of recurrent hepatic encephalopathy (secondary prophylaxis) [2], mainly based on the pivotal RCT by Bass et al. in 2010 [83]. However, both observational studies and a few small-scale RCTs showed an association between rifaximin treatment and important clinical outcomes, including better control of ascites [84,85], a reduced incidence of decompensation, hospitalizations, variceal bleeding, SBP, and HRS with a decreased risk of renal replacement therapy [86–93]. Some studies even suggested an improvement in mortality [85,87,89]. However, several metanalyses [94–96] highlighted the overall low quality of these studies precluding any generalization on the beneficial impact of rifaximin on the clinical course of decompensated cirrhosis. Therefore, before using rifaximin as a DMAC can be advocated in clinical practice, well-designed RCTs with hard endpoints and adequate sample size are needed.

3.4. Statins

The first proposal of statins for treating portal hypertension in cirrhosis dates back to the early 2000s [97] since they reduce intrahepatic vascular resistance by enhancing nitric oxide (NO) production in liver sinusoids. Subsequent investigations in experimental cirrhosis also unveiled anti-inflammatory and hepatoprotective properties [98–102]. Statins exert their effects on liver inflammation and fibrogenesis by upregulating the endothelial Kruppel-like factor 2 (KLF2) [101]. This transcription factor regulates the expression of several vasoprotective genes controlling apoptosis, inflammation, oxidative stress, thrombosis, and vasodilation. Furthermore, it inhibits RhoA/Rho-kinase signaling, which is partly responsible for the contractility of hepatic stellate cells [102].

Several observational studies reported the beneficial effects of statins on various clinical aspects of advanced liver disease. They include lower rates of decompensation, liver cancer, and bacterial infections along with increased survival [103,104]. However, these results require caution due to potential flaws in observational studies [105]. Different RCTs convincingly showed that simvastatin decreases portal pressure [106,107]. Further studies compared the lowering effect on portal pressure induced by combining statins with beta-blockers vs. beta-blockers alone, providing discordant results [108,109].

Only one randomized trial evaluated the effects of statins on the complications of cirrhosis [110]. This trial included patients with recent variceal bleeding and assessed the effects of adding simvastatin 40 mg daily or placebo to the standard therapy to prevent rebleeding (NSBBs and endoscopic variceal ligation). Simvastatin did not significantly influence the primary endpoint, which was a composite of rebleeding and death. Nevertheless, it was associated with a significant survival benefit, mainly related to decreased mortality from bleeding and bacterial infections. Patient subgroup analysis showed that this result was limited to patients belonging to Child-Pugh classes A and B. This apparent contradiction (no prevention of complications but improved survival) suggests that the effect on portal pressure might be less relevant than the non-hemodynamic effects of statins, attenuating the intense inflammatory response triggered by infections or bleeding events [99,100,111,112] that plays a major role in the development of ACLF and mortality [6,113].

In conclusion, although there is a robust rationale suggesting that statins might be beneficial for patients with cirrhosis, the evidence from randomized trials is scarce, limited to a single study with a positive result on a secondary endpoint. Non-hemodynamic effects of statins might be more important than the effects of portal pressure.

The currently ongoing LiverHope Efficacy study, a multicenter double-blind trial comparing the effects of simvastatin plus rifaximin vs. placebo in the prevention of ACLF and mortality (www.liverhope-h2020.eu, accessed on 4 October 2021), should clarify whether statins are effective and safe in advanced cirrhosis. Growing evidence support the role of bacterial translocation and systemic inflammation as key drivers of cirrhosis progression and ACLF development. On this pathophysiological background, the association of an agent effective in preventing bacterial translocation (rifaximin) and a drug with anti-inflammatory properties (simvastatin) could provide a dual effect able to counteract disease progression. It is important to emphasize that although there have been no safety issues in patients with compensated cirrhosis, statin pharmacokinetic is markedly altered in patients with decompensated liver disease [110], with a very high risk of muscle toxicity compared to the general population [110]. Very recent data from the LiverHope double-blind dose-finding safety trial showed that a dose of 20 mg/day was associated with no muscle toxicity [114].

3.5. Human Albumin

The well-established recommendations for human albumin (HA) use in patients with decompensated cirrhosis pertain to conditions characterized by an acute worsening of effective volemia. Indeed, one-shot or short-term HA administration is employed to prevent paracentesis-induced circulatory dysfunction (PICD), prevent renal dysfunction induced by SBP, and diagnose and treat HRS in association with vasoconstrictors [2,115].

The oncotic properties of HA make it an optimal candidate to correct or attenuate effective hypovolemia. However, HA exerts several functions not related to its oncotic properties. These pleiotropic functions include binding of damaging molecules, modulating inflammation and immune responses, exerting antioxidant activity, improving cardiac function, and restoring endothelial integrity [116]. Therefore, from a pathophysiological perspective, HA could act as a multitarget agent, potentially modifying the clinical course of decompensated cirrhosis. Such an approach would imply long-term HA administration.

In 2018, two RCTs and one prospective observational study evaluated the efficacy of long-term HA in patients with ascites, opening new perspectives for the treatment of decompensated cirrhosis [117–119]. The ANSWER study [117], a multicenter open-label RCT, enrolled patients with uncomplicated grade 2 or 3 ascites. Those patients included in the active arm of the study received 40 g of HA per week for the initial two weeks, then 40 g weekly for a maximal duration of 18 months. The primary endpoint of the study was reached, as patients receiving HA had a significantly better 18-month overall survival, with a 38% reduction in mortality hazard ratio. Moreover, the management of ascites became easier, as the need for paracentesis and the incidence of refractory ascites were reduced by about 50%. HA administration also lowered the incidence rate of the major complications of cirrhosis. As a result, patients receiving albumin needed fewer and shorter liver-related hospitalizations and preserved their quality of life. Similar results were also reported by a single-center, prospective, non-randomized study in patients with refractory ascites [118]. In contrast, the MACHT study [119], a multicenter placebo-controlled RCT performed in patients with ascites waitlisted for liver transplantation, showed no differences in either the probability of developing complications or death between patients treated or not with HA.

These divergent results should not advise against long-term HA use in decompensated patients. Contrariwise, their comparison provides essential information about patients to be treated and, mainly, the dose and schedule of HA administration. The ANSWER and the MACHT studies differed in terms of design, baseline patient characteristics, length of follow-up, and dosage and timing of albumin administration. A consequence of the lower amount of HA given to patients enrolled in the MACHT trial was that serum albumin concentration remained steady throughout the follow-up [119]. In contrast, serum albumin concentration rose by 0.7–0.8 g/L to almost 4 g/dL in the ANSWER study [117]. A post-hoc analysis of the latter trial showed that on-treatment serum albumin concentration at one month predicts the probability of 18-month overall survival, which was greater than 90% in patients whose serum albumin concentration reached levels 4 g/dL [120]. Baseline serum albumin and MELD score value independently predicted the achievement of this threshold. This would imply that patients with severe hypoalbuminema and very high MELD score should receive greater amounts of HA to achieve the best results [120]. Two other pieces of evidence support the importance of steadily increasing serum albumin concentration beyond a certain level. First, in the pilot-PRECIOSA study, only a "high dose" of HA (1.5 g/kg b.w. every week) made serum albumin rise to a concentration close to 4 g/dl, while a lower dose (1 g/kg b.w. every 10 days) failed to normalize serum albumin in most cases. Notably, only patients who received the high HA dose improved their cardiocirculatory function [121]. Second, a serum albumin concentration greater than 4 g/dL is physiologically present in more than 90% of healthy adult individuals [122].

The recently published ATTIRE Trial [123], an open-label, multicenter RCT which included hospitalized patients with acute decompensation of cirrhosis (with or without ACLF) deserves some comments. In this study, albumin was administered for up to 14 days with the goal to maintain a serum albumin level >3.0 g/dL. No differences were observed in the incidence of infections, renal dysfunction, and death between the two study arms. Moreover, some safety concerns have been raised, mainly due to a higher incidence of fluid overload and pulmonary edema in treated patients. Therefore, albumin administration does not appear to modify the short-term course of cirrhosis in severely ill patients admitted to hospital for an acute complication, at least with the dose and schedule of administration chosen in the ATTIRE study. So far, indeed, the efficacy of short-term albumin use has been demonstrated only in patients with SBP or HRS. Acutely ill hospitalized patients, however, represent a completely different clinical setting compared to chronic administration to stable decompensated patients.

In conclusion, there is growing evidence that long-term HA administration can modify the natural history of decompensated cirrhosis, thus acting as a DMAC rather than a specific treatment for ascites and their acute complications. Future studies are warranted to better characterize patient subgroups who could benefit the most from this novel approach. There is also a need to go beyond a fixed dosage and schedule of HA administration, ideally tending to an individualized and patient-tailored approach. Future investigations should prove or challenge this hypothesis and other open issues, including the definition of stopping rules and the cost-effectiveness (in settings other than Italy [117]) of this relatively demanding treatment in terms of logistics and patient adherence.

3.6. Granulocyte Colony-Stimulating Factor

Several RCTs assessed the effects of granulocyte colony-stimulating factor (G-CSF), either alone or in combination with bone marrow stem cell transplantation, in patients with acute alcoholic hepatitis (AH) and/or ACLF and in patients with more stable decompensated cirrhosis. Among the pleiotropic effects of GCS-F, the stimulation of liver regeneration and the improvement in immune dysfunction have been proposed as the mechanisms of action [124]. A recent meta-analysis including 7 RCTs [125–131] in patients with AH and/or ACLF showed a significant benefit of 90-day survival in favor of G-CSF [132]. However, these results were not confirmed by another analysis [133]. Conclusions are also challenging due to the high heterogeneity of the studies and by the different outcomes found in Europe and Asia [132].

Similar results have been reported in RCTs assessing G-CSF in patients with more stable decompensated cirrhosis. Studies from India provided positive results [134–137]. In contrast, a trial performed in the United Kingdom showed no improvement in MELD score at three months with G-CSF, with or without hematopoietic stem-cell infusion (CD133+) [138]. Moreover, there was an increase in adverse events and sepsis.

RCTs demonstrating the efficacy of G-CSF in European and US cohorts are needed if G-CSF is to be considered a therapeutic option in the future. Aspects to be evaluated include the ideal dose and schedule of administration, the duration of therapy, the use of combinatorial therapies, the identification of the most appropriate target population, a better understanding of the mechanisms of action, including those potentially adverse, and, finally, understanding whether geographical differences affect the response.

4. Controversial Areas and Future Perspectives

Based on the data reported above, no treatments are so far available to effectively manage patients with cirrhosis, especially in the decompensated stage of the disease. Besides various etiological treatments, that in patients with compensated cirrhosis can often prevent decompensations and complications, no solid data support the efficacy as a DMAC of any currently available treatment for decompensated patients. Indeed, some interventions given to treat/prevent a specific complication or comorbidities appear to act as a DMAC (i.e., albumin or TIPS) or have the potential to act (i.e., rifaximin, NSBBs, statins, G-CSF) in certain subgroups of patients.

Since the goal of a DMAC is to halt or at least slow down the progression of the disease, or even partially revert decompensation, its efficacy should be tested by RCTs with patients' survival as a primary endpoint. However, the very large sample size required to reveal statistically significant differences forces researchers to use alternative "surrogate primary endpoints", such as the incidence of complications and/or ACLF. These latter events, however, would work better as secondary endpoints, which should also include hospitalizations, quality of life, and cost-effectiveness of treatment [11,12]. Unfortunately, up to now, very few published RCTs have addressed the above endpoints. Examples of such trials are the ANSWER and MACTH trials on albumin [117,119] or the NORFLOCIR trial on norfloxacin [77]. In contrast, the low-quality data generated by a long series of observational studies and small-scale RCTs, which even fairly consistently show an improvement in survival and incidence of complications [84–93], have to date precluded the use of rifaximin beyond the evidence-based indication of the prevention of HE recurrence. As a result, in the future reliable and conclusive data on DMACs can only derive from multicenter, possibly international, well-designed and adequately powered RCTs, thus highlighting the importance of scientific consortia for promoting and coordinating these research projects.

Moreover, due to the complexity and heterogeneity of patients included in the definition of decompensated cirrhosis, some interventions could act as DMAC only in well-defined subgroups of patients. An example is given by albumin, which has been found effective in the ANSWER trial, if administered long-term in patients with stable decompensated cirrhosis and persistent grade 2 or 3 uncomplicated ascites [117], but not in the ATTIRE study, which enrolled severe and acutely decompensated patients admitted to hospital, with or without ACLF [123]. In addition to the target population, other open issues for any intervention include transferability to daily clinical practice, the definition of dosage and schedule of administration, factors guiding treatment, temporary or permanent stopping rules, the use of combinatorial approaches, cost-effectiveness for healthcare systems, and access to treatment worldwide. Hopefully, some ongoing RCTs will clarify whether the course of decompensated cirrhosis could be positively impacted in well-defined groups of patients by drugs or interventions that are currently used for more limited indications (NCT04072601, NCT03780673, NCT02401490, NCT03451292).

The increasing understanding of the pathophysiological mechanisms underlying decompensated cirrhosis and leading to hepatic and extra-hepatic organ failure could potentially provide new interventions, drugs, and biological substances. Novel candidate DMACs should be able to target gut microbiota or key mechanisms in the pathogenetic network of gut-liver axis, systemic inflammation, and immune dysfunction. One such approach, which is already under development, aims to antagonize a crucial upstream step of the inflammatory cascade by TAK-242, an inhibitor of toll-like receptor 4

(TLR4) [139], which binds the circulating pathogen-associated molecular patterns (PAMPs), such as lipopolysaccharides (LPS) and gram-negative endotoxins [140], as well as damage-associated molecular patterns (DAMPs), such as cleaved nucleosomes, histones, and high-mobility group box 1 proteins (HMGB1) [141].

In the context of acutely decompensated disease with an abnormal burst of systemic inflammation, interesting perspectives could derive from studies assessing albumin-based extracorporeal liver assist devices. The molecular adsorbent recirculating system (MARS) and Prometheus provided proof of concept that such a strategy could be successful but did not show improvement in survival [142–144]. A novel device, DIALIVE, has been developed to remove and replace the damaged albumin while also removing DAMPs and PAMPs [145]. A multicenter RCT (NCT03065699) aiming to assess the safety and performance of DIALIVE in patients with ACLF has been recently completed and positive results have been publicly announced. Moreover, as an extension of this concept, another phase III, multicenter, RCT on plasma exchange in patients with ACLF (NCT03702920) is currently ongoing. Their results are eagerly needed to improve the management of these severe acute patients.

The identification of new DMACs will be also aided by innovative research technologies and approaches, such as high throughput -omics techniques and systems medicine analysis. When applied to large cohorts of patients with detailed clinical data, treatment history and outcome as well as biological samples, these approaches will support the identification or development of new DMACs and biomarkers to predict patient prognosis and response to therapies, such as the DECISION project (www.decision-for-liver.eu, accessed on 4 October 2021) is currently pursuing in the perspective of personalized medicine.

The next decade will reveal whether patients with cirrhosis, especially in its decompensated stage, could benefit from treatments that globally manage their disease by reducing the occurrence of complications and ACLF, preventing hospitalization, and ultimately improving survival and quality of life, as already occurs for other impactful diseases.

Author Contributions: Writing—Original draft preparation, G.Z.; writing—review and editing, M.T.; writing—review and editing, M.B.; writing—review and editing, P.C. All authors have read and agreed to the published version of the manuscript.

Funding: This project has received funding from the European Union's Horizon 2020 Research and Innovation Programme under Grant Agreement No 731875.

Institutional Review Board Statement: Not applicable.

Informed Consent Statement: Not applicable.

Data Availability Statement: No new data were created or analyzed in this study. Data sharing is not applicable to this article.

Conflicts of Interest: Zaccherini is part of the speakers' bureau for Grifols SA and Octapharma SA, outside the submitted work. Tufoni is part of the speakers' bureau for Grifols SA and Octapharma SA, outside the submitted work. Bernardi is part of the speakers' bureau for Grifols SA, Octapharma AG, Takeda, CSL Behring GmbH, and PPTA, and is a consultant for CLS Behring GmbH, Grifols SA and Takeda, outside the submitted work. Caraceni is part of the speakers' bureau for Grifols SA, Octapharma SA, Kedrion Biopharma SpA, Mallinkrodt SA, Gilead SA and Takeda SA, outside the submitted work.

References

1. D'Amico, G.; Morabito, A.; D'Amico, M.; Pasta, L.; Malizia, G.; Rebora, P.; Valsecchi, M.G. Clinical states of cirrhosis and competing risks. *J. Hepatol.* **2018**, *68*, 563–576. [CrossRef]
2. Angeli, P.; Bernardi, M.; Villanueva, C.; Francoz, C.; Mookerjee, R.; Trebicka, J.; Krag, A.; Laleman, W.; Gines, P. EASL Clinical practice guidelines for the management of patients with decompensated cirrhosis. *J. Hepatol.* **2018**, *69*, 406–460. [CrossRef]
3. Bernardi, M.; Caraceni, P.; Navickis, R.J.; Wilkes, M.M. Albumin infusion in patients undergoing large-volume paracentesis: A meta-analysis of randomized trials. *Hepatology* **2012**, *55*, 1172–1181. [CrossRef]
4. Bai, M.; Qi, X.S.; Yang, Z.P.; Yang, M.; Fan, D.M.; Han, G.H. TIPS improves liver transplantation-free survival in cirrhotic patients with refractory ascites: An updated meta-analysis. *World J. Gastroenterol.* **2014**, *20*, 2704–2714. [CrossRef]

5. Bernardi, M.; Caraceni, P. Novel perspectives in the management of decompensated cirrhosis. *Nat. Rev. Gastroenterol. Hepatol.* **2018**, *15*, 753–764. [CrossRef]

6. Caraceni, P.; Abraldes, J.G.; Ginès, P.; Newsome, P.N.; Sarin, S.K. The search for disease-modifying agents in decompensated cirrhosis: From drug repurposing to drug discovery. *J. Hepatol.* **2021**, *75*, S118–S134. [CrossRef]

7. Lens, S.; Baiges, A.; Alvarado-Tapias, E.; Llop, E.; Martinez, J.; Fortea, J.I.; Ibáñez-Samaniego, L.; Mariño, Z.; Rodríguez-Tajes, S.; Gallego, A.; et al. Clinical outcome and hemodynamic changes following HCV eradication with oral antiviral therapy in patients with clinically significant portal hypertension. *J. Hepatol.* **2020**, *73*, 1415–1424. [CrossRef] [PubMed]

8. Verna, E.C.; Morelli, G.; Terrault, N.A.; Lok, A.S.; Lim, J.K.; Di Bisceglie, A.M.; Zeuzem, S.; Landis, C.S.; Kwo, P.; Hassan, M.; et al. DAA therapy and long-term hepatic function in advanced/decompensated cirrhosis: Real-world experience from HCV-TARGET cohort. *J. Hepatol.* **2020**, *73*, 540–548. [CrossRef] [PubMed]

9. Bernardi, M.; Moreau, R.; Angeli, P.; Schnabl, B.; Arroyo, V. Mechanisms of decompensation and organ failure in cirrhosis: From peripheral arterial vasodilation to systemic inflammation hypothesis. *J. Hepatol.* **2015**, *63*, 1272–1284. [CrossRef] [PubMed]

10. Engelmann, C.; Clària, J.; Szabo, G.; Bosch, J.; Bernardi, M. Pathophysiology of decompensated cirrhosis: Portal hypertension, circulatory dysfunction, inflammation, metabolism and mitochondrial dysfunction. *J. Hepatol.* **2021**, *75*, S49–S66. [CrossRef]

11. Solà, E.; Pose, E.; Campion, D.; Piano, S.; Roux, O.; Simon-Talero, M.; Uschner, F.; de Wit, K.; Zaccherini, G.; Alessandria, C.; et al. Endpoints and design of clinical trials in patients with decompensated cirrhosis: Position paper of the LiverHope Consortium. *J. Hepatol.* **2020**, *74*, 200–219. [CrossRef]

12. Abraldes, J.G.; Trebicka, J.; Chalasani, N.; D'Amico, G.; Rockey, D.C.; Shah, V.H.; Bosch, J.; Garcia-Tsao, G. Prioritization of therapeutic targets and trial design in cirrhotic portal hypertension. *Hepatology* **2018**, *69*, 1287–1299. [CrossRef] [PubMed]

13. Trebicka, J.; Fernández, J.; Papp, M.; Caraceni, P.; Laleman, W.; Gambino, C.; Giovo, I.; Uschner, F.E.; Jimenez, C.; Mookerjee, R.; et al. The PREDICT study uncovers three clinical courses of acutely decompensated cirrhosis that have distinct pathophysiology. *J. Hepatol.* **2020**, *73*, 842–854. [CrossRef]

14. Moreau, R.; Jalan, R.; Gines, P.; Pavesi, M.; Angeli, P.; Cordoba, J.; Durand, F.; Gustot, T.; Saliba, F.; Domenicali, M.; et al. Acute-on-chronic liver failure is a distinct syndrome that develops in patients with acute decompensation of cirrhosis. *Gastroenterology* **2013**, *144*, 1426–1437.e9. [CrossRef]

15. Mandorfer, M.; Simbrunner, B. Prevention of first decompensation in advanced chronic liver disease. *Clin. Liver Dis.* **2021**, *25*, 291–310. [CrossRef] [PubMed]

16. Lok, A.S.; McMahon, B.J.; Brown, R.S., Jr.; Wong, J.B.; Ahmed, A.T.; Farah, W.; Almasri, J.; Alahdab, F.; Benkhadra, K.; Mouchli, M.A.; et al. Antiviral therapy for chronic hepatitis B viral infection in adults: A systematic review and meta-analysis. *Hepatology* **2015**, *63*, 284–306. [CrossRef] [PubMed]

17. Peng, C.-Y.; Chien, R.-N.; Liaw, Y.-F. Hepatitis B virus-related decompensated liver cirrhosis: Benefits of antiviral therapy. *J. Hepatol.* **2012**, *57*, 442–450. [CrossRef]

18. Jang, J.W.; Choi, J.Y.; Kim, Y.S.; Yoo, J.-J.; Woo, H.Y.; Choi, S.K.; Jun, C.H.; Lee, C.H.; Sohn, J.H.; Tak, W.Y.; et al. Effects of virologic response to treatment on short- and long-term outcomes of patients with chronic hepatitis b virus infection and decompensated cirrhosis. *Clin. Gastroenterol. Hepatol.* **2018**, *16*, 1954–1963.e3. [CrossRef]

19. Ju, Y.C.; Jun, D.W.; Choi, J.; Saeed, W.K.; Lee, H.Y.; Oh, H.W. Long term outcome of antiviral therapy in patients with hepatitis B associated decompensated cirrhosis. *World J. Gastroenterol.* **2018**, *24*, 4606–4614. [CrossRef]

20. Mendizabal, M.; Piñero, F.; Ridruejo, E.; Herz Wolff, F.; Anders, M.; Reggiardo, V.; Ameigeiras, B.; Palazzo, A.; Alonso, C.; Schinoni, M.I.; et al. Disease progression in patients with hepatitis C virus infection treated with Direct-Acting Antiviral agents. *Clin. Gastroenterol. Hepatol.* **2020**, *28*, 30263–30269. [CrossRef]

21. Belli, L.S.; Berenguer, M.; Cortesi, P.A.; Strazzabosco, M.; Rockenschaub, S.-R.; Martini, S.; Morelli, C.; Donato, F.; Volpes, R.; Pageaux, G.-P.; et al. Delisting of liver transplant candidates with chronic hepatitis C after viral eradication: A European study. *J. Hepatol.* **2016**, *65*, 524–531. [CrossRef]

22. El-Sherif, O.; Jiang, Z.G.; Tapper, E.B.; Huang, K.; Zhong, A.; Osinusi, A.; Charlton, M.; Manns, M.; Afdhal, N.; Mukamal, K.; et al. Baseline factors associated with improvements in decompensated cirrhosis after direct-acting antiviral therapy for hepatitis C virus infection. *Gastroenterology* **2018**, *154*, 2111–2121.e8. [CrossRef]

23. European Association for the Study of the Liver. EASL Clinical Practice Guidelines: Liver transplantation. *J. Hepatol.* **2016**, *64*, 433–485. [CrossRef]

24. Terrault, N.A.; Mccaughan, G.; Curry, M.P.; Gane, E.; Fagiuoli, S.; Fung, J.; Agarwal, K.; Lilly, L.; Strasser, S.I.; Brown, K.A.; et al. International liver transplantation society consensus statement on Hepatitis C management in liver transplant candidates. *Transplantation* **2017**, *101*, 945–955. [CrossRef] [PubMed]

25. Altamirano, J.; López-Pelayo, H.; Michelena, J.; Jones, P.D.; Ortega, L.; Ginès, P.; Caballería, J.; Gual, A.; Bataller, R.; Lligoña, A. Alcohol abstinence in patients surviving an episode of alcoholic hepatitis: Prediction and impact on long-term survival. *Hepatology* **2017**, *66*, 1842–1853. [CrossRef] [PubMed]

26. Degré, D.; Stauber, R.E.; Englebert, G.; Sarocchi, F.; Verset, L.; Rainer, F.; Spindelboeck, W.; Njimi, H.; Trépo, E.; Gustot, T.; et al. Long-term outcomes in patients with decompensated alcohol-related liver disease, steatohepatitis and Maddrey's discriminant function <32. *J. Hepatol.* **2020**, *72*, 636–642. [CrossRef] [PubMed]

27. El Sherif, O.; Dhaliwal, A.; Newsome, P.N.; Armstrong, M.J. Sarcopenia in nonalcoholic fatty liver disease: New challenges for clinical practice. *Expert Rev. Gastroenterol. Hepatol.* **2020**, *14*, 197–205. [CrossRef]

28. Tandon, P.; Ney, M.; Irwin, I.; Ma, M.M.; Gramlich, L.; Bain, V.G.; Esfandiari, N.; Baracos, V.; Montano-Loza, A.J.; Myers, R.P. Severe muscle depletion in patients on the liver transplant wait list: Its prevalence and independent prognostic value. *Liver Transplant.* **2012**, *18*, 1209–1216. [CrossRef]

29. Berzigotti, A.; Albillos, A.; Villanueva, C.; Genescá, J.; Ardevol, A.; Augustín, S.; Calleja, J.L.; Bañares, R.; García-Pagán, J.C.; Mesonero, F.; et al. Effects of an intensive lifestyle intervention program on portal hypertension in patients with cirrhosis and obesity: The SportDiet study. *Hepatology* **2017**, *65*, 1293–1305. [CrossRef]

30. Hoeroldt, B.; McFarlane, E.; Dube, A.; Basumani, P.; Karajeh, M.; Campbell, M.J.; Gleeson, D. Long-term outcomes of patients with auto-immune hepatitis managed at a nontransplant center. *Gastroenterology* **2011**, *140*, 1980–1989. [CrossRef]

31. De Franchis, R.; Baveno, V.I.F. Expanding consensus in portal hypertension: Report of the Baveno VI Consensus Workshop: Stratifying risk and individualizing care for portal hypertension. *J. Hepatol.* **2015**, *63*, 743–752. [CrossRef]

32. Garcia-Tsao, G.; Abraldes, J.G.; Berzigotti, A.; Bosch, J. Portal hypertensive bleeding in cirrhosis: Risk stratification, diagnosis, and management: 2016 practice guidance by the American Association for the study of liver diseases. *Hepatology* **2016**, *65*, 310–335. [CrossRef] [PubMed]

33. Bendtsen, F.; Henriksen, J.H.; Sørensen, T.I. Propranolol and haemodynamic response in cirrhosis. *J. Hepatol.* **1991**, *13*, 144–148. [CrossRef]

34. Rodrigues, S.G.; Mendoza, Y.P.; Bosch, J. Beta-blockers in cirrhosis: Evidence-based indications and limitations. *JHEP Rep.* **2019**, *2*, 100063. [CrossRef] [PubMed]

35. Bañares, R.; Moitinho, E.; Matilla, A.; García-Pagán, J.C.; Lampreave, J.L.; Piera, C.; Abraldes, J.G.; De Diego, A.; Albillos, A.; Bosch, J. Randomized comparison of long-term carvedilol and propranolol administration in the treatment of portal hypertension in cirrhosis. *Hepatology* **2002**, *36*, 1367–1373. [CrossRef]

36. Reiberger, T.; Ferlitsch, A.; Payer, B.A.; Mandorfer, M.; Heinisch, B.B.; Hayden, H.; Lammert, F.; Trauner, M.; Peck-Radosavljevic, M.; Vogelsang, H. Non-selective betablocker therapy decreases intestinal permeability and serum levels of LBP and IL-6 in patients with cirrhosis. *J. Hepatol.* **2012**, *58*, 911–921. [CrossRef]

37. Poynard, T.; Calès, P.; Pasta, L.; Ideo, G.; Pascal, J.P.; Pagliaro, L.; Lebrec, D.; Franco–Italian Multicenter Study Group. Beta-adrenergic-antagonist drugs in the prevention of gas-trointestinal bleeding in patients with cirrhosis and esophageal varices. An analysis of data and prognostic factors in 589 patients from four randomized clinical trials. Franco-Italian Multicenter Study Group. *N. Engl. J. Med.* **1991**, *324*, 1532–1538. [PubMed]

38. Albillos, A.; Zamora, J.; Martínez, J.; Arroyo, D.; Ahmad, I.; De-La-Peña, J.; Garcia-Pagán, J.-C.; Lo, G.-H.; Sarin, S.; Sharma, B.; et al. Stratifying risk in the prevention of recurrent variceal hemorrhage: Results of an individual patient meta-analysis. *Hepatology* **2017**, *66*, 1219–1231. [CrossRef]

39. Ripoll, C.; Augustin, S.; Reiberger, T.; Moreau, R.; Salerno, F.; Albillos, A.; Abraldes, J.G.; García-Tsao, G. *Effect of Current Therapies Aimed at Preventing Variceal Rebleeding on Other Complications of Cirrhosis*; Springer: Berlin/Heidelberg, Germany, 2016; pp. 333–339. [CrossRef]

40. Turco, L.; Villanueva, C.; La Mura, V.; García-Pagán, J.C.; Reiberger, T.; Genescà, J.; Groszmann, R.J.; Sharma, B.C.; Merkel, C.; Bureau, C.; et al. Lowering portal pressure improves out-comes of patients with cirrhosis, with or without ascites: A meta-analysis. *Clin. Gastroenterol. Hepatol.* **2020**, *18*, 313–327. [CrossRef]

41. Villanueva, C.; Albillos, A.; Genescà, J.; Garcia-Pagan, J.C.; Calleja, J.L.; Aracil, C.; Bañares, R.; Morillas, R.M.; Poca, M.; Peñas, B.; et al. beta blockers to prevent decompensation of cirrhosis in patients with clinically significant portal hypertension (PREDESCI): A randomised, double-blind, placebo-controlled, multicentre trial. *Lancet* **2019**, *393*, 1597–1608. [CrossRef]

42. Kumar, M.; Kainth, S.; Choudhury, A.; Maiwall, R.; Mitra, L.G.; Saluja, V.; Agarwal, P.M.; Shasthry, S.M.; Jindal, A.; Bhardwaj, A.; et al. Treatment with carvedilol improves survival of patients with acute-on-chronic liver failure: A randomized controlled trial. *Hepatol. Int.* **2019**, *13*, 800–813. [CrossRef] [PubMed]

43. Sarin, S.K.; APASL ACLF Research Consortium (AARC) for APASL ACLF Working Party; Choudhury, A.; Sharma, M.K.; Maiwall, R.; Al Mahtab, M.; Rahman, S.; Saigal, S.; Saraf, N.; Soin, A.S.; et al. Acute-on-chronic liver failure: Consensus recommendations of the Asian Pacific association for the study of the liver (APASL): An update. *Hepatol. Int.* **2019**, *13*, 353–390. [CrossRef]

44. Conn, H.O.; Pope, A. Propranolol in the treatment of portal hypertension: A caution. *Hepatology* **2007**, *2*, 641S–644S. [CrossRef]

45. Sersté, T.; Melot, C.; Francoz, C.; Durand, F.; Rautou, P.-E.; Valla, D.; Moreau, R.; Lebrec, D. Deleterious effects of beta-blockers on survival in patients with cirrhosis and refractory ascites. *Hepatology* **2010**, *52*, 1017–1022. [CrossRef]

46. Mandorfer, M.; Bota, S.; Schwabl, P.; Bucsics, T.; Pfisterer, N.; Kruzik, M.; Hagmann, M.; Blacky, A.; Ferlitsch, A.; Sieghart, W.; et al. Nonselective beta blockers increase risk for hepato-renal syndrome and death in patients with cirrhosis and spontaneous bacterial peritonitis. *Gastroenterology* **2014**, *146*, 1680–1690. [CrossRef] [PubMed]

47. Krag, A.; Wiest, R.; Albillos, A.; Gluud, L.L. The window hypothesis: Haemodynamic and non-haemodynamic effects of be-ta-blockers improve survival of patients with cirrhosis during a window in the disease. *Gut* **2012**, *61*, 967–969. [CrossRef]

48. Chirapongsathorn, S.; Valentin, N.; Alahdab, F.; Krittanawong, C.; Erwin, P.J.; Murad, M.H.; Kamath, P.S. Nonselective beta-blockers and survival in patients with cirrhosis and ascites: A systematic review and meta-analysis. *Clin. Gastroenterol. Hepatol.* **2016**, *14*, 1096–1104. [CrossRef]

49. Téllez, L.; Ibáñez-Samaniego, L.; del Villar, C.P.; Yotti, R.; Martínez, J.; Carrión, L.; de Santiago, E.R.; Rivera, M.; González-Mansilla, A.; Pastor, O.; et al. Non-selective beta-blockers impair global circulatory homeostasis and renal function in cirrhotic patients with refractory ascites. *J. Hepatol.* **2020**, *73*, 1404–1414. [CrossRef]

50. Tergast, T.L.; Kimmann, M.; Laser, H.; Gerbel, S.; Manns, M.P.; Cornberg, M.; Maasoumy, B. Systemic arterial blood pressure determines the therapeutic window of non-selective beta blockers in decompensated cirrhosis. *Aliment. Pharmacol. Ther.* **2019**, *50*, 696–706. [CrossRef]

51. Garcia-Pagan, J.C.; Saffo, S.; Mandorfer, M.; Garcia-Tsao, G. Where does TIPS fit in the management of patients with cirrhosis? *J. Hep. Rep.* **2020**, *2*, 100122.

52. Monescillo, A.; Martínez-Lagares, F.; Ruiz-Del-Arbol, L.; Sierra, A.; Guevara, C.; Jiménez, E.; Marrero, J.M.; Buceta, E.; Sánchen, J.; Castellot, A.; et al. Influence of portal hypertension and its early decompression by TIPS placement on the outcome of variceal bleeding. *Hepatology* **2004**, *40*, 793–801. [CrossRef] [PubMed]

53. Garcia-Pagan, J.C.; Caca, K.; Bureau, C.; Laleman, W.; Appenrodt, B.; Luca, A.; Gonzalez-Abraldes, J.; Nevens, F.; Vinel, J.P.; Mössner, J.; et al. Early use of TIPS in patients with cirrhosis and variceal bleeding. *N. Engl. J. Med.* **2010**, *362*, 2370–2379. [CrossRef] [PubMed]

54. Lv, Y.; Yang, Z.; Liu, L.; Li, K.; He, C.; Wang, Z.; Bai, W.; Guo, W.; Yu, T.; Yuan, X.; et al. Early TIPS with covered stents versus standard treatment for acute variceal bleeding in patients with advanced cirrhosis: A randomised controlled trial. *Lancet Gastroenterol. Hepatol.* **2019**, *4*, 587–598. [CrossRef]

55. Trebicka, J.; Gu, W.; Ibáñez-Samaniego, L.; Hernández-Gea, V.; Pitarch, C.; Garcia, E.; Procopet, B.; Giráldez, A.; Amitrano, L.; Villanueva, C.; et al. Rebleeding and mortality risk are increased by ACLF but reduced by pre-emptive TIPS. *J. Hepatol.* **2020**, *73*, 1082–1091. [CrossRef]

56. Kumar, R.; Kerbert, A.J.; Sheikh, M.F.; Roth, N.; Calvao, J.A.; Mesquita, M.D.; Barreira, A.I.; Gurm, H.S.; Ramsahye, K.; Mookerjee, R.P.; et al. Determinants of mortality in patients with cirrhosis and uncontrolled variceal bleeding. *J. Hepatol.* **2020**, *74*, 66–79. [CrossRef] [PubMed]

57. Lebrec, D.; Giuily, N.; Hadengue, A.; Vilgrain, V.; Moreau, R.; Poynard, T.; Gadano, A.; Lassen, C.; Benhamou, J.-P.; Erlinger, S. Transjugular intrahepatic portosystemic shunts: Comparison with paracentesis in patients with cirrhosis and refractory ascites: A randomized trial. *J. Hepatol.* **1996**, *25*, 135–144. [CrossRef]

58. Rössle, M.; Ochs, A.; Gülberg, V.; Siegerstetter, V.; Holl, J.; Deibert, P.; Olschewski, M.; Reiser, M.; Gerbes, A.L. A comparison of paracentesis and transjugular intrahepatic portosystemic shunting in patients with ascites. *New Engl. J. Med.* **2000**, *342*, 1701–1707. [CrossRef]

59. Ginès, P.; Uriz, J.; Calahorra, B.; Garcia–Tsao, G.; Kamath, P.S.; Del Arbol, L.R.; Planas, R.; Bosch, J.; Arroyo, V.; Rodés, J. Transjugular intrahepatic portosystemic shunting versus paracentesis plus albumin for refractory ascites in cirrhosis. *Gastroenterology* **2002**, *123*, 1839–1847. [CrossRef]

60. Sanyal, A.J.; Genning, C.; Reddy, K.; Wong, F.; Kowdley, K.V.; Benner, K.; McCashland, T. The North American study for the treatment of refractory ascites. *Gastroenterology* **2003**, *124*, 634–641. [CrossRef]

61. Salerno, F.; Merli, M.; Riggio, O.; Cazzaniga, M.; Valeriano, V.; Pozzi, M.; Nicolini, A.; Salvatori, F.; GIST. Randomized controlled study of TIPS versus para-centesis plus albumin in cirrhosis with severe ascites. *Hepatology* **2004**, *40*, 629–635. [CrossRef] [PubMed]

62. Narahara, Y.; Kanazawa, H.; Fukuda, T.; Matsushita, Y.; Harimoto, H.; Kidokoro, H.; Katakura, T.; Atsukawa, M.; Taki, Y.; Kimura, Y.; et al. Transjugular intrahepatic portosystemic shunt versus paracentesis plus albumin in patients with refractory ascites who have good hepatic and renal function: A prospective randomized trial. *J. Gastroenterol.* **2011**, *46*, 78–85. [CrossRef]

63. Bureau, C.; Thabut, D.; Oberti, F.; Dharancy, S.; Carbonell, N.; Bouvier, A.; Mathurin, P.; Otal, P.; Cabarrou, P.; Péron, J.M.; et al. Transjugular intrahepatic portosystemic shunts with covered stents increase transplant-free survival of patients with cirrhosis and recurrent ascites. *Gastroenterology* **2017**, *152*, 157–163. [CrossRef] [PubMed]

64. Miraglia, R.; Maruzzelli, L.; Tuzzolino, F.; Petridis, I.; D'Amico, M.; Luca, A. Transjugular intrahepatic portosystemic shunts in patients with cirrhosis with refractory ascites: Comparison of clinical outcomes by using 8- and 10-mm PTFE-covered stents. *Radiology* **2017**, *284*, 281–288. [CrossRef] [PubMed]

65. Trebicka, J.; Bastgen, D.; Byrtus, J.; Praktiknjo, M.; Terstiegen, S.; Meyer, C.; Thomas, D.; Fimmers, R.; Treitl, M.; Euringer, W.; et al. Smaller-diameter covered transjugular intrahepatic portosystemic shunt stents are associated with increased survival. *Clin. Gastroenterol. Hepatol.* **2019**, *17*, 2793–2799.e1. [CrossRef] [PubMed]

66. Brensing, K.A.; Textor, J.; Perz, J.; Schiedermaier, P.; Raab, P.; Strunk, H.; Klehr, H.U.; Kramer, H.J.; Spengler, U.; Schild, H.; et al. Long term outcome after transjugular intrahepatic portosystemic stentshunt in non-transplant cirrhotics with hepatorenal syndrome: A phase II study. *Gut* **2000**, *47*, 288–295. [CrossRef] [PubMed]

67. Guevara, M.; Ginès, P.; Bandi, J.C.; Gilabert, R.; Sort, P.; Jiménez, W.; Garcia-Pagán, J.C.; Bosch, J.; Arroyo, V.; Rodés, J. Transjugular intrahepatic portosystemic shunt in hepato-renal syndrome: Effects on renal function and vasoactive systems. *Hepatology* **1998**, *28*, 416–422. [CrossRef]

68. Testino, G.; Ferro, C.; Sumberaz, A.; Messa, P.; Morelli, N.; Guadagni, B.; Ardizzone, G.; Valente, U. Type-2 hepatorenal syndrome and refractory ascites: Role of transjugular intrahepatic portosystemic stent-shunt in eighteen patients with advanced cirrhosis awaiting orthotopic liver transplantation. *Hepatogastroenterology* **2003**, *50*, 1753–1755.

69. Conn, H.O.; Fessel, J.M. Spontaneous bacterial peritonitis: Variations on a theme. *Medicine* **1971**, *50*, 161–197. [CrossRef]

70. Rimola, A.; Soto, R.; Bory, F.; Arroyo, V.; Piera, C.; Rodes, J. Reticuloendothelial system phagocytic activity in cirrhosis and its relation to bacterial infections and prognosis. *Hepatology* **1984**, *4*, 53–58. [CrossRef]

71. Jalan, R.; Fernandez, J.; Wiest, R.; Schnabl, B.; Moreau, R.; Angeli, P.; Stadlbauer, V.; Gustot, T.; Bernardi, M.; Canton, R.; et al. Bacterial infections in cirrhosis: A position statement based on the EASL Special Conference. *J. Hepatol.* **2014**, *60*, 1310–1324. [CrossRef]

72. Ginés, P.; Rimola, A.; Planas, R.; Vargas, V.; Marco, F.; Almela, M.; Forne, M.; Miranda, M.L.; Llach, J.; Salmerón, J.M.; et al. Norfloxacin prevents spontaneous bacterial peritonitis re-currence in cirrhosis: Results of a double-blind, placebo-controlled trial. *Hepatology* **1990**, *12*, 716–724. [CrossRef]

73. Facciorusso, A.; Papagiouvanni, I.; Cela, M.; Buccino, V.R.; Sacco, R. Comparative efficacy of long-term antibiotic treatments in the primary prophylaxis of spontaneous bacterial peritonitis. *Liver Int.* **2019**, *39*, 1448–1458. [CrossRef] [PubMed]

74. Mücke, M.M.; Mücke, V.T.; Graf, C.; Schwarzkopf, K.M.; Ferstl, P.G.; Fernandez, J.; Zeuzem, S.; Trebicka, J.; Lange, C.M.; Herrmann, E. Efficacy of norfloxacin prophylaxis to prevent spontaneous bacterial peritonitis: A systematic review and meta-analysis. *Clin. Transl. Gastroenterol.* **2020**, *11*, e00223. [CrossRef] [PubMed]

75. Albillos, A.; de la Hera, A.; González, M.; Moya, J.; Calleja, J.; Monserrat, J.; Ruiz-Del-Arbol, L.; Alvarez-Mon, M. Increased lipopolysaccharide binding protein in cirrhotic patients with marked immune and hemodynamic derangement. *Hepatology* **2003**, *37*, 208–217. [CrossRef]

76. Fernández, J.; Navasa, M.; Planas, R.; Montoliu, S.; Monfort, D.; Soriano, G.; Vila, C.; Pardo, A.; Quintero, E.; Vargas, V.; et al. Primary prophylaxis of spontaneous bacterial peritonitis delays hepatorenal syndrome and improves survival in cirrhosis. *Gastroenterology* **2007**, *133*, 818–824. [CrossRef] [PubMed]

77. Moreau, R.; Elkrief, L.; Bureau, C.; Perarnau, J.-M.; Thévenot, T.; Saliba, F.; Louvet, A.; Nahon, P.; Lannes, A.; Anty, R.; et al. Effects of long-term norfloxacin therapy in patients with advanced cirrhosis. *Gastroenterology* **2018**, *155*, 1816–1827.e9. [CrossRef] [PubMed]

78. Piano, S.; Singh, V.; Caraceni, P.; Maiwall, R.; Alessandria, C.; Fernandez, J.; Soares, E.C.; Kim, D.J.; Kim, S.E.; Marino, M.; et al. Epidemiology and effects of bacterial infections in patients with cirrhosis worldwide. *Gastroenterology* **2019**, *156*, 1368–1380. [CrossRef]

79. Scarpignato, C.; Pelosini, I. Rifaximin, a poorly absorbed antibiotic: Pharmacology and clinical potential. *Chemotherapy* **2005**, *51*, 36–66. [CrossRef]

80. Bajaj, J.S. Review article: Potential mechanisms of action of rifaximin in the management of hepatic encephalopathy and other complications of cirrhosis. *Aliment. Pharmacol. Ther.* **2015**, *43*, 11–26. [CrossRef] [PubMed]

81. Vlachogiannakos, J.; Saveriadis, A.S.; Viazis, N.; Theodoropoulos, I.; Foudoulis, K.; Manolakopoulos, S.; Raptis, S.; Karamanolis, D.G. Intestinal decontami-nation improves liver haemodynamics in patients with alcohol-related decompensated cirrhosis. *Aliment. Pharmacol. Ther.* **2009**, *29*, 992–999. [CrossRef]

82. Esposito, G.; Nobile, N.; Gigli, S.; Seguella, L.; Pesce, M.; d'Alessandro, A.; Bruzzese, E.; Capoccia, E.; Steardo, L.; Cuomo, R.; et al. Rifaximin improves Clostridium difficile toxin A-induced toxicity in Caco-2 cells by the PXR-dependent TLR4/MyD88/NF-κB pathway. *Front. Pharmacol.* **2016**, *7*, 1–8. [CrossRef] [PubMed]

83. Bass, N.M.; Mullen, K.D.; Sanyal, A.; Poordad, F.; Neff, G.; Leevy, C.B.; Sigal, S.; Sheikh, M.Y.; Beavers, K.; Frederick, T.; et al. Rifaximin treatment in hepatic encephalopathy. *N. Engl. J. Med.* **2010**, *362*, 1071–1081. [CrossRef] [PubMed]

84. Hanafy, A.; Hassaneen, A.M. Rifaximin and midodrine improve clinical outcome in refractory ascites including renal function, weight loss, and short-term survival. *Eur. J. Gastroenterol. Hepatol.* **2016**, *28*, 1455–1461. [CrossRef]

85. Lv, X.-Y.; Ding, H.-G.; Zheng, J.-F.; Fan, C.-L.; Li, L. Rifaximin improves survival in cirrhotic patients with refractory ascites: A real-world study. *World J. Gastroenterol.* **2020**, *26*, 199–218. [CrossRef] [PubMed]

86. Kang, S.H.; Lee, Y.B.; Lee, J.-H.; Nam, J.Y.; Chang, Y.; Cho, H.; Yoo, J.-J.; Cho, Y.Y.; Cho, E.J.; Yu, S.J.; et al. Rifaximin treatment is associated with reduced risk of cirrhotic complications and prolonged overall survival in patients experiencing hepatic encephalopathy. *Aliment. Pharmacol. Ther.* **2017**, *46*, 845–855. [CrossRef] [PubMed]

87. Flamm, S.L.; Mullen, K.D.; Heimanson, Z.; Sanyal, A.J. Rifaximin has the potential to prevent complications of cirrhosis. *Ther. Adv. Gastroenterol.* **2018**, *11*. [CrossRef]

88. Salehi, S.; Tranah, T.H.; Lim, S.; Heaton, N.; Heneghan, M.; Aluvihare, V.; Patel, V.; Shawcross, D.L. Rifaximin reduces the incidence of spontaneous bacterial peritonitis, variceal bleeding and all-cause admissions in patients on the liver transplant waiting list. *Aliment. Pharmacol. Ther.* **2019**, *50*, 435–441. [CrossRef]

89. Vlachogiannakos, J.; Viazis, N.; Vasianopoulou, P.; Vafiadis, I.; Karamanolis, D.G.; Ladas, S.D. Long-term administration of rifaximin improves the prognosis of patients with decompensated alcoholic cirrhosis. *J. Gastroenterol. Hepatol.* **2013**, *28*, 450–455. [CrossRef]

90. Ibrahim, E.-S.; Alsebaey, A.; Zaghla, H.; Abdelmageed, S.M.; Gameel, K.; Abdelsameea, E. Long-term rifaximin therapy as a primary prevention of hepatorenal syndrome. *Eur. J. Gastroenterol. Hepatol.* **2017**, *29*, 1247–1250. [CrossRef]

91. Dong, T.; Aronsohn, A.; Reddy, K.G.; Te, H.S. Rifaximin decreases the incidence and severity of acute kidney injury and hepatorenal syndrome in cirrhosis. *Dig. Dis. Sci.* **2016**, *61*, 3621–3626. [CrossRef]

92. Assem, M.; Elsabaawy, M.; Abdelrashed, M.; Elemam, S.; Khodeer, S.; Hamed, W.; Abdelaziz, A.; El-Azab, G. Efficacy and safety of alternating norfloxacin and rifaximin as primary prophylaxis for spontaneous bacterial peritonitis in cirrhotic ascites: A prospective randomized open-label comparative multicenter study. *Hepatol. Int.* **2015**, *10*, 377–385. [CrossRef]

93. Elfert, A.; Ali, L.A.; Soliman, S.; Ibrahim, S.; Abd-Elsalam, S. Randomized-controlled trial of rifaximin versus norfloxacin for secondary prophylaxis of spontaneous bacterial peritonitis. *Eur. J. Gastroenterol. Hepatol.* **2016**, *28*, 1450–1454. [CrossRef]

94. Kamal, F.; Khan, M.A.; Cholankeril, G.; Khan, Z.; Lee, W.M.; Gadiparthi, C.; Ahmed, A.; Howden, C.W.; Nair, S.; Satapathy, S.K. Rifaximin for prevention of spontaneous bacterial peritonitis and hepatorenal syndrome in cirrhosis: A systematic review and meta-analysis. *Gastroenterology* **2017**, *152*, S1151–S1152. [CrossRef]
95. Goel, A.; Rahim, U.; Nguyen, L.; Stave, C. Systematic review with meta-analysis: Rifaximin for the prophylaxis of spontaneous bacterial peritonitis. *Aliment. Pharmacol. Ther.* **2017**, *46*, 1029–1036. [CrossRef] [PubMed]
96. Komolafe, O.; Roberts, D.; Freeman, S.C.; Wilson, P.; Sutton, A.J.; Cooper, N.J.; Pavlov, C.S.; Milne, E.J.; Hawkins, N.; Cowlin, M.; et al. Antibiotic prophylaxis to prevent spontaneous bacterial peritonitis in people with liver cirrhosis: A network meta-analysis. *Cochrane Database Syst. Rev.* **2020**, *1*, CD013125. [CrossRef]
97. Zafra, C.; Abraldes, J.G.; Turnes, J.; Berzigotti, A.; Fernández, M.; Garcia-Pagán, J.C.; Rodés, J.; Bosch, J. Simvastatin enhances hepatic nitric oxide production and decreases the hepatic vascular tone in patients with cirrhosis. *Gastroenterology* **2004**, *126*, 749–755. [CrossRef] [PubMed]
98. Bosch, J.; Gracia-Sancho, J.; Abraldes, J.G. Cirrhosis as new indication for statins. *Gut* **2020**, *69*, 953–962. [CrossRef] [PubMed]
99. Meireles, C.Z.; Pasarin, M.; Lozano, J.J.; García-Calderó, H.; Gracia-Sancho, J.; Garcia-Pagan, J.C.; Bosch, J.; Abraldes, J.G. Simvastatin attenuates liver injury in rodents with biliary cirrhosis submitted to hemorrhage/resuscitation. *Shock* **2017**, *47*, 370–377. [CrossRef] [PubMed]
100. Tripathi, D.M.; Vilaseca, M.; Lafoz, E.; García-Calderó, H.; Haute, G.V.; Fernández-Iglesias, A.; de Oliveira, J.R.; Garcia-Pagan, J.C.; Bosch, J.; Gracia-Sancho, J. Simvastatin prevents progression of acute on chronic liver failure in rats with cirrhosis and portal hypertension. *Gastroenterology* **2018**, *155*, 1564–1577. [CrossRef]
101. Marrone, G.; Maeso-Díaz, R.; García-Cardena, G.; Abraldes, J.G.; Garcia-Pagan, J.C.; Bosch, J.; Gracia-Sancho, J. KLF2 exerts antifibrotic and vasoprotective effects in cirrhotic rat livers: Behind the molecular mechanisms of statins. *Gut* **2014**, *64*, 1434–1443. [CrossRef]
102. Trebicka, J.; Hennenberg, M.; Laleman, W.; Shelest, N.; Biecker, E.; Schepke, M.; Nevens, F.; Sauerbruch, T.; Heller, J. Atorvastatin lowers portal pressure in cirrhotic rats by inhibition of RhoA/Rho-kinase and activation of endothelial nitric oxide synthase. *Hepatology* **2007**, *46*, 242–253. [CrossRef] [PubMed]
103. Kim, R.G.; Loomba, R.; Prokop, L.J.; Singh, S. Statin use and risk of cirrhosis and related complications in patients with chronic liver diseases: A systematic review and meta-analysis. *Clin. Gastroenterol. Hepatol.* **2017**, *15*, 1521–1530.e8. [CrossRef] [PubMed]
104. Pose, E.; Trebicka, J.; Mookerjee, R.P.; Angeli, P.; Gines, P. Statins: Old drugs as new therapy for liver diseases? *J. Hepatol.* **2019**, *70*, 194–202. [CrossRef] [PubMed]
105. Dickerman, B.A.; Garcia-Albeniz, X.; Logan, R.W.; Denaxas, S.; Hernan, M.A. Avoidable flaws in observational analyses: An application to statins and cancer. *Nat. Med.* **2019**, *25*, 1601–1606. [CrossRef]
106. Abraldes, J.G.; Albillos, A.; Bañares, R.; Turnes, J.; González, R.; Garcia-Pagan, J.C.; Bosch, J. Simvastatin lowers portal pressure in patients with cirrhosis and portal hypertension: A randomized controlled trial. *Gastroenterology* **2009**, *136*, 1651–1658. [CrossRef]
107. Pollo-Flores, P.; Soldan, M.; Santos, U.C.; Kunz, D.G.; Mattos, D.E.; da Silva, A.C.; Marchiori, R.C.; Rezende, G.F.D.M. Three months of simvastatin therapy vs. placebo for severe portal hypertension in cirrhosis: A randomized controlled trial. *Dig. Liver Dis.* **2015**, *47*, 957–963. [CrossRef] [PubMed]
108. Bishnu, S.; Ahammed, S.K.; Sarkar, A.; Hembram, J.; Chatterjee, S.; Das, K.; Dhali, G.K.; Chowdhury, A.; Das, K. Effects of atorvastatin on portal hemodynamics and clinical outcomes in patients with cirrhosis with portal hypertension: A proof-of-concept study. *Eur. J. Gastroenterol. Hepatol.* **2018**, *30*, 54–59. [CrossRef]
109. Vijayaraghavan, R.; Jindal, A.; Arora, V.; Choudhary, A.; Kumar, G.; Sarin, S.K. Hemodynamic effects of adding simvastatin to carvedilol for primary prophylaxis of variceal bleeding: A randomized controlled trial. *Am. J. Gastroenterol.* **2020**, *115*, 729–737. [CrossRef]
110. Abraldes, J.G.; Villanueva, C.; Aracil, C.; Turnes, J.; Hernandez-Guerra, M.; Genesca, J.; Rodriguez, M.; Castellote, J.; Garcia-Pagan, J.C.; Torres, F.; et al. Addition of simvastatin to standard therapy for the prevention of variceal rebleeding does not reduce rebleeding but increases survival in patients with cirrhosis. *Gastroenterology* **2016**, *150*, 1160–1170.e3. [CrossRef]
111. La Mura, V.; Pasarín, M.; Meireles, C.Z.; Miquel, R.; Rodríguez-Vilarrupla, A.; Hide, D.; Gracia-Sancho, J.; García-Pagán, J.C.; Bosch, J. Effects of simvastatin administration on rodents with lipopolysaccharide-induced liver microvascular dysfunction. *Hepatology* **2013**, *57*, 1172–1181. [CrossRef]
112. Hide, D.; Ribera, M.O.; Garcia-Pagan, J.C.; Peralta, C.; Bosch, J.; Gracia-Sancho, J. Effects of warm ischemia and reperfusion on the liver microcirculatory phenotype of rats: Underlying mechanisms and pharmacological therapy. *Sci. Rep.* **2016**, *6*, 22107. [CrossRef] [PubMed]
113. Arroyo, V.; Moreau, R.; Jalan, R. Acute-on-chronic liver failure. *N. Engl. J. Med.* **2020**, *382*, 2137–2145. [CrossRef] [PubMed]
114. Pose, E.; Napoleone, L.; Amin, A.; Campion, D.; Jimenez, C.; Piano, S.; Roux, O.; Uschner, F.E.; de Wit, K.; Zaccherini, G.; et al. Safety of two different doses of simvastatin plus rifaximin in decompensated cirrhosis (LIVERHOPE-SAFETY): A randomised, double-blind, placebo-controlled, phase 2 trial. *Lancet Gastroenterol. Hepatol.* **2019**, *5*, 31–41. [CrossRef]
115. Biggins, S.W.; Angeli, P.; Garcia-Tsao, G.; Ginès, P.; Ling, S.C.; Nadim, M.K.; Wong, F.; Kim, W.R. Diagnosis, Evaluation, and Management of Ascites, Spontaneous Bacterial Peritonitis and Hepatorenal Syndrome: 2021 Practice Guidance by the American Association for the Study of Liver Diseases. *Hepatology* **2021**, *74*, 1014–1048. [CrossRef] [PubMed]
116. Bernardi, M.; Angeli, P.; Claria, J.; Moreau, R.; Gines, P.; Jalan, R.; Caraceni, P.; Fernandez, J.; Gerbes, A.L.; O'Brien, A.J.; et al. Albumin in decompensated cirrhosis: New concepts and perspectives. *Gut* **2020**, *69*, 1127–1138. [CrossRef]

117. Caraceni, P.; Riggio, O.; Angeli, P.; Alessandria, C.; Neri, S.; Foschi, F.G.; Levantesi, F.; Airoldi, A.; Boccia, S.; Svegliati-Baroni, G.; et al. Long-term albumin administration in decompensated cirrhosis (ANSWER): An open-label randomised trial. *Lancet* **2018**, *391*, 2417–2429. [CrossRef]

118. Di Pascoli, M.; Fasolato, S.; Piano, S.; Bolognesi, M.; Angeli, P. Faculty opinions recommendation of long-term administration of human albumin improves survival in patients with cirrhosis and refractory ascites. *Liver Int.* **2021**, *39*, 98–105. [CrossRef]

119. Solà, E.; Solé, C.; Simón-Talero, M.; Martín-Llahí, M.; Castellote, J.; Martinez, R.G.; Moreira, R.; Torrens, M.; Márquez, F.; Fabrellas, N.; et al. Midodrine and albumin for prevention of complications in patients with cirrhosis awaiting liver transplantation. A randomized placebo-controlled trial. *J. Hepatol.* **2018**, *69*, 1250–1259. [CrossRef]

120. Caraceni, P.; Tufoni, M.; Zaccherini, G.; Riggio, O.; Angeli, P.; Alessandria, C.; Neri, S.; Foschi, F.G.; Levantesi, F.; Airoldi, A.; et al. On-treatment serum albumin level can guide long-term treatment in patients with cirrhosis and uncomplicated ascites. *J. Hepatol.* **2020**, *74*, 340–349. [CrossRef]

121. Fernández, J.; Clària, J.; Amorós, A.; Aguilar, F.; Castro, M.; Casulleras, M.; Acevedo, J.; Duran-Güell, M.; Nuñez, L.; Costa, M.; et al. Effects of albumin treatment on systemic and portal hemodynamics and systemic inflammation in patients with decompensated cirrhosis. *Gastroenterology* **2019**, *157*, 149–162. [CrossRef]

122. Campion, E.W.; Delabry, L.O.; Glynn, R.J. The effect of age on serum albumin in healthy males: Report from the normative aging study. *J. Gerontol.* **1988**, *43*, M18–M20. [CrossRef] [PubMed]

123. China, L.; Freemantle, N.; Forrest, E.; Kallis, Y.; Ryder, S.D.; Wright, G.; Portal, A.J.; Becares Salles, N.; Gilroy, D.W.; O'Brien, A. A randomized trial of albumin infusions in hospitalized patients with cirrhosis. *N. Engl. J. Med.* **2021**, *384*, 808–817. [CrossRef] [PubMed]

124. Gustot, T. Beneficial role of G-CSF in acute-on-chronic liver failure: Effects on liver regeneration, inflammation/immunoparalysis or both? *Liver Int.* **2014**, *34*, 484–486. [CrossRef]

125. Spahr, L.; Lambert, J.-F.; Rubbia-Brandt, L.; Chalandon, Y.; Frossard, J.-L.; Giostra, E.; Hadengue, A. Granulocyte-colony stimulating factor induces proliferation of hepatic progenitors in alcoholic steatohepatitis: A randomized trial. *Hepatology* **2008**, *48*, 221–229. [CrossRef]

126. Garg, V.; Garg, H.; Khan, A.; Trehanpati, N.; Kumar, A.; Sharma, B.C.; Sakhuja, P.; Sarin, S.K. granulocyte colony–stimulating factor mobilizes CD34+ cells and improves survival of patients with acute-on-chronic liver failure. *Gastroenterology* **2012**, *142*, 505–512. [CrossRef]

127. Singh, V.; Sharma, A.K.; Narasimhan, L.R.; Bhalla, A.; Sharma, N.; Sharma, R. Granulocyte colony-stimulating factor in severe alcoholic hepatitis: A randomized pilot study. *Am. J. Gastroenterol.* **2014**, *109*, 1417–1423. [CrossRef]

128. Sharma, A.; Setia, A.; Rai, R.R. Effect of granulocyte colony-stimulating factor (G-CSF) on mortality and complications viz. sepsis, encephalopathy, hepatorenal syndrome, and gastrointestinal bleed in severe alcoholic hepatitis: A randomized con-trolled study. *United Eur. Gastroenterol. J.* **2017**, *5*, A17.

129. Singh, V.; Keisham, A.; Bhalla, A.; Sharma, N.; Agarwal, R.; Sharma, R.; Singh, A. Efficacy of granulocyte colony-stimulating factor and N-acetylcysteine therapies in patients with severe alcoholic hepatitis. *Clin. Gastroenterol. Hepatol.* **2018**, *16*, 1650–1656. [CrossRef]

130. Shasthry, S.M.; Sharma, M.K.; Shasthry, V.; Pande, A.; Sarin, S.K. Efficacy of granulocyte colony-stimulating factor in the management of steroid- nonresponsive severe alcoholic hepatitis: A double-blind randomized controlled trial. *Hepatology* **2019**, *70*, 802–811. [CrossRef]

131. Engelmann, C.H.A.; Bruns, T.; Schiefke, I.; Zipprich, A.; Schiedeknecht, A.; Zeuzem, S.; Goeser, T.; Canbay, A.E.; Trebicka, C.; Berg, J. Granulocyte-Colony Stimulating Factor (G-CSF) to Treat Acute-on-Chronic Liver Failure (Graft Trial): Interim Analysis of the First Randomised European Multicentre Trial. In Proceedings of the American Association for the Study of Liver Diseases: The Liver Meeting 2019, Boston, MA, USA, 8–12 November 2019.

132. Marot, A.; Singal, A.K.; Moreno, C.; Deltenre, P. Granulocyte colony-stimulating factor for alcoholic hepatitis: A systematic review and meta-analysis of randomised controlled trials. *JHEP Rep.* **2020**, *2*, 100139. [CrossRef] [PubMed]

133. Philips, C.A.; Augustine, P.; Rajesh, S.K.; Ahamed, R.; George, T.; Padsalgi, G.; Paramaguru, R.; Valiathan, G.; John, S.K. Granulocyte colony-stimulating factor use in decompensated cirrhosis: Lack of survival benefit. *J. Clin. Exp. Hepatol.* **2019**, *10*, 124–134. [CrossRef] [PubMed]

134. Prajapati, R.; Arora, A.; Sharma, P.; Bansal, N.; Singla, V.; Kumar, A. Granulocyte colony-stimulating factor improves survival of patients with decompensated cirrhosis: A randomized-controlled trial. *Eur. J. Gastroenterol. Hepatol.* **2017**, *29*, 448–455. [CrossRef]

135. Kedarisetty, C.K.; Anand, L.; Bhardwaj, A.; Bhadoria, A.S.; Kumar, G.; Vyas, A.K.; David, P.; Trehanpati, N.; Rastogi, A.; Bihari, C.; et al. Combination of granulocyte colo-ny-stimulating factor and erythropoietin improves outcomes of patients with decompensated cirrhosis. *Gastroenterology* **2015**, *148*, 1362–1370. [CrossRef]

136. Verma, N.; Kaur, A.; Sharma, R.; Bhalla, A.; Sharma, N.; De, A.; Singh, V. Outcomes after multiple courses of granulocyte colo-ny-stimulating factor and growth hormone in decompensated cirrhosis: A randomized trial. *Hepatology* **2018**, *68*, 1559–1573. [CrossRef]

137. De, A.; Kumari, S.; Singh, A.; Kaur, A.; Sharma, R.; Bhalla, A.; Sharma, N.; Kalra, N.; Singh, V. Multiple cycles of granulo-cyte colony-stimulating factor increase survival times of patients with decompensated cirrhosis in a randomized trial. *Clin. Gastroenterol. Hepatol.* **2020**, *19*, 375–383.e5. [CrossRef] [PubMed]

138. Newsome, P.N.; Fox, R.; King, A.L.; Barton, D.; Than, N.-N.; Moore, J.; Corbett, C.; Townsend, S.; Thomas, J.; Guo, K.; et al. Granulocyte colony-stimulating factor and autologous CD133-positive stem-cell therapy in liver cirrhosis (REALISTIC): An open-label, randomised, controlled phase 2 trial. *Lancet Gastroenterol. Hepatol.* **2017**, *3*, 25–36. [CrossRef]

139. Engelmann, C.; Sheikh, M.; Sharma, S.; Kondo, T.; Loeffler-Wirth, H.; Zheng, Y.B.; Novelli, S.; Hall, A.; Kerbert, A.J.; Macnaughtan, J.; et al. Toll-like receptor 4 is a therapeutic target for prevention and treatment of liver failure. *J. Hepatol.* **2020**, *73*, 102–112. [CrossRef] [PubMed]

140. Poltorak, A.; He, X.; Smirnova, I.; Liu, M.-Y.; Van Huffel, C.; Du, X.; Birdwell, D.; Alejos, E.; Silva, M.; Galanos, C.; et al. Defective LPS signaling in C3H/HeJ and C57BL/10ScCr mice: Mutations in Tlr4 gene. *Science* **1998**, *282*, 2085–2088. [CrossRef] [PubMed]

141. Wang, J.; He, G.Z.; Wang, Y.K.; Zhu, Q.K.; Chen, W.; Guo, T. TLR4-HMGB1-, MyD88- and TRIF-dependent signaling in mouse in-testinal ischemia/reperfusion injury. *World J. Gastroenterol.* **2015**, *21*, 8314–8325. [CrossRef]

142. Kribben, A.; Gerken, G.; Haag, S.; Herget–Rosenthal, S.; Treichel, U.; Betz, C.; Sarrazin, C.; Hoste, E.; Van Vlierberghe, H.; Escorsell, A.; et al. Effects of fractionated plasma separation and adsorption on survival in patients with acute-on-chronic liver failure. *Gastroenterology* **2012**, *142*, 782–789.e3. [CrossRef]

143. Bañares, R.; Nevens, F.; Larsen, F.S.; Jalan, R.; Albillos, A.; Dollinger, M.; Saliba, F.; Sauerbruch, T.; Klammt, S.; Ockenga, J.; et al. Extracorporeal albumin dialysis with the molecular adsorbent recirculating system in acute-on-chronic liver failure: The RELIEF trial. *Hepatology* **2012**, *57*, 1153–1162. [CrossRef] [PubMed]

144. Hassanein, T.I.; Tofteng, F.; Brown, R.S.; McGuire, B.; Lynch, P.; Mehta, R.; Larsen, F.S.; Gornbein, J.; Stange, J.; Blei, A.T. Randomized controlled study of extracorporeal albumin dialysis for hepatic encephalopathy in advanced cirrhosis. *Hepatology* **2007**, *46*, 1853–1862. [CrossRef] [PubMed]

145. Lee, K.C.; Baker, L.A.; Stanzani, G.; Alibhai, H.; Chang, Y.M.; Palacios, C.J.; Leckie, P.J.; Giordano, P.; Priestnall, S.; Antoine, D.J.; et al. Extracorporeal liver assist device to exchange albumin and remove endotoxin in acute liver failure: Results of a pivotal pre-clinical study. *J. Hepatol.* **2015**, *63*, 634–642. [CrossRef] [PubMed]

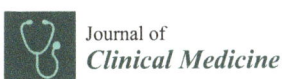

Review

Management of Ascites in Patients with Cirrhosis: An Update

Giacomo Zaccherini [1], Manuel Tufoni [2], Giulia Iannone [1] and Paolo Caraceni [1,2,3,*]

1   Department of Medical and Surgical Sciences, University of Bologna, 40138 Bologna, Italy;
    giacomo.zaccherini@unibo.it (G.Z.); giulia.iannone@studio.unibo.it (G.I.)
2   IRCCS AOU di Bologna—Policlinico di S. Orsola, 40138 Bologna, Italy; manuel.tufoni@aosp.bo.it
3   Center for Biomedical Applied Research, University of Bologna, 40126 Bologna, Italy
*   Correspondence: paolo.caraceni@unibo.it

Abstract: Ascites represents a critical event in the natural history of liver cirrhosis. From a prognostic perspective, its occurrence marks the transition from the compensated to the decompensated stage of the disease, leading to an abrupt worsening of patients' life expectancy. Moreover, ascites heralds a turbulent clinical course, characterized by acute events and further complications, frequent hospitalizations, and eventually death. The pathophysiology of ascites classically relies on hemodynamic mechanisms, with effective hypovolemia as the pivotal event. Recent discoveries, however, integrated this hypothesis, proposing systemic inflammation and immune system dysregulation as key mechanisms. The mainstays of ascites treatment are represented by anti-mineralocorticoids and loop diuretics, and large volume paracentesis. When ascites reaches the stage of refractoriness, however, diuretics administration should be cautious due to the high risk of adverse events, and patients should be treated with periodic execution of paracentesis or with the placement of a trans-jugular intra-hepatic portosystemic shunt (TIPS). TIPS reduces portal hypertension, eases ascites control, and potentially modify the clinical course of the disease. Further studies are required to expand its indications and improve the management of complications. Long-term human albumin administration has been studied in two RCTs, with contradictory results, and remains a debated issue worldwide, despite a potential effectiveness both in ascites control and long-term survival. Other treatments (vaptans, vasoconstrictors, or implantable drainage systems) present some promising aspects but cannot be currently recommended outside clinical protocols or a case-by-case evaluation.

Keywords: decompensated cirrhosis; portal hypertension; effective hypovolemia; anti-mineralocorticoids; loop diuretics; vaptans; TIPS; human albumin

Citation: Zaccherini, G.; Tufoni, M.; Iannone, G.; Caraceni, P. Management of Ascites in Patients with Cirrhosis: An Update. *J. Clin. Med.* **2021**, *10*, 5226. https://doi.org/10.3390/jcm10225226

Academic Editor: Pierluigi Toniutto

Received: 30 August 2021
Accepted: 6 November 2021
Published: 10 November 2021

Publisher's Note: MDPI stays neutral with regard to jurisdictional claims in published maps and institutional affiliations.

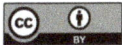
1. Introduction

The development of ascites is the most frequent decompensation event in patients with liver cirrhosis. Five to ten percent of patients with compensated cirrhosis per year develop ascites, an event that represents a cornerstone in the natural history of the disease, so that it has become accustomed considering it the hallmark of the transition to decompensated cirrhosis [1]. Indeed, it often marks the border between a stable and a turbulent clinical course, burdened with acute events of decompensation, including acute-on-chronic liver failure (ACLF), bacterial infections, and frequent hospitalizations, thus determining a dramatic worsening in quality of life and prognosis [2]. Consequently, 5-year survival drops from ~80% in compensated patients to ~30% after ascites onset, and the overall median survival is around two years [1].

Such unfavorable prognosis can be explained—at least partially—by considering that ascites development results from the concurrence of multiple and interrelated pathogenetic mechanisms, involving splanchnic and systemic hemodynamics, along with liver and extrahepatic organs dysfunction (mainly kidney and heart) [3]. Therefore, the onset of ascites presupposes that such abnormalities have reached a critical threshold.

In this context, an appropriate treatment of ascites is a crucial goal in managing patients with cirrhosis [4]. Preventing ascites onset and controlling its evolution means offering the patients a better quality of life, reducing the incidence of acute decompensations and emergency hospitalizations, and improving survival, thus also leading to a more appropriate long-term allocation of healthcare resources [4].

The present review, after a brief recall of the main pathogenetic mechanisms underlying decompensation and ascites formation in patients with cirrhosis, will discuss the currently available approaches for ascites management, along with some emerging perspectives and areas for future research.

2. Pathophysiology of Ascites and Decompensation

The classical pathophysiological paradigm of ascites formation in patients with liver cirrhosis relies on the so-called peripheral arterial vasodilatation hypothesis [5]. The primary event is the progressive disruption of the normal structure of the liver that leads to portal hypertension as a result of the increased intrahepatic vascular resistance and sinusoidal pressure. In turn, portal hypertension favors the production of endogenous vasodilating substances, such as nitric oxide (NO), endocannabinoids, and carbon monoxide (CO), that exert their action on systemic vascular resistances, mainly affecting the splanchnic arteriolar bed which becomes abnormally dilated. Because of this dysregulated splanchnic vasodilation, effective hypovolemia develops. Effective hypovolemia is the crucial event in the pathogenetic cascade of decompensation in patients with liver cirrhosis, as it causes the activation of neuro-humoral systems able to promote vasoconstriction and renal retention of sodium and water, such as the renin–angiotensin–aldosterone (RAA) axis, the sympathetic nervous system (SNS), arginine–vasopressin (ADH), thus producing a compensatory increase in cardiac output. As the disease progresses and these mechanisms are sustained over time, the exhaustion of left ventricular function and the development of cirrhotic cardiomyopathy could lead to an impairment of cardiac output and a further decrease of effective volemia, thus leading to peripheral hypoperfusion and contributing to multi-organ failure [5].

This pathophysiological interpretation, however, does not fully explain all the clinical manifestations of decompensated cirrhosis, with the subsequent need to integrate it with new fundamental discoveries. In recent years, indeed, newly available evidence led to consider systemic inflammation and immune system activation as major drivers of organ impairment and failure in decompensated cirrhosis [3]. The key event is a dysregulated activation of the immune system from two major drivers: first, portal hypertension increases intestinal mucosal permeability and favors the translocation from gut lumen of pathogen-associated molecular patterns (PAMPs), such as bacterial products, lipopolysaccharide (LPS), and bacterial DNA [6], and, second, the chronic liver damage with hepatocyte necrosis releases circulating damage-associated molecular patterns (DAMPs), intracellular components released by dying or damaged host cells [7]. The resulting increased production of cytokines and other proinflammatory molecules, reactive oxygen species (ROS) and vasodilating substances can cause peripheral organ damage and failure via tissue hypoperfusion, immune-mediated tissue damage, and mitochondrial dysfunction [3]. The detailed discussion of these complex mechanisms, however, falls beyond the scope of this review.

3. Diagnosis of Ascites

Cirrhosis and portal hypertension are the main causes of ascites, accounting for about 80% of cases in Western countries, but many other etiologies, such as malignancies, congestive heart failure, nephrotic syndrome, or tuberculosis, may be responsible of ascites formation [8]. Previous patient's history, physical examination, laboratory tests, abdominal ultrasound and diagnostic paracentesis are therefore recommended in all patients with new onset ascites [4].

A serum–ascites albumin gradient (SAAG) of 1.1 mg/dL or above is suggestive of the presence of portal hypertension and helps to discriminate the underlying condition when the causative disease is unclear [9]. Therefore, in case of paracentesis, ascitic total protein and albumin concentration should be measured. Moreover, neutrophil count and ascitic fluid culture should be routinely performed to exclude spontaneous bacterial peritonitis (SBP), a severe and potentially life-threatening complication in patients with decompensated cirrhosis [4,10]. To notice, an ascitic total protein concentration below 1.5 mg/dL may identify patients at high risk for SBP development, so that a long-term antibiotic prophylaxis could be considered [11,12]. Other ascitic fluid analysis (e.g., cytology or culture for mycobacteria) could be performed, depending on clinical suspicion [4].

As regards a quantitative classification, ascites could be graded as mild, moderate, or severe (grade 1 to 3) according to the total amount of fluid in the abdomen [8].

4. Management of Uncomplicated Ascites

With the term "uncomplicated ascites" it is generally defined any ascites that is not refractory, not infected nor associated with renal failure (i.e., hepatorenal syndrome) [8]. Grade 1 (or mild) ascites does not generally require a specific treatment since only few data on its long-term evolution and prognosis are available, nor clear evidence on the effects of therapies on its natural history [4,13]. In patients developing grade 2 (moderate) ascites, a specific treatment should be initiated [4].

4.1. Dietary Salt Restriction

As a positive sodium balance is a major determinant of ascites accumulation, the reduction of dietary salt intake and the increase of renal sodium excretion are the two cornerstones of moderate ascites management. Dietary salt restriction should be suggested with caution and carefully supervised: although low-sodium diets can induce or support ascites resolution in a portion of patients [14], an extreme or exaggerated salt restriction could even favor hyponatremia and renal failure [15], along with a worsening in nutritional status, due to a reduced calories intake and impaired food palatability [16]. Therefore, international guidelines currently recommend a moderate salt restriction (medium intake of 80–120 mmol/day), mainly to avoid excessive intake [4].

4.2. Diuretic Therapy

The initiation of a diuretic therapy has the goal to induce natriuresis and consequently a negative sodium balance. From a mechanistic point of view, diuretics can be considered symptomatic treatments, not clearly affecting the general course of the disease, since they act downstream in the pathophysiological cascade. As already reported, the main pathogenetic mechanism of renal sodium retention in patients with decompensated cirrhosis and preserved renal perfusion is secondary hyperaldosteronism [17]. Therefore, the mainstays of ascites treatment so far are the anti-mineralocorticoid drugs, such as spironolactone, canrenone or potassium-canrenoate, at the initial dose of 100 mg/day, up to a maximum of 400 mg/day [4]. These drugs block the aldosterone pathway in the distal convoluted tubule through a slow action (involving cytosolic and nuclear receptors), so that the natriuretic effect begins after 72 h from the first dose and dose changes should be managed accordingly. If patients could not be treated with anti-mineralocorticoids due to intolerance or severe adverse effects, amiloride could be used. Amiloride acts on aldosterone pathway in the renal collecting duct, but it is less effective than spironolactone [18].

As a second step, in non-responder patients (defined as subjects presenting a weight loss of less than 2 kg/week or side effects such as hyperkalemia) or in patients with long lasting ascites, a combination therapy should be considered, adding loop diuretics (furosemide at a starting dose of 25–40 mg, and up to 160 mg in 25–40 mg steps) to anti-mineralocorticoids [4]. Indeed, as portal hypertension progresses, proximal tubule sodium reabsorption becomes relatively prevalent due to the activation of RAAS and SNS and reduced renal perfusion [19]. Therefore, combining loop diuretics to anti-mineralocorticoids has been demonstrated to be more effective in controlling ascites than anti-mineralocorticoids alone, also preventing serum potassium alterations [20]. In patients showing an inadequate response to furosemide, torasemide can be considered, as it showed a more effective natriuresis in one randomized trial [21].

The target of therapy in patients with moderate to severe ascites is a weight loss of maximum 0.5 kg/day in patients without peripheral edema, and of maximum 1 kg/day in patient with peripheral edema, to avoid the development of renal impairment and adverse effects, such as hyponatremia [22]. In parallel with the effective mobilization of ascites (i.e., its consistent reduction until resolution), diuretic therapy dosage should be gradually reduced to the minimal effective dose [4].

In case of high dose diuretic therapy, especially at the beginning, patients should be frequently monitored to notice adverse effect (Table 1). The most common side effects of furosemide are hyponatremia and hypokalemia, while anti-mineralocorticoids can lead to hyperkalemia and painful gynecomastia. Moreover, diuretic-induced rapid reduction of extracellular volume or electrolyte imbalance can favor the occurrence of other severe complications such as overt HE, acute kidney injury (AKI) until renal failure, and muscle cramps. According to the severity of side effects, dose reduction or even temporary interruption of diuretic therapy could be necessary [4] (Table 1).

Table 1. Complications and adverse events related to diuretic therapy and recommendations on diuretics management according to major international guidelines [4].

Adverse Event/Complication	Recommendations
Renal failure or acute kidney injury Overt hepatic encephalopathy Severe hyponatremia (<125 mmol/L) Incapacitating muscle cramps	Discontinuation (or at least reduction) of diuretic therapy
Severe hyperkalemia (>6 mmol/L)	Anti-mineralocorticoids withdrawal
Severe hypokalemia (<3 mmol/L)	Loop diuretics withdrawal

4.3. Therapeutic Paracentesis

In patients developing grade 3 (severe/tense) ascites, large volume paracentesis (LVP) represents the treatment of choice due to its efficacy and low rate of complications [4]. The procedure is associated with a very low risk of bleeding, even in patients with altered international normalized ratio (INR > 1.5) and platelet count < 50,000/microl [23]. LVP should be avoided in patients with disseminated intravascular coagulation; moreover, no evidence supports the routine use of fresh frozen plasma or pooled platelets before LVP execution in case of mild or moderate coagulopathy [4]. Although not routinely recommended by international guidelines, the use of bedside ultrasound guidance can reduce the incidence of adverse events, particularly in settings where LVPs are performed by non-physician healthcare providers [24].

After drainage of large volumes of ascitic fluid (especially > 5 L), plasma volume expansion is recommended to avoid paracentesis-induced circulatory dysfunction (PICD), a severe syndrome due to the acute worsening of effective hypovolemia and the consequent increase in plasma renin activity, leading to renal failure, severe hyponatremia, hepatic encephalopathy (HE), and eventually death [25]. Human albumin, at the recommended dose of 8 g per liter of tapped ascites, has been demonstrated to be the plasma expander of choice and should be administered to all patients undergoing LVP [4,25]. Other plasma expanders (such as dextran-70, polygeline, or saline solution) show similar efficacy in preventing PICD compared to albumin only in case of small volume paracentesis (<5 L) [26,27]. Drainage of less than 5 L could require human albumin administration in case of concomitant of acute-on-chronic liver failure (ACLF) or in patients at high risk of renal failure development [24,28].

4.4. Referral for Liver Transplantation

All patients with cirrhosis and grade 2 or 3 ascites should be considered for liver transplantation (LT) [4,24]. The presence of hyponatremia, a reduced renal sodium excretion and glomerular filtration rate, and hypotension are all predictors of mortality in these patients [29]. Therefore, a major issue in this setting is the appropriate prioritization for organ allocation, since nor Child–Pugh score, nor MELD/MELD-Na score fully reflects the potentially poor prognosis of patients with ascites [30,31]. Indeed, in case of an excessive time on waitlist for LT, decompensated patients could develop further complications and severe acute events (mainly infections) leading to a significant clinical deterioration. The development of innovative and specific prognostic tools for patients with ascites is a major objective for future research.

5. Management of Refractory Ascites

Refractory ascites (RA) is generally defined as "ascites that cannot be mobilized or the early recurrence of which (i.e., after LVP) cannot be satisfactorily prevented by medical treatment" [8], both for a progressive lack of response to diuretic therapy (diuretic-resistant RA) and for the development of diuretics-related complications (diuretic-intractable RA). To notice, the diagnostic criteria for RA should be evaluated in clinically stable patients, without recent acute complications. Recurrent ascites, which is defined as ascites that recurs at least three times within 1 year despite dietary sodium restriction and adequate diuretic dosage, could be a forerunner of RA, although its natural history and prognostic significance are only partially known [8,13].

Besides challenges in the therapeutic management of patients, RA also dramatically worsen patients' prognosis, reducing the median survival to about six months. Therefore, a prompt evaluation for LT or the immediate referral to a transplant center are strongly recommended for any patients with RA [4,32]. In this regard, as already reported, a major problem is the appropriate patient prioritization on the waitlist. Indeed, the main liver function parameters could often be only moderately altered, so that the main prognostic scores (Child-Pugh and MELD/MELD-Na) do not fully reflect patient urgency. Some proposals have been made to refine patients' priority and improve organ allocation. This is the case, for example, of the Italian Score for Organ allocation (ISO), that introduce some "MELD exceptions" and provide additional points to patients, based on specific complications that heavily affect prognosis and ease further complications [33].

Periodic execution of LVPs is generally agreed to be the treatment of choice—both effective and safe—for patients with RA [4,32]. Plasma volume expansion with albumin (8 g/L of tapped ascites) should always follow any LVP to prevent PICD [34]. A lower dose of albumin (4 g/L of tapped ascites) has been proposed in patients undergoing paracentesis of less than 5 L of ascites drained [35]. According to the major guidelines, in these cases the use of albumin could be administered on a case-by-case basis (e.g., patients at risk of renal impairment or failure) [4,32].

As regards diuretic therapy, it should be modulated or withdrawn due the high risk of diuretic-related adverse effects, such as worsening in glomerular filtration rate and electrolytes disturbances [8]. Instead, non-selective beta-blockers (NSBBs) could be administered unless severe hypotension, hyponatremia or renal failure develop, as clarified in the BAVENO VI consensus [36]; to note, carvedilol is not recommended at this stage [4,37].

6. Trans-Jugular Intra-Hepatic Portosystemic Shunt

Currently recommended therapeutic strategies for patients with decompensated cirrhosis and ascites act downstream on the complex pathophysiological cascade leading from portal hypertension to ascites development. Indeed, the mainstays of ascites treatment, anti-mineralocorticoids, loop diuretics and LVPs, can be considered symptomatic treatments from a mechanistic point of view. The trans-jugular intra-hepatic portosystemic shunt (TIPS), conversely, addresses portal hypertension, a key upstream event in the pathophysiology of decompensated cirrhosis.

TIPS consists of creating an artificial shunt between portal and hepatic vein, thus decreasing portal hypertension. Currently, the main clinical settings for the use of TIPS are the management of variceal bleeding and the control of refractory ascites [38]. TIPS leads to an increase in cardiac output and a decrease in systemic vascular resistance. Therefore, it causes an improvement in effective hypovolemia and renal perfusion, thus inducing natriuresis [39]. In clinical practice, however, the main contentious points on TIPS placement remain the identification of target patients and appropriate timing for its use. The main side effect of TIPS is the occurrence or worsening of HE [40]; moreover, major possible complications are related to dysfunction due to stent stenosis or thrombosis [41]. The introduction of polytetrafluoroethylene (PTFE)-covered stent, currently the standard of care, instead of bare stent grafts has been shown to significantly reduce these risks [42,43]. Absolute and relative contraindications to TIPS placement are reported in Table 2.

Table 2. Contraindications to TIPS placement.

Absolute Contraindications	Relative Contraindications
Very advanced disease (Child-Pugh > 13)	Hepatic tumors (especially if centrally located)
Overt or recurrent hepatic encephalopathy	Obstruction of all hepatic veins
Congestive heart failure	History of episodic hepatic encephalopathy
Severe tricuspid regurgitation	Portal vein thrombosis
Severe pulmonary hypertension (mean pulmonary pressure > 45 mmHg)	Severe thrombocytopenia (<20,000/microL)
Polycystic liver disease	Mild/moderate pulmonary hypertension
Active systemic infection or sepsis	
Unrelieved biliary obstruction	

In patients with decompensated cirrhosis and ascites, seven RCTs [44–50] compared TIPS to LVPs plus albumin, the standard of care for patients with RA, showing a superior efficacy in controlling ascites in all of them. However, beyond a beneficial effect on ascites, the trials showed slightly different results. Indeed, TIPS positively affected survival when performed using PTFE-covered stents [50] and in patients with a less advanced disease [49] or recurrent'/recidivant' ascites not fulfilling criteria for refractory ascites [45,48,50]. At the same time, TIPS placement requires great caution and a careful selection of target patients, because of the high risk of adverse events, such as hepatic encephalopathy, liver failure, and cardiac dysfunction [38]. The use of smaller diameter stents (6–8 mm of diameter instead of standard 10 mm) seems promising for the expansion of TIPS indications, since they showed a similar efficacy with a lower incidence of adverse events, likely by preventing excessive shunting [42,43].

In summary, addressing a key pathophysiological mechanism as portal hypertension, TIPS eases ascites control and shows a great potential in increasing patients' survival. However, two factors currently limit its widespread use in clinical practice: First, available studies evaluated TIPS efficacy in patients with portal hypertensive bleeding or difficult-to-treat/refractory ascites; its impact in patients with clinically significant portal hypertension but without these complications has never been assessed. Second, the occurrence of severe TIPS-related complications often prevents its placement in patients with RA refractory ascites. The use of small diameter covered stent may help in overcoming these limitations.

7. Long-Term Human Albumin Administration

Albumin use in patients with cirrhosis is currently recommended for the treatment or prevention of conditions characterized by an acute worsening of effective volemia: its well-established indications are the prevention of paracentesis-induced circulatory dysfunction (PICD), of renal dysfunction induced by SBP, and the diagnosis and treatments of HRS in association with vasoconstrictors [4,32]. Indeed, with its oncotic properties, albumin can counteract effective hypovolemia, a central event in cirrhosis pathophysiology. At the same time, albumin molecule exerts several functions not related to its oncotic power (the so called non-oncotic properties), including antioxidant activities, binding with many endogenous and exogenous substances, modulation of immune response and inflammation, restoration of endothelial integrity, and cardiac function [51]. These pleiotropic effects make it a multitarget agent in a mechanistic perspective, thus supporting a potential role in modifying the long-term clinical course of decompensated cirrhosis.

Recently, the ANSWER trial [52] showed for the first time that long-term albumin administration, on top of a standard diuretic therapy, could be a novel therapeutic approach for patients with cirrhosis and grade 2–3 uncomplicated ascites. Indeed, albumin administration obtained a 38% reduction in 18-month mortality hazard ratio, eased the management of ascites (with a 50% reduction in the need for LVPs and RA diagnosis) and reduced the incidence of major complications of cirrhosis [52]. Following the positive results of the ANSWER trial, a single-center non-randomized trial showed that long-term human albumin administration could improve 24-month survival in patients with RA [53]. The results of the ANSWER trial have been challenged by the MACHT trial, that did not obtain differences between the two arms, both in survival and in the incidence of complications of cirrhosis [54]. However, instead of simply advise against long-term albumin use, the careful comparison of the two studies can provide essential information for its appropriate use [55]. The different results could be at least partially explained by differences in disease severity of patients enrolled (slightly less severe in the ANSWER trial), and dosage and duration of albumin treatment (higher and longer, respectively, in the ANSWER trial) (Table 3).

Table 3. Comparison of the two available RCTs on long-term albumin use for decompensated cirrhosis and ascites [52,54].

Feature of the Study	Answer Trial [51]	Macht Trial [53]
Study design	Randomized Open label	Randomized Placebo-controlled
Number of patients	431 (218 HA/213 SMT)	173 (87 HA/86 SMT)
Baseline MELD score	12/13	17/18
Albumin dose	40 g weekly (with a loading dose of 40 g twice a week for the first 2 weeks)	40 g every 2 weeks (+midodrine)
Duration of treatment	17.6 (8.0–18.0) months [§]	63 days [‡]
Effects on albumin concentration	Increase in SA level (0.6–0.8 g/dL) in about 4 weeks	No changes in SA levels
Outcomes of the interventional arm	Reduction of mortality and complications of cirrhosis	No effect on mortality or complications

[§] duration of follow-up in the treated group according to reverse Kaplan–Meier method; [‡] median duration of follow up in the treated group. HA, human albumin; SMT, standard medical treatment; MELD, model for end-stage liver disease; SA, serum albumin.

One of the most important findings of the ANSWER trial was the increase of serum albumin concentration (by approximately 0.6–0.8 g/dL), leading to the normalization of albuminemia (up to close 4 g/dL) in treated patients [52]. This result was further explored in a post hoc analysis [56] that showed two interesting findings: first, the best 18-month survival probability (greater than 90%) was obtained by patients reaching an on-treatment serum albumin concentration of at least 4 g/dL (not only a normalization above 3.5 g/dL); second, baseline MELD score and serum albumin value independently predicted the achievement of this threshold. Consequently, it could be assumed that patients with severe hypoalbuminemia and high MELD score could require greater amounts of albumin to obtain long-term beneficial effects. Last, the serum albumin threshold of 4 g/dL was not arbitrarily assumed, as such a concentration represents the normal serum albumin level in healthy individuals in their eighth or even ninth decade [57].

In summary, growing evidence support long-term albumin use in patients with decompensated cirrhosis and ascites, showing a potential role in modifying the natural history of the disease, beyond the treatment of ascites or other specific complications. Further studies are needed to better characterize target subgroups, who could benefit the most from this innovative approach, and to establish different dosages and schedules of albumin administration, ideally tending to an individualization of treatment. However, the effectiveness of chronic albumin administration is still a debated issue worldwide, and the major international guidelines do not recommend long-term albumin as an established treatments [4,32]. The only exception, so far, is represented by the recently released Italian clinical practice guidelines [58], that include albumin among the medical treatment options for decompensated patients with ascites.

8. Other Proposed Treatments for Ascites

8.1. Vaptans

Vaptans antagonize vasopressin by blocking V2 receptors in the renal collecting ducts, thus inducing diuresis without excretion of electrolytes [59]. Their use in managing ascites with hyponatremia is controversial. Indeed, these drugs improved serum sodium concentration in patients with hyponatremia and eased ascites control, according to two metanalyses [60,61], although no benefits were demonstrated on cirrhosis complications or mortality. However, a small single-center real-life study did not show the effectiveness of vaptans in patients with severe hyponatremia [62], perhaps due to reduced response to the treatment related to renal impairment, common in advanced cirrhosis. So far, the available studies did not demonstrate a clear survival benefit of vaptans in patients with ascites. Interestingly, a non-randomized single-center clinical trial showed an improvement in survival in a subgroup of patients, treated with Tolvaptan and a low-dose of furosemide [63]. Although interesting, these results need further confirmations to be generalized.

The European Medicines Agency (EMA) approved the administration of vaptans only for the syndrome of inappropriate antidiuretic hormone secretion (SIADH). On the other hand, the Food and Drug Administration (FDA) also included heart failure and cirrhosis, until 2013. In 2013, indeed, cases of severe hepatic damage occurred in patients with autosomal dominant polycystic renal disease treated with vaptans in a trial [64], so that FDA currently do not recommend the use of vaptans in patients with liver disease.

In conclusion, no evidence currently supports the routine use of vaptans in patients with cirrhosis and ascites. Moreover, according to some clinical practice guidelines, vaptans should only be administered for a short period of time in hospital setting with strict electrolytes monitoring, due to the risks of a rapid sodium correction [4,65].

8.2. Midodrine and Clonidine

Splanchnic vasodilation plays a major role in the development and maintenance of effective hypovolemia, a key step in the pathophysiology of ascites in cirrhosis. Therefore, the use of vasopressor such as midodrine, an alfa-adrenergic agonist, could theoretically help in the management of ascites. Indeed, in non-azotemic patients with ascites, midodrine showed an increase in mean arterial pressure and in renal sodium excretion, with a decrease in plasma renin activity and aldosterone [66]. Two small RCTs showed benefits of midodrine in the control of ascites [67,68], although larger studies are needed to confirm these findings. A possible alternative is clonidine, an alfa-2-adrenergic agonist which blocks RAA and SNS activity and, in association with diuretics, may enhance diuretic response [69,70]. Based on the currently available evidence, however, the use of midodrine or clonidine in patients with cirrhosis and ascites could not be recommended and should be considered only on a case-by-case basis.

8.3. Automated Low-Flow Ascites Pump (Alfapump)

The Alfapump is a subcutaneously implanted battery-powered programmable pump connected to catheters that move ascites from the peritoneal cavity to the bladder, from which it is eliminated with urine. It could be considered, in experienced centers, for patients with RA and contraindications to TIPS placement. The available evidence shows that Alfapump can reduce the need for LVPs and improve patients' quality of life and nutritional status [71,72]. However, important side effects have been reported and deserve consideration. First, device-related infective complications are relatively frequent (mainly SBPs and urinary tract infections) [73]; the routine use of antibiotic prophylaxis reduced their occurrence, but long-term antibiotic administration remains a debated issue in patients with decompensated cirrhosis. Second, renal impairment or failure develop in a proportion of patients [73,74], probably as a form of PICD due to the continuous ascites tapping without albumin use. Intermittent albumin administration has been proposed but its efficacy (as well as its dose and timing) needs to be demonstrated in clinical trials. Moreover, no survival benefit of Alfapump has been showed so far [73]. In conclusion the routine use of Alfapump is currently not an established option in patients with cirrhosis and refractory ascites.

9. Conclusions

Currently recommended treatments for ascites are based on symptomatic measures, aiming to excrete the excess of water and sodium by the kidney (with diuretics) or directly drain ascites from the abdomen (with LVPs). Alternative approaches, like vasoconstrictors (i.e., midodrine) or automated drainage systems (i.e., alfapump) present some promising aspects but did not show clear and undoubted beneficial effects, so far.

Future research should focus on pathophysiological treatments, able to treat or prevent ascites in a wider context, ideally modifying the long-term clinical course of the disease, thus improving survival and quality of life for patients [75]. Such measures could derive from a better knowledge—and extended use—of currently available treatment (e.g., TIPS and albumin administration), from the repurposing or repositioning of existing drugs [76], or even from the development of innovative approaches or molecules.

Author Contributions: Writing—original draft preparation, G.Z.; writing—review and editing, M.T.; writing—review and editing, G.I.; writing—review and editing, P.C. All authors have read and agreed to the published version of the manuscript.

Funding: This research has received funding from the European Union's Horizon 2020 Research and Innovation Programme under Grant Agreement No 731875 "Simvastatin and Rifaximin as new therapy for patients with decompensated cirrhosis—LIVERHOPE Project".

Institutional Review Board Statement: Not applicable.

Informed Consent Statement: Not applicable.

Data Availability Statement: No new data were created or analyzed in this study. Data sharing is not applicable to this article.

Conflicts of Interest: Zaccherini is part of the speakers' bureau for Grifols SA and Octapharma SA, outside the submitted work. Tufoni is part of the speakers' bureau for Grifols SA and Octapharma SA, outside the submitted work. Iannone has nothing to disclose. Caraceni is part of the speakers' bureau for Grifols SA, Octapharma SA, Kedrion Biopharma SpA, Mallinkrodt SA, Gilead SA and Takeda SA, outside the submitted work.

References

1.   D'Amico, G.; Garcia-Tsao, G.; Pagliaro, L. Natural history and prognostic indicators of survival in cirrhosis: A systematic review of 118 studies. *J. Hepatol.* **2006**, *44*, 217–231. [CrossRef]
2.   D'Amico, G.; Morabito, A.; D'Amico, M.; Pasta, L.; Malizia, G.; Rebora, P.; Valsecchi, M.G. Clinical states of cirrhosis and competing risks. *J. Hepatol.* **2018**, *68*, 563–576. [CrossRef]

3. Bernardi, M.; Moreau, R.; Angeli, P.; Schnabl, B.; Arroyo, V. Mechanisms of decompensation and organ failure in cirrhosis: From peripheral arterial vasodilation to systemic inflammation hypothesis. *J. Hepatol.* **2015**, *63*, 1272–1284. [CrossRef] [PubMed]
4. Angeli, P.; Bernardi, M.; Villanueva, C.; Francoz, C.; Mookerjee, R.; Trebicka, J.; Krag, A.; Laleman, W.; Gines, P. EASL Clinical Practice Guidelines for the management of patients with decompensated cirrhosis. *J. Hepatol.* **2018**, *69*, 406–460. [CrossRef] [PubMed]
5. Schrier, R.W.; Arroyo, V.; Bernardi, M.; Epstein, M.; Henriksen, J.H.; Rodes, J. Peripheral arterial vasodilation hypothesis: A proposal for the initiation of renal sodium and water retention in cirrhosis. *Hepatology* **1988**, *8*, 1151–1157. [CrossRef] [PubMed]
6. Wiest, R.; Lawson, M.; Geuking, M. Pathological bacterial translocation in liver cirrhosis. *J. Hepatol.* **2014**, *60*, 197–209. [PubMed]
7. Kubes, P.; Mehal, W.Z. Sterile Inflammation in the Liver. *Gastroenterology* **2012**, *143*, 1158–1172. [CrossRef]
8. Moore, K.P.; Wong, F.; Ginès, P.; Bernardi, M.; Ochs, A.; Salerno, F.; Angeli, P.; Porayko, M.; Moreau, R.; Garcia-Tsao, G.; et al. The management of ascites in cirrhosis: Report on the consensus conference of the International Ascites Club. *Hepatology* **2003**, *38*, 258–266. [CrossRef]
9. Runyon, B.A.; Montano, A.A.; Akriviadis, E.A.; Antillon, M.R.; Irving, M.A.; McHutchison, J.G. The serum-ascites albumin gradient is superior to the exudate-transudate concept in the differential diagnosis of ascites. *Ann. Intern. Med.* **1992**, *117*, 215–220. [CrossRef]
10. Wiest, R.; Krag, A.; Gerbes, A. Spontaneous bacterial peritonitis: Recent guidelines and beyond. *Gut* **2012**, *61*, 297–310. [CrossRef]
11. Rimola, A.; García-Tsao, G.; Navasa, M.; Piddock, L.J.; Planas, R.; Bernard, B.; Inadomi, J. Diagnosis, treatment and prophylaxis of spontaneous bacterial peritonitis: A consensus document. International Ascites Club. *J. Hepatol.* **2000**, *32*, 142–153. [CrossRef]
12. Bruns, T.; Lutz, P.; Stallmach, A.; Nischalke, H.D. Low ascitic fluid protein does not indicate an increased risk for spontaneous bacterial peritonitis in current cohorts. *J. Hepatol.* **2015**, *63*, 527–528. [CrossRef] [PubMed]
13. Tonon, M.; Piano, S.; Gambino, C.G.; Romano, A.; Pilutti, C.; Incicco, S.; Brocca, A.; Sticca, A.; Bolognesi, M.; Angeli, P. Outcomes and mortality of grade 1 ascites and recurrent ascites in patients with cirrhosis. *Clin. Gastroenterol. Hepatol.* **2021**, *19*, 358–366.e8. [CrossRef] [PubMed]
14. Bernardi, M.; Laffi, G.; Salvagnini, M.; Azzena, G.; Bonato, S.; Marra, F.; Trevisani, F.; Gasbarrini, G.; Naccarato, R.; Gentilini, P. Efficacy and safety of the stepped care medical treatment of ascites in liver cirrhosis: A randomized controlled clinical trial comparing two diets with different sodium content. *Liver* **1993**, *13*, 156–162. [CrossRef]
15. Reynolds, T.B.; Lieberman, F.L.; Goodman, A.R. Advantages of treatment of ascites without sodium restriction and without complete removal of excess fluid. *Gut* **1978**, *19*, 549–553. [CrossRef] [PubMed]
16. Morando, F.; Rosi, S.; Gola, E.; Nardi, M.; Piano, S.; Fasolato, S.; Stanco, M.; Cavallin, M.; Romano, A.; Sticca, A.; et al. Adherence to a moderate sodium restriction diet in outpatients with cirrhosis and ascites: A real-life cross-sectional study. *Liver Int.* **2015**, *35*, 1508–1515. [CrossRef]
17. Bernardi, M.; Trevisani, F.; Gasbarrini, A.; Gasbarrini, G. Hepatorenal disorders: Role of the renin-angiotensin-aldosterone system. *Semin. Liver Dis.* **1994**, *14*, 23–34. [CrossRef]
18. Angeli, P.; Dalla Pria, M.; De Bei, E.; Albino, G.; Caregaro, L.; Merkel, C.; Ceolotto, G.; Gatta, A. Randomized clinical study of the efficacy of amiloride and potassium canrenoate in nonazotemic cirrhotic patients with ascites. *Hepatology* **1994**, *19*, 72–79. [CrossRef]
19. Angeli, P.; Gatta, A.; Caregaro, L.; Menon, F.; Sacerdoti, D.; Merkel, C.; Rondana, M.; DE Toni, R.; Ruol, A. Tubular site of renal sodium retention in ascitic liver cirrhosis evaluated by lithium clearance. *Eur. J. Clin. Investig.* **1990**, *20*, 111–117. [CrossRef]
20. Angeli, P.; Fasolato, S.; Mazza, E.; Okolicsanyi, L.; Maresio, G.; Velo, E.; Galioto, A.; Salinas, F.; D'Aquino, M.; Sticca, A.; et al. Combined vs. sequential diuretic treatment of ascites in non-azotaemic patients with cirrhosis: Results of an open randomised clinical trial. *Gut* **2010**, *59*, 98–104. [CrossRef]
21. Gerbes, A.L.; Bertheau-Reitha, U.; Falkner, C.; Jüngst, D.; Paumgartner, G. Advantages of the new loop diuretic torasemide over furosemide in patients with cirrhosis and ascites. A randomized, double blind crossover trial. *J. Hepatol.* **1993**, *17*, 353–358. [CrossRef]
22. Pockros, P.J.; Reynolds, T.B. Rapid diuresis in patients with ascites from chronic liver disease: The importance of peripheral edema. *Gastroenterology* **1986**, *90*, 1827–1833. [CrossRef]
23. Lin, C.H.; Shih, F.Y.; Ma, M.H.; Chiang, W.C.; Yang, C.W.; Ko, P.C. Should bleeding tendency deter abdominal paracentesis? *Dig. Liver Dis.* **2005**, *37*, 946–951. [CrossRef] [PubMed]
24. Aithal, G.P.; Palaniyappan, N.; China, L.; Härmälä, S.; Macken, L.; Ryan, J.M.; Wilkes, E.A.; Moore, K.; Leithead, J.A.; Hayes, P.C.; et al. Guidelines on the management of ascites in cirrhosis. *Gut* **2021**, *70*, 9–29. [CrossRef]
25. Ginès, P.; Tító, L.; Arroyo, V.; Planas, R.; Panes, J.; Viver, J.; Torres, M.; Humbert, P.; Rimola, A.; Llach, J.; et al. Randomized comparative study of therapeutic paracentesis with and without intravenous albumin in cirrhosis. *Gastroenterology* **1988**, *94*, 1493–1502. [CrossRef]
26. Gines, A.; Fernandez-Esparrach, G.; Monescillo, A.; Vila, C.; Domenech, E.; Abecasis, R.; Angeli, P.; Ruiz-Del-Arbol, L.; Planas, R.; Sola, R.; et al. Randomized trial comparing albumin, dextran 70, and polygeline in cirrhotic patients with ascites treated by paracentesis. *Gastroenterology* **1996**, *111*, 1002–1010. [CrossRef]

27. Sola-Vera, J.; Minana, J.S.; Miñana, J.; Ricart, E.; Planella, M.; González, B.; Torras, X.; Rodríguez, J.; Such, J.; Pascual, S.; et al. Randomized trial comparing albumin and saline in the prevention of paracentesis-induced circulatory dysfunction in cirrhotic patients with ascites. *Hepatology* 2003, *37*, 1147–1153. [CrossRef] [PubMed]

28. Arora, V.; Vijayaraghavan, R.; Maiwall, R.; Sahney, A.; Thomas, S.S.; Ali, R.; Jain, P.; Kumar, G.; Sarin, S.K. Paracentesis-Induced Circulatory Dysfunction with Modest-Volume Paracentesis Is Partly Ameliorated by Albumin Infusion in Acute-on-Chronic Liver Failure. *Hepatology* 2020, *72*, 1043–1055. [CrossRef]

29. Llach, J.; Ginès, P.; Arroyo, V.; Rimola, A.; Tító, L.; Badalamenti, S.; Jiménez, W.; Gaya, J.; Rivera, F.; Rodés, J. Prognostic value of arterial pressure, endogenous vasoactive systems, and renal function in cirrhotic patients admitted to the hospital for the treatment of ascites. *Gastroenterology* 1988, *94*, 482–487. [CrossRef]

30. Caregaro, L.; Menon, F.; Angeli, P.; Amodio, P.; Merkel, C.; Bortoluzzi, A.; Alberino, F.; Gatta, A. Limitations of serum creatinine level and creatinine clearance as filtration markers in cirrhosis. *Arch. Intern. Med.* 1994, *154*, 201–205. [CrossRef]

31. Bernardi, M.; Gitto, S.; Biselli, M. The MELD score in patients awaiting liver transplant: Strengths and weaknesses. *J. Hepatol.* 2011, *54*, 1297–1306. [CrossRef] [PubMed]

32. Biggins, S.W.; Angeli, P.; Garcia-Tsao, G.; Ginès, P.; Ling, S.; Nadim, M.K.; Wong, F.; Kim, W.R. Diagnosis, evaluation, and management of ascites and hepatorenal syndrome. *Hepatology* 2021. [CrossRef]

33. Cillo, U.; Burra, P.; Mazzaferro, V.; Belli, L.; Pinna, A.D.; Spada, M.; Costa, A.N.; Toniutto, P.; On Behalf of the I-BELT (Italian Board of Experts in the Field of Liver Transplantation). A Multistep, Consensus-Based Approach to Organ Allocation in Liver Transplantation: Toward a "Blended Principle Model". *Am. J. Transplant.* 2015, *15*, 2552–2561. [CrossRef] [PubMed]

34. Bernardi, M.; Caraceni, P.; Navickis, R.J.; Wilkes, M.M. Albumin infusion in patients undergoing large-volume paracentesis: A meta-analysis of randomized trials. *Hepatology* 2012, *55*, 1172–1181. [CrossRef]

35. Alessandria, C.; Elia, C.; Mezzabotta, L.; Risso, A.; Andrealli, A.; Spandre, M.; Morgando, A.; Marzano, A.; Rizzetto, M. Prevention of paracentesis-induced circulatory dysfunction in cirrhosis: Standard vs. half albumin doses. A prospective, randomized, unblinded pilot study. *Dig. Liver Dis.* 2011, *43*, 881–886. [CrossRef] [PubMed]

36. De Franchis, R.; Baveno VI Faculty. Expanding consensus in portal hypertension: Report of the Baveno VI Consensus Workshop: Stratifying risk and individualizing care for portal hypertension. *J. Hepatol.* 2015, *63*, 743–752. [CrossRef] [PubMed]

37. Reiberger, T.; Mandorfer, M. Beta adrenergic blockade and decompensated cirrhosis. *J. Hepatol.* 2017, *66*, 849–859. [CrossRef]

38. Garcia-Pagan, J.C.; Saffo, S.; Mandorfer, M.; Garcia-Tsao, G. Where does TIPS fit in the management of patients with cirrhosis? *JHEP Rep.* 2020, *2*, 100122. [CrossRef]

39. Wong, F.; Sniderman, K.; Liu, P.; Allidina, Y.; Sherman, M.; Blendis, L. Transjugular intrahepatic portosystemic stent shunt: Effects on hemodynamics and sodium homeostasis in cirrhosis and refractory ascites. *Ann. Intern. Med.* 1995, *122*, 816–822. [CrossRef]

40. Riggio, O.; Angeloni, S.; Salvatori, F.M.; De Santis, A.; Cerini, F.; Farcomeni, A.; Attili, A.F.; Merli, M. Incidence, natural history, and risk factors of hepatic encephalopathy after transjugular intrahepatic portosystemic shunt with polytetrafluoroethylene-covered stent grafts. *Am. J. Gastroenterol.* 2008, *103*, 2738–2746. [CrossRef]

41. Casado, M.; Bosch, J.; Garcia-Pagan, J.C.; Bru, C.; Bañares, R.; Bandi, J.C.; Escorsell, A.; Rodríguez-Láiz, J.M.; Gilabert, R.; Feu, F.; et al. Clinical events after transjugular intrahepatic portosystemic shunt: Correlation with hemodynamic findings. *Gastroenterology* 1998, *114*, 1296–1303. [CrossRef]

42. Miraglia, R.; Maruzzelli, L.; Tuzzolino, F.; Petridis, I.; D'Amico, M.; Luca, A. Transjugular intrahepatic portosystemic shunts in patients with cirrhosis with refractory ascites: Comparison of clinical outcomes by using 8- and 10-mm PTFE-covered stents. *Radiology* 2017, *284*, 281–288. [CrossRef] [PubMed]

43. Trebicka, J.; Bastgen, D.; Byrtus, J.; Praktiknjo, M.; Terstiegen, S.; Meyer, C.; Thomas, D.; Fimmers, R.; Treitl, M.; Euringer, W.; et al. Smaller-diameter covered transjugular intrahepatic portosystemic shunt stents are associated with increased survival. *Clin. Gastroenterol. Hepatol.* 2019, *17*, 2793–2799. [CrossRef] [PubMed]

44. Lebrec, D.; Giuily, N.; Hadengue, A.; Vilgrain, V.; Moreau, R.; Poynard, T.; Gadano, A.; Lassen, C.; Benhamou, J.-P.; Erlinger, S. Transjugular intrahepatic portosystemic shunts: Comparison with paracentesis in patients with cirrhosis and refractory ascites: A randomized trial. French Group of Clinicians and a Group of Biologists. *J. Hepatol.* 1996, *25*, 135–144. [CrossRef]

45. Rössle, M.; Ochs, A.; Gülberg, V.; Siegerstetter, V.; Holl, J.; Deibert, P.; Olschewski, M.; Reiser, M.; Gerbes, A.L. A comparison of paracentesis and transjugular intrahepatic portosystemic shunting in patients with ascites. *N. Engl. J. Med.* 2000, *342*, 1701–1707. [CrossRef]

46. Ginès, P.; Uriz, J.; Calahorra, B.; Garcia-Tsao, G.; Kamath, P.S.; Del Arbol, L.R.; Planas, R.; Bosch, J.; Arroyo, V.; Rodés, J. Transjugular intrahepatic portosystemic shunting versus paracentesis plus albumin for refractory ascites in cirrhosis. *Gastroenterology* 2002, *123*, 1839–1847. [CrossRef]

47. Sanyal, A.J.; Genning, C.; Reddy, K.; Wong, F.; Kowdley, K.V.; Benner, K.; McCashland, T. The North American study for the treatment of refractory ascites. *Gastroenterology* 2003, *124*, 634–641. [CrossRef]

48. Salerno, F.; Merli, M.; Riggio, O.; Cazzaniga, M.; Valeriano, V.; Pozzi, M.; Nicolini, A.; Salvatori, F. Randomized controlled study of TIPS versus paracentesis plus albumin in cirrhosis with severe ascites. *Hepatology* 2004, *40*, 629–635. [CrossRef]

49. Narahara, Y.; Kanazawa, H.; Fukuda, T.; Matsushita, Y.; Harimoto, H.; Kidokoro, H.; Katakura, T.; Atsukawa, M.; Taki, Y.; Kimura, Y.; et al. Transjugular intrahepatic portosystemic shunt versus paracentesis plus albumin in patients with refractory ascites who have good hepatic and renal function: A prospective randomized trial. *J. Gastroenterol.* 2011, *46*, 78–85. [CrossRef]

50. Bureau, C.; Thabut, D.; Oberti, F.; Dharancy, S.; Carbonell, N.; Bouvier, A.; Mathurin, P.; Otal, P.; Cabarrou, P.; Péron, J.M.; et al. Transjugular intrahepatic portosystemic shunts with covered stents increase transplant-free survival of patients with cirrhosis and recurrent ascites. *Gastroenterology* **2017**, *152*, 157–163. [CrossRef]
51. Bernardi, M.; Angeli, P.; Claria, J.; Moreau, R.; Gines, P.; Jalan, R.; Caraceni, P.; Fernandez, J.; Gerbes, A.L.; O'Brien, A.J.; et al. Albumin in decompensated cirrhosis: New concepts and perspectives. *Gut* **2020**, *69*, 1127–1138. [CrossRef]
52. Caraceni, P.; Riggio, O.; Angeli, P.; Alessandria, C.; Neri, S.; Foschi, F.G.; Levantesi, F.; Airoldi, A.; Boccia, S.; Svegliati-Baroni, G.; et al. Long-term albumin administration in decompensated cirrhosis (ANSWER): An open-label randomised trial. *Lancet* **2018**, *391*, 2417–2429. [CrossRef]
53. Di Pascoli, M.; Fasolato, S.; Piano, S.; Bolognesi, M.; Angeli, P. Long-term administration of human albumin improves survival in patients with cirrhosis and refractory ascites. *Liver Int.* **2019**, *39*, 98–105. [CrossRef] [PubMed]
54. Solà, E.; Solé, C.; Simón-Talero, M.; Martín-Llahí, M.; Castellote, J.; Martinez, R.G.; Moreira, R.; Torrens, M.; Márquez, F.; Fabrellas, N.; et al. Midodrine and albumin for prevention of complications in patients with cirrhosis awaiting liver transplantation. A randomized placebo-controlled trial. *J. Hepatol.* **2018**, *69*, 1250–1259. [CrossRef] [PubMed]
55. Tufoni, M.; Zaccherini, G.; Caraceni, P. Prolonged albumin administration in patients with decompensated cirrhosis: The amount makes the difference. *Ann. Transl. Med.* **2019**, *7* (Suppl. S6), S201. [CrossRef] [PubMed]
56. Caraceni, P.; Tufoni, M.; Zaccherini, G.; Riggio, O.; Angeli, P.; Alessandria, C.; Neri, S.; Foschi, F.G.; Levantesi, F.; Airoldi, A.; et al. On-treatment serum albumin level as guide for long-term albumin treatment of patients with cirrhosis and uncomplicated ascites. *J. Hepatol.* **2021**, *74*, 340–349. [CrossRef] [PubMed]
57. Campion, E.W.; deLabry, L.O.; Glynn, R.J. The effect of age on serum albumin in healthy males: Report from the Normative Aging Study. *J. Gerontol.* **1988**, *43*, M18–M20. [CrossRef]
58. Italian Association for the Study of the Liver (AISF). Portal Hypertension and Ascites: Patient- and Population-centered Clinical Practice Guidelines by the Italian Association for the Study of the Liver (AISF). *Dig. Liver Dis.* **2021**, *53*, 1089–1104. [CrossRef] [PubMed]
59. Decaux, G.; Soupart, A.; Vassart, G. Non-peptide arginine-vasopressin antagonists: The vaptans. *Lancet* **2008**, *371*, 1624–1632. [CrossRef]
60. Dahl, E.; Gluud, L.L.; Kimer, N.; Krag, A. Meta-analysis: The safety and efficacy of vaptans (tolvaptan, satavaptan and lixivaptan) in cirrhosis with ascites or hyponatraemia. *Aliment. Pharmacol. Ther.* **2012**, *36*, 619–626. [CrossRef] [PubMed]
61. Yan, L.; Xie, F.; Lu, J.; Ni, Q.; Shi, C.; Tang, C.-X.; Yang, J. The treatment of vasopressin V2-receptor antagonists in cirrhosis patients with ascites: A meta-analysis of randomized controlled trials. *BMC Gastroenterol.* **2015**, *15*, 65. [CrossRef]
62. Pose, E.; Solà, E.; Piano, S.; Gola, E.; Graupera, I.; Guevara, M.; Cárdenas, A.; Angeli, P.; Ginès, P. Limited Efficacy of Tolvaptan in Patients with Cirrhosis and Severe Hyponatremia: Real-Life Experience. *Am. J. Med.* **2017**, *130*, 372–375. [CrossRef] [PubMed]
63. Hosui, A.; Tanimoto, T.; Okahara, T.; Ashida, M.; Ohnishi, K.; Wakahara, Y.; Kusumoto, Y.; Yamaguchi, T.; Sueyoshi, Y.; Hirao, M.; et al. Early Administration of Tolvaptan Can Improve Survival in Patients with Cirrhotic Ascites. *J. Clin. Med.* **2021**, *10*, 294. [CrossRef]
64. Torres, V.E.; Chapman, A.B.; Devuyst, O.; Gansevoort, R.T.; Grantham, J.J.; Higashihara, E.; Perrone, R.D.; Krasa, H.B.; Ouyang, J.; Czerwiec, F.S. Tolvaptan in patients with autosomal dominant polycystic kidney disease. *N. Engl. J. Med.* **2012**, *367*, 2407–2418. [CrossRef] [PubMed]
65. Spasovski, G.; Vanholder, R.; Allolio, B.; Annane, D.; Ball, S.; Bichet, D.-G.; Decaux, G.; Fenske, W.; Hoorn, E.J.; Ichai, C.; et al. Clinical practice guideline on diagnosis and treatment of hyponatraemia. *Intensive Care Med.* **2014**, *40*, 320–331. [CrossRef]
66. Kalambokis, G.; Fotopoulos, A.; Economou, M.; Pappas, K.; Tsianos, E.V. Effects of a 7-day treatment with midodrine in non-azotemic cirrhotic patients with and without ascites. *J. Hepatol.* **2007**, *46*, 213–221. [CrossRef]
67. Singh, V.; Dhungana, S.P.; Singh, B.; Vijayvergiya, R.; Nain, C.K.; Sharma, N.; Bhalla, A.; Gupta, P.K. Midodrine in patients with cirrhosis and refractory or recurrent ascites: A randomized pilot study. *J. Hepatol.* **2012**, *56*, 348–354. [CrossRef]
68. Ali, A.; Farid, S.; Amin, M.; Kassem, M.; Al-Garem, N. Clinical study on the therapeutic role of midodrine in non azotemic cirrhotic patients with tense ascites: A double-blind, placebo-controlled, randomized trial. *Hepatogastroenterology* **2014**, *61*, 1915–1924.
69. Lenaerts, A.; Codden, T.; Meunier, J.C.; Henry, J.P.; Ligny, G. Effects of clonidine on diuretic response in ascitic patients with cirrhosis and activation of sympathetic nervous system. *Hepatology* **2006**, *44*, 844–849. [CrossRef]
70. Singh, V.; Singh, A.; Singh, B.; Vijayvergiya, R.; Sharma, N.; Ghai, A.; Bhalla, A. Midodrine and clonidine in patients with cirrhosis and refractory or recurrent ascites: A randomized pilot study. *Am. J. Gastroenterol.* **2013**, *108*, 560–567. [CrossRef] [PubMed]
71. Bellot, P.; Welker, M.-W.; Soriano, G.; von Schaewen, M.; Appenrodt, B.; Wiest, R.; Whittaker, S.; Tzonev, R.; Handshiev, S.; Verslype, C.; et al. Automated low flow pump system for the treatment of refractory ascites: A multi-center safety and efficacy study. *J. Hepatol.* **2013**, *58*, 922–927. [CrossRef] [PubMed]
72. Bureau, C.; Adebayo, D.; de Rieu, M.C.; Elkrief, L.; Valla, D.; Peck-Radosavljevic, M.; McCune, A.; Vargas, V.; Simon-Talero, M.; Cordoba, J.; et al. Alfapump® system vs. large volume paracentesis for refractory ascites: A multicenter randomized controlled study. *J. Hepatol.* **2017**, *67*, 940–949. [CrossRef] [PubMed]
73. Lepida, A.; Marot, A.; Trépo, E.; Degré, D.; Moreno, C.; Deltenre, P. Systematic review with meta-analysis: Automated low-flow ascites pump therapy for refractory ascites. *Aliment. Pharmacol. Ther.* **2019**, *50*, 978–987. [CrossRef]

74. Solà, E.; Sánchez-Cabús, S.; Rodriguez, E.; Elia, C.; Cela, R.; Moreira, R.; Pose, E.; Sánchez-Delgado, J.; Cañete, N.; Morales-Ruiz, M.; et al. Effects of alfapump system on kidney and circulatory function in patients with cirrhosis and refractory ascites. *Liver Transpl.* **2017**, *23*, 583–593. [CrossRef]

75. Bernardi, M.; Caraceni, P. Novel perspectives in the management of decompensated cirrhosis. *Nat. Rev. Gastroenterol. Hepatol.* **2018**, *15*, 753–764. [CrossRef] [PubMed]

76. Caraceni, P.; Abraldes, J.G.; Ginès, P.; Newsome, P.N.; Sarin, S.K. The search for disease-modifying agents in decompensated cirrhosis: From drug repurposing to drug discovery. *J. Hepatol.* **2021**, *75* (Suppl. S1), S118–S134. [CrossRef] [PubMed]

Journal of
Clinical Medicine

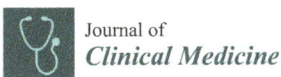

Article

Early Administration of Tolvaptan Can Improve Survival in Patients with Cirrhotic Ascites

Atsushi Hosui *, Takafumi Tanimoto, Toru Okahara, Munehiro Ashida, Kohsaku Ohnishi, Yuhhei Wakahara, Yukihiro Kusumoto, Toshio Yamaguchi, Yuka Sueyoshi, Motohiro Hirao , Takuya Yamada and Naoki Hiramatsu

Department of Gastroenterology and Hepatology, Osaka-Rosai Hospital, 1179-3 Nagasone, Kitaku, Sakai, Osaka 591-8025, Japan; aijyousaizu@yahoo.co.jp (T.T.); t.okahara@osakah.johas.go.jp (T.O.); mashida1013@yahoo.co.jp (M.A.); k-ohnishi@osakah.johas.go.jp (K.O.); youu0805hey@yahoo.co.jp (Y.W.); yukizarulucky_3lib@yahoo.co.jp (Y.K.); yamaguchi-to@osakah.johas.go.jp (T.Y.); sueyoshi@osakah.johas.go.jp (Y.S.); snowmotty@yahoo.co.jp (M.H.); yamada@osakah.johas.go.jp (T.Y.); hiramatsu@osakah.johas.go.jp (N.H.)
* Correspondence: hosui@osakah.johas.go.jp; Tel.: +81-72-252-3561; Fax: +81-72-255-3349

Abstract: (1) Backgrounds and aim: Tolvaptan, a selective vasopressin type 2 receptor antagonist, was approved for ascites, and its short-term efficacy and safety have been confirmed. However, it is still unclear whether this novel drug may improve long-term survival rates in cirrhotic patients with ascites. (2) Patients and methods: A total of 206 patients who responded insufficiently to conventional diuretics and were hospitalized for refractory ascites for the first time were retrospectively enrolled in this study. Among them, the first 57 consecutive patients were treated with conventional diuretics (the conventional therapy group); the latter 149 consecutive patients were treated with tolvaptan in addition to the conventional therapy (the tolvaptan group). (3) Results: The exacerbation of renal function was significantly milder in the tolvaptan group than in the conventional therapy group. The prognostic factors for survival in the tolvaptan group were being male, having hyperbilirubinemia, having a high blood urea nitrogen (BUN), and receiving high-dose furosemide at the start of tolvaptan treatment. The one-year and three-year cumulative survival rates were 67.8 and 45.3%, respectively, in patients with low-dose furosemide (<40 mg/day) at the start of tolvaptan treatment. The prognosis was significantly better in the tolvaptan group with low-dose furosemide than in the conventional therapy group ($p < 0.001$). (4) Conclusion: Tolvaptan can improve survival in patients with cirrhotic ascites, especially when tolvaptan is started before high-dose furosemide administration.

Keywords: tolvaptan; cirrhotic ascites; survival rate; furosemide

Citation: Hosui, A.; Tanimoto, T.; Okahara, T.; Ashida, M.; Ohnishi, K.; Wakahara, Y.; Kusumoto, Y.; Yamaguchi, T.; Sueyoshi, Y.; Hirao, M.; et al. Early Administration of Tolvaptan Can Improve Survival in Patients with Cirrhotic Ascites. *J. Clin. Med.* **2021**, *10*, 294. https://doi.org/ 10.3390/jcm10020294

Received: 14 December 2020
Accepted: 11 January 2021
Published: 14 January 2021

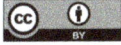
1. Introduction

Progression of liver diseases is characterized by a large decrease in the excretion of urinary sodium and accumulation of retained fluid within the abdominal cavity. For patients with liver cirrhosis who have ascites, current guidelines recommend the administration of a diuretic drug if the efficacy of sodium intake restriction is inadequate [1,2]. Conventional diuretics are natriuretic drugs that block sodium reabsorption in the nephrons, increasing renal sodium excretion to achieve a negative sodium balance [3,4]. Although ascites can be controlled through the restriction of sodium intake and administration of a natriuretic medication, some patients with ascites develop resistance to conventional therapy, which is referred to as refractory ascites (RA). For the treatment of diuretic-intractable ascites, an effective diuretic dosage has not yet been determined because of the development of severe diuretic-related side effects [5]. The strategy for treating ascites refractory to diuretic therapy has still not been established.

Recently, several studies have evaluated the effects of aquaretic drugs, such as tolvaptan, for treating ascites resistant to conventional diuretics [6,7]. Tolvaptan, which blocks arginine vasopressin (AVP) from binding to V_2 receptors in the distal nephrons and thus restricts water reabsorption, is an ideal aquaretic drug for the treatment of hyponatremia in conditions associated with increased circulating levels of antidiuretic hormones, such as decompensated liver cirrhosis [8,9]. Tolvaptan was approved on September 2013 in Japan, and many investigators have reported that tolvaptan is effective against RA for a short time and have shown many parameters predictive of its effectiveness [10–12]. However, it remains unclear whether a combination therapy with natriuretic and aquaretic medications is more effective than the conventional therapy with a natriuretic medication for patients with liver cirrhosis who have ascites for an extended time. It is also unknown when tolvaptan should be used in combination with conventional diuretics. Administration of conventional diuretics for an extended time causes activation of the renin-aldosterone system and, finally, worsens renal function. The one-year probability of survival after developing RA was reported to be approximately 30%, and the mean survival was only seven ± two days in patients developing hepatorenal syndrome [13]. It is important that patients with RA do not develop renal dysfunction. To clarify these issues, we compared the effects of combination diuretic therapy with conventional diuretic therapy in cirrhotic ascites patients.

2. Materials and Methods

The primary outcome was the overall survival, and the secondary outcomes were the prognostic factors for survival and contributing factors to a good response to tolvaptan. A total of 206 patients who responded insufficiently to conventional diuretics and who were hospitalized for RA for the first time were retrospectively enrolled in this study. The first 57 consecutive patients were treated with conventional diuretics and intravenous albumin administration between January 2010 and November 2013 (for approximately four years) in the conventional therapy group; a historical control was used for the group without administration of tolvaptan, which we treated only with conventional diuretics. The latter 149 consecutive patients were treated with tolvaptan in addition to the conventional therapy between December 2013 and December 2018 (for five years) in the tolvaptan group. In the conventional therapy group, the dose of furosemide or spironolactone was basically increased; sometimes, ascitic fluid was removed and a human serum albumin preparation was dripped intravenously. In the tolvaptan group, tolvaptan was administered without increasing conventional diuretics, and all other treatments were identical to those in the conventional therapy group. The initial administration dose of tolvaptan was 3.75 mg, and the dose was increased to 7.5 mg if ascites was not improved. We usually continue to treat tolvaptan, thus, the duration of treatment is the same as the observation period. The initial therapeutic effect of tolvaptan is defined as the "body weight [decreasing] by 1.5 kg or more within a week from the start of tolvaptan administration" [14]. The tolvaptan group was next divided into two groups according to the administration dose of furosemide on admission (<40 mg/day, low-dose furosemide group; ≥40 mg/day, high-dose furosemide group) (Figure 1).

The study observation period was from 1 January 2010 to 31 December 2019. The starting point was the hospitalization day. The conventional therapy group was treated with increasing conventional diuretics and/or administration of intravenous albumin and/or removing ascites ($n = 57$). The tolvaptan group was started on tolvaptan without increasing conventional therapy ($n = 149$).

Liver function was examined at least every two months, and imaging (computed tomography, ultrasound, or magnetic resonance imaging) results were evaluated every three months. This study was approved by the ethics committee of Osaka-Rosai Hospital.

Data were analyzed using the statistical software JMP 11.0.1 (SAS Institute, Tokyo, Japan), and the data are presented as means ± SEs. Data from the two groups were compared using unpaired *t*-tests. Multiple comparisons were performed by the Cox proportional hazards regression test; $p < 0.05$ was considered statistically significant. The log-rank test was used to assess the cumulative incidence rates for survival.

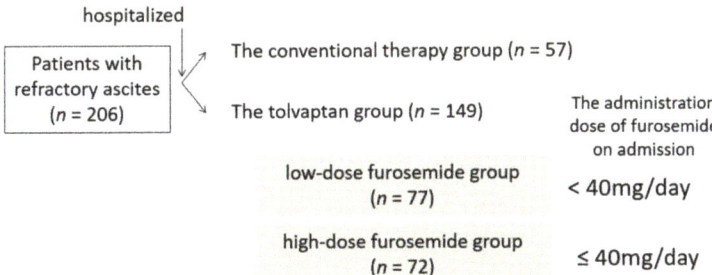

Figure 1. Scheme of this study.

3. Results

3.1. Changes in Renal Function after Hospitalization for the First Time in the Conventional Therapy Group and the Tolvaptan Group

The characteristics of the 206 patients with ascites treated with diuretics are shown in Table 1. A higher BUN value and lower sodium concentration were observed in the tolvaptan group than in the conventional group, and no significant differences aside from these factors were found in the clinical backgrounds of patients in the two groups. For safety, adverse events (AEs) were found to be similar in approximately 20% of the patients in each group, but different types of AEs were observed; the conventional group had renal dysfunction (12.2%), hepatic encephalopathy (5.2%), and general fatigue (3.5%), while the tolvaptan group had thirst (8.7%), general fatigue (5.3%), and appetite loss (4.0%). We next evaluated changes in renal function after hospital admission due to RA, because patients with ascites gradually become unresponsive to conventional diuretics, followed by renal dysfunction after administration of furosemide and spironolactone. Both the BUN and creatinine values gradually increased in the conventional therapy group over the course of one year, but they remained at an almost normal range in the tolvaptan group (Figure 2). The occurrence of hepatorenal syndrome was 58% and 11% during one year, in the control group and the tolvaptan group, respectively ($p < 0.001$). Tolvaptan was reported to cause hypernatremia after treatment, and thus, changes in sodium were examined, but sodium levels did not change at all in these two groups.

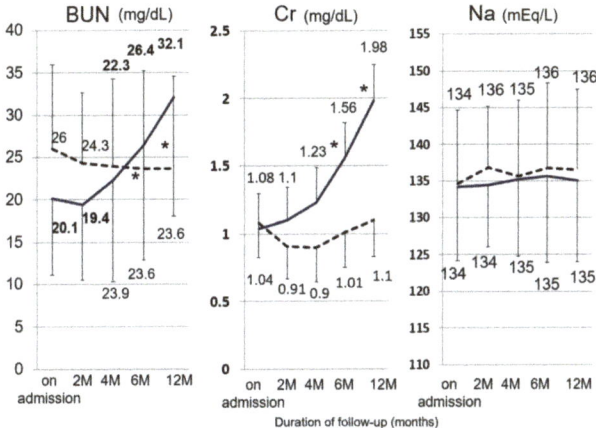

Figure 2. Serial changes in the serum concentration of BUN, creatinine, and sodium in the conventional therapy group and the tolvaptan group. Solid line: the conventional therapy group; dotted line: the tolvaptan group. Asterisks indicate significant differences (* $p < 0.01$ compared with the value recorded before treatment).

Table 1. Clinical backgrounds in the conventional therapy group and the tolvaptan group enrolled in this study.

	Conventional Group	Tolvaptan Group	*p*-Value
Cases	57	149	
Mean Age	70.7 ± 11.3	72.6 ± 10.4	0.26
Gender (Male/Female)	33/24	94/55	0.47
AST (U/L)	67.1 ± 33.2	66.3 ± 20.0	0.97
ALT (U/L)	44.2 ± 30.3	44.5 ± 50.7	0.98
gGTP (U/L)	87.1 ± 104.5	61.9 ± 80.0	0.44
ALP (IU/mL)	418 ± 183	486 ± 280	0.43
Total Bilirubin (mg/dL)	1.92 ± 1.40	2.67 ± 4.51	0.23
Albumin (g/dL)	2.79 ± 0.42	2.69 ± 0.45	0.15
PT Activity (%)	57.8 ± 16.7	59.9 ± 17.4	0.45
Creatinine (mg/dL)	1.04 ± 0.91	1.08 ± 0.53	0.70
BUN (mg/dL)	20.1 ± 11.9	26.0 ± 18.9	**0.028**
Na (mEq/L)	137.1 ± 2.4	134.3 ± 3.9	**0.021**
K (mEq/L)	3.96 ± 0.72	4.09 ± 0.82	0.63
AFP (ng/mL) Median	232	159	0.78
PIVKA-2 (mAU/mL) Median	227	274	0.40
Child-Pugh Score	8.8 ± 1.3	8.7 ± 1.3	0.75
Child-Pugh Status (B/C)	31/26	83/66	0.75
Administration Dose of Furosemide (mg)	34.2 ± 35.6 (0–240)	29.3 ± 22.3 (0–120)	0.23
Administration Dose of Spironolactone (mg)	34.7 ± 25.8 (0–100)	28.8 ± 22.2 (0–100)	0.11
Administration Period of Conventional Diuretics (Months)	24.2 ± 21.3	22.8 ± 29.2	0.43
HCC (Past History)	19	41	0.13
HCC (First Six Months)	3	8	0.95
HCC (Presence/Absence)	33/24	89/60	0.06

Marked with bold the *p*-value of BUN and Na are significantly different among two groups. Abbreviations: AST, aspartate aminotransferase; ALT, alanine amino transferase; gGTP, γ-glutamyl transpeptidase; ALP, alkaline phosphatase; PT, prothrombin; BUN, blood urea nitrogen; AFP, α-fetoprotein; PIVKA-2, protein induced by vitamin K absence; HCC, hepatocellular carcinoma.

3.2. Overall Survival in the Conventional Therapy Group and the Tolvaptan Group

We investigated the overall survival (OS) regarding the admission day as the starting point in the two groups and found that OS at one and two years in all patients were 43.6% and 30.6%, respectively. As shown in Figure 3, OS at one and two years in the tolvaptan group and in the conventional therapy group were 46.2% and 35.4%, and 36.8% and 19.9%, respectively. The prognosis was statistically insignificant between these two groups (*p* = 0.38).

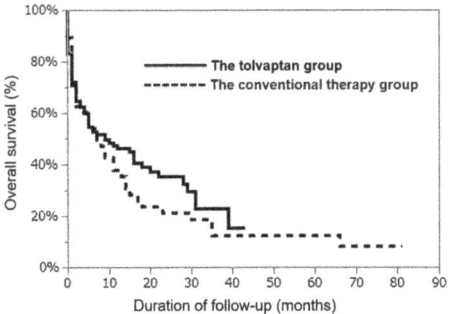

Figure 3. Comparison of cumulative survival rates between the conventional therapy group and the tolvaptan group.

3.3. A Critical Contributory Factor to the Good Response to Tolvaptan

Not all patients with ascites respond to tolvaptan, and many predictive factors have been reported. A good response to tolvaptan is defined as a 1.5 kg decrease in body weight after one week of treatment, as shown above. The good response rate based on this definition was 65.8%. We investigated predictive factors and univariately analyzed age, gender, and laboratory data (including AVP, aldosterone, renin, urine osmolality (U osm), and plasma osmolality (P osm), and found that five factors (creatinine, BUN, potassium, Child-Pugh score, and administration period of conventional diuretics) were positively associated (Table 2). A multivariate analysis revealed that only low BUN (<20 mg/dL: $p = 0.005$) was a critical contributory factor to the good response to tolvaptan, which was consistent with the findings of the START study [11].

Table 2. Contributing factors to a good response to tolvaptan. A good response to tolvaptan is defined as a 1.5 kg decrease in body weight after one week of treatment.

	Univariate Analysis		Multivariate Analysis	
	OR	*p*-Value	OR	*p*-Value
Age (Older Than 70 Years)	2.02	0.07		
Gender (Female)	1.16	0.675		
Total Bilirubin (<2 mg/dL)	1.97	0.234		
Albumin (>2.8 g/dL)	1.82	0.10		
PT Activity (>70%)	1.23	0.56		
Creatinine (<1.1 mg/dL)	3.12	0.0015	1.42	0.46
BUN (<25 mg/dL)	4.43	<0.0001	3.59	0.005
Na (>135 mEq/L)	2.10	0.1050		
K (<4.0 mEq/L)	2.58	0.0416	1.12	0.65
U osm ($\leq$400 mOSM/L)	1.71	0.3049		
P osm (>280 mOSM/L)	1.04	0.9398		
AVP ($\leq$2.5 pg/mL)	1.83	0.3967		
Aldosterone ($\leq$200 pg/mL)	1.40	0.6128		
Renin Activity ($\leq$5.0 ng/mL/h)	1.08	0.9021		
Child-Pugh Score ($\leq$10)	2.34	0.0297	1.94	0.20
Administration Dose of Furosemide ($\leq$40 mg)	1.48	0.267		
Administration Dose of Spironolactone ($\leq$50 mg)	1.02	0.967		
Administration Period of Conventional Diuretics (<Two Years)	2.76	0.0462	1.72	0.24
HCC (Presence)	2.03	0.058		

Abbreviations. PT, prothrombin; BUN, blood urea nitrogen; U osm, urine osmolality; P osm, plasma osmolality; AVP, arginine vasopressin; HCC, hepatocellular carcinoma.

3.4. The Prognostic Factors for Survival in the Tolvaptan Group

We next examined the prognostic factors among age, gender, renal and liver functions, administration dose of furosemide or spironolactone, and the presence/absence of HCC in the tolvaptan group. As shown in Table 3, a univariate analysis revealed that the prognostic factors were being male, having hyperbilirubinemia, having a high BUN, receiving high-dose furosemide at the start of tolvaptan treatment, and the presence of hepatocellular carcinoma (HCC). Finally, a multivariate analysis of these five factors clarified that the prognostic factors were being male (OR 1.59, $p = 0.049$), having hyperbilirubinemia (>2 mg/dL, OR 1.89, $p = 0.009$), having a high BUN (>25 mg/dL, OR 1.67, $p = 0.031$), and receiving high-dose furosemide ($\geq$40 mg/day, OR 2.63, $p < 0.001$).

Table 3. The prognostic factors for survival in the tolvaptan group.

	Univariate Analysis		Multivariate Analysis	
	OR	*p*-Value	OR	*p*-Value
Age (Older Than 70 Years)	1.40	0.16		
Gender (Male)	1.42	0.013	1.59	0.049
Total Bilirubin (>2 mg/dL)	1.73	0.0158	1.89	0.009
Albumin (<2.8 g/dL)	1.39	0.15		
PT Activity (<70%)	1.56	0.076		
Creatinine (>1.1 mg/dL)	1.43	0.12		
BUN (>25 mg/dL)	1.67	0.024	1.67	0.031
Administration Dose of Furosemide ($\geq$40 mg)	3.20	< 0.001	2.63	< 0.001
Administration Dose of Spironolactone ($\geq$50 mg)	1.32	0.22		
HCC (Presence)	1.73	0.0164	1.47	0.11

Abbreviations: PT, prothrombin; BUN, blood urea nitrogen; HCC, hepatocellular carcinoma.

3.5. The Prognosis in the Tolvaptan Group with Low- or High-Dose Furosemide and the Conventional Therapy Group

The dose of furosemide administered was one of the most important prognostic factors, thus, the tolvaptan group was divided into two groups according to the dose of furosemide at the start of tolvaptan treatment (<40 mg/day, low-dose furosemide group; $\geq$40 mg/day, high-dose furosemide group). The clinical backgrounds of these two groups and the conventional therapy group are shown in Table 4. Renal function had already worsened in the high-dose furosemide group compared to that in the other groups, and there were no differences except renal function between the low-dose furosemide group and the conventional therapy group.

As shown in Figure 4, OS at one and two years in the tolvaptan group with low-dose furosemide and in the conventional therapy group were 67.8% and 52.8% and 36.8% and 19.9%, respectively. The prognosis was significantly better in the low-dose furosemide group than in the conventional therapy group (log-rank test $p < 0.0001$).

This result shows the possibility that tolvaptan can improve survival in patients with cirrhotic ascites, especially in those whose tolvaptan treatment was started before high-dose furosemide administration.

The overall survival rate was better in the tolvaptan group with low-dose furosemide than in the conventional therapy group or in the tolvaptan group with high-dose furosemide (log-rank test $p < 0.001$).

Table 4. Clinical backgrounds in the two tolvaptan groups. The tolvaptan group was divided into two groups according to the dose of furosemide administered on admission (<40 mg/day, low-dose furosemide group; ≥40 mg/day, high-dose furosemide group).

	Tolvaptan Group		*p*-Value
	High-Dose Furosemide	Low-Dose Furosemide	
Cases	72	77	
Mean Age	72.8 ± 10.3	72.3 ± 10.5	ns
Gender (Male/Female)	44/28	50/27	ns
Total Bilirubin (mg/dL)	2.69 ± 3.43	2.66 ± 5.34	ns
Albumin (g/dL)	2.64 ± 0.49	2.73 ± 0.39	ns
PT Activity (%)	59.3 ± 17.1	60.4 ± 17.7	ns
Creatinine (mg/dL)	1.14 ± 0.54	1.02 ± 0.52	ns
BUN (mg/dL)	29.9 ± 21.1	22.4 ± 15.8	0.014
Administration Dose of Furosemide (mg)	45.8 ± 15.2	16.5 ± 7.4	<0.001
Administration Dose of Spironolactone (mg)	33.3 ± 26.2	24.5 ± 16.5	0.0015
HCC (Presence/Absence)	49/23	40/37	ns

Abbreviations: PT, prothrombin; BUN, blood urea nitrogen; HCC, hepatocellular carcinoma.

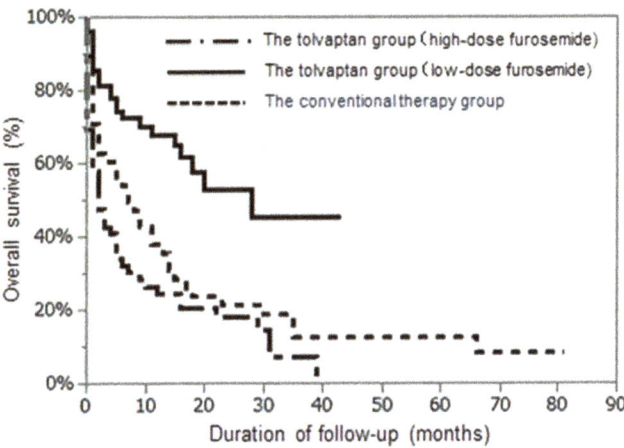

Figure 4. Comparison of cumulative survival rates among the conventional therapy group and the tolvaptan groups with low- or high-dose furosemide.

4. Discussion

We have experienced difficulties with and inadequacies in conventional diuretic treatments in patients with cirrhotic ascites. Although the deterioration of renal function is frequently observed with conventional diuretic therapy, renal dysfunction has been shown to be related to poor prognosis. The therapeutic strategy for cirrhotic ascites has changed drastically since tolvaptan was approved in 2013 [15]. Tolvaptan, an oral AVP V2 receptor antagonist, has been used as a new diuretic for ascites in combination with conventional diuretics. It is unknown whether this novel drug may help with the maintenance of renal function and improve long-term survival rates in cirrhotic patients with ascites. Tolvaptan has been reported to be quite effective against RA for a short time [7,15]. Thus, it was difficult to do a randomized controlled trial for a longer time.

The prognosis was statistically insignificant between the conventional therapy group and the tolvaptan group in this study. There were two reasons for the negative result. First, the tolvaptan group had a higher BUN value and lower serum sodium than those in the conventional therapy group. A higher BUN was associated with renal dysfunction. Low serum sodium was also related to an increased risk of death in patients with cirrhosis [16]. These clinical backgrounds might adversely affect the result. Second, a higher BUN showed not only renal dysfunction, but also unresponsiveness to tolvaptan. Tolvaptan is quite effective, but not all patients with cirrhotic ascites respond to this new drug. As BUN values worsened, patients were less likely to respond to tolvaptan [11]. The patients with higher BUN levels are presumed not to have enough water in their blood vessels to be excreted by tolvaptan, or to have worse renal perfusion, thus, tolvaptan is not effective in patients with higher BUN levels [17].

OS among patients with HCC and without HCC in this cohort was investigated, and we found that it is significantly better in the HCC (−) group than in the HCC (+) group (Supplementary Figure S1). However, the prognostic factor among patients with refractory ascites was gender (male), liver function (high value of total bilirubin), renal function (high value of BUN), and administration dose of furosemide (high dose of furosemide), but not the presence of HCC in the multivariate analysis. Patients with refractory ascites have poor liver and renal function, and, in that case, the prognosis might not depend on the presence/absence of HCC.

Tolvaptan can control RA, and, as a result, it leads to a good prognosis when it is started before high-dose furosemide administration. There are some reasons why tolvaptan improves OS in patients with ascites. First, it can decrease hepatic ascites and body fluid retention without worsening renal function, as shown in this manuscript. Before tolvaptan can be used, we had to increase the dose of conventional diuretics, which was finally followed by renal dysfunction. Second, tolvaptan can control RA more quickly than the conventional therapy, and, as a result, the nutritional status of patients may rapidly improve. Skeletal muscle mass decreases with age, especially in patients with liver cirrhosis (LC). Sarcopenia is characterized by the loss of muscle mass and is significantly associated with mortality in patients with LC [18]. Improvement in nutritional status can suppress the reduction of muscle mass, and it might be related to a good prognosis. On the other hand, loop diuretics directly suppress the differentiation of myofibroblasts, and sarcopenia in patients with LC may be attributable to treatment with loop diuretics [19]. Third, as tolvaptan can control ascites, the number of complications of decompensated cirrhosis (such as spontaneous bacterial peritonitis) decreases, and patients do not need to be in the hospital.

Not all patients with ascites respond to tolvaptan. The effectiveness rate has been reported to be approximately 50–60%, and non-responders have a poor prognosis, which is similar to those who are treated with conventional diuretics [11]. The present study showed that tolvaptan should be started before the BUN value becomes too high in order to reduce the number of non-responders. This high BUN value implies not only renal dysfunction, but also the deterioration of osmotic pressure in the renal interstitium, which is mainly caused by the administration of high-dose loop diuretics. Thus, we should be careful not to give high-dose loop diuretics in order to obtain a good response to tolvaptan.

Some investigators have already reported the efficacy and safety of tolvaptan. Uchida has shown that the ascites-related events-free duration was prolonged following tolvaptan treatment compared with that before treatment [20]. Kogiso also explained the impact of continued administration of tolvaptan and proved that long-term tolvaptan treatment increased serum levels of albumin, decreased ammonia levels, and preserved renal function [21]. We have never found a study in which the OS was compared between the tolvaptan group and the conventional therapy group in more than 200 patients with refractory ascites for more than four years.

5. Conclusions

This is the first report to reveal that tolvaptan can improve survival, especially when tolvaptan treatment is started before high-dose furosemide administration. Therapy for RA has drastically changed, and clinicians give tolvaptan early for RA rather than increasing the doses of conventional diuretics. The limitations of this study are the small number of patients and the retrospective nature of this study. Prospective and double-blind studies should be better, but tolvaptan has been reported to be quite effective in short-term and long-term administration. It might be difficult to prove it by prospective study.

Supplementary Materials: The following are available online at https://www.mdpi.com/2077-0383/10/2/294/s1, Figure S1: Comparison of cumulative survival rates between the tolvaptan group with HCC and without HCC.

Author Contributions: A.H.: study concept and design, acquisition of data; T.T., T.O., M.A., K.O., Y.W., Y.K., T.Y. (Toshio Yamaguchi), Y.S., M.H., and T.Y. (Takuya Yamada), acquisition of data; N.H., analysis and interpretation of data, funding procurement. All authors have read and agreed to the published version of the manuscript.

Funding: This research received no external funding.

Institutional Review Board Statement: The study was conducted according to the guidelines of the Declaration of Helsinki and approved by the ethics committee of Osaka-Rosai Hospital (protocol 20150024, the date of approval; 5 September 2015).

Informed Consent Statement: Informed consent was obtained from all subjects involved in the study.

Data Availability Statement: Data is contained within the article or Supplementary Materials.

Acknowledgments: We are grateful to Shokura H, Izutani Y and Kuyama Y (our medical assistants) for collecting the large amounts of data analyzed in this study. This study was supported by a Grant-in-Aid for Research on Hepatitis from the Ministry of Health, Labor, and Welfare of Japan and the Japan Agency for Medical Research and Development (17fk0210106h0901).

Conflicts of Interest: The authors declare no conflict of interest.

References

1. Runyon, B.A. Introduction to the revised American Association for the Study of Liver Diseases Practice Guideline management of adult patients with ascites due to cirrhosis 2012. *Hepatology* **2013**, *57*, 1651–1653. [CrossRef]
2. Fukui, H. Gut-liver axis in liver cirrhosis: How to manage leaky gut and endotoxemia. *World J. Hepatol.* **2015**, *7*, 425–442. [CrossRef]
3. Schuppan, D.; Afdhal, N.H. Liver cirrhosis. *Lancet* **2008**, *371*, 838–851. [CrossRef]
4. Gines, P.; Cardenas, A.; Arroyo, V.; Rodes, J. Management of cirrhosis and ascites. *N. Engl. J. Med.* **2004**, *350*, 1646–1654. [CrossRef]
5. Salerno, F.; Guevara, M.; Bernardi, M.; Moreau, R.; Wong, F.; Angeli, P.; Garcia-Tsao, G.; Lee, S.S. Refractory ascites: Pathogenesis, definition and therapy of a severe complication in patients with cirrhosis. *Liver Int.* **2010**, *30*, 937–947. [CrossRef]
6. Okita, K.; Kawazoe, S.; Hasebe, C.; Kajimura, K.; Kaneko, A.; Okada, M.; Sakaida, I. Dose-finding trial of tolvaptan in liver cirrhosis patients with hepatic edema: A randomized, double-blind, placebo-controlled trial. *Hepatol. Res.* **2014**, *44*, 83–91. [CrossRef]
7. Sakaida, I.; Kawazoe, S.; Kajimura, K.; Saito, T.; Okuse, C.; Takaguchi, K.; Okada, M.; Okita, K. Tolvaptan for improvement of hepatic edema: A phase 3, multicenter, randomized, double-blind, placebo-controlled trial. *Hepatol. Res.* **2014**, *44*, 73–82. [CrossRef] [PubMed]
8. Jaber, B.L.; Almarzouqi, L.; Borgi, L.; Seabra, V.F.; Balk, E.M.; Madias, N.E. Short-term efficacy and safety of vasopressin receptor antagonists for treatment of hyponatremia. *Am. J. Med.* **2011**, *124*, 977.e1–977.e9. [CrossRef]
9. Schrier, R.W.; Gross, P.; Gheorghiade, M.; Berl, T.; Verbalis, J.G.; Czerwiec, F.S.; Orlandi, C.; Investigators, S. Tolvaptan, a selective oral vasopressin V2-receptor antagonist, for hyponatremia. *N. Engl. J. Med.* **2006**, *355*, 2099–2112. [CrossRef] [PubMed]
10. Kawaratani, H.; Fukui, H.; Moriya, K.; Noguchi, R.; Namisaki, T.; Uejima, M.; Kitade, M.; Takeda, K.; Okura, Y.; Kaji, K.; et al. Predictive parameter of tolvaptan effectiveness in cirrhotic ascites. *Hepatol. Res.* **2017**, *47*, 854–861. [CrossRef] [PubMed]
11. Sakaida, I.; Terai, S.; Kurosaki, M.; Yasuda, M.; Okada, M.; Bando, K.; Fukuta, Y. Effectiveness and safety of tolvaptan in liver cirrhosis patients with edema: Interim results of post-marketing surveillance of tolvaptan in liver cirrhosis (START study). *Hepatol. Res.* **2017**, *47*, 1137–1146. [CrossRef] [PubMed]

12. Atsukawa, M.; Tsubota, A.; Kato, K.; Abe, H.; Shimada, N.; Asano, T.; Ikegami, T.; Koeda, M.; Okubo, T.; Arai, T.; et al. Analysis of factors predicting the response to tolvaptan in patients with liver cirrhosis and hepatic edema. *J. Gastroenterol. Hepatol.* **2018**, *33*, 1256–1263. [CrossRef] [PubMed]
13. Planas, R.; Montoliu, S.; Balleste, B.; Rivera, M.; Miquel, M.; Masnou, H.; Galeras, J.A.; Gimenez, M.D.; Santos, J.; Cirera, I.; et al. Natural history of patients hospitalized for management of cirrhotic ascites. *Clin. Gastroenterol. Hepatol.* **2006**, *4*, 1385–1394. [CrossRef] [PubMed]
14. Hiramine, Y.; Uojima, H.; Nakanishi, H.; Hiramatsu, A.; Iwamoto, T.; Kimura, M.; Kawaratani, H.; Terai, S.; Yoshiji, H.; Uto, H.; et al. Response criteria of tolvaptan for the treatment of hepatic edema. *J. Gastroenterol.* **2018**, *53*, 258–268. [CrossRef]
15. Sakaida, I.; Yamashita, S.; Kobayashi, T.; Komatsu, M.; Sakai, T.; Komorizono, Y.; Okada, M.; Okita, K. Efficacy and safety of a 14-day administration of tolvaptan in the treatment of patients with ascites in hepatic oedema. *J. Int. Med. Res.* **2013**, *41*, 835–847. [CrossRef]
16. Londono, M.C.; Cardenas, A.; Guevara, M.; Quinto, L.; de Las Heras, D.; Navasa, M.; Rimola, A.; Garcia-Valdecasas, J.C.; Arroyo, V.; Gines, P. MELD score and serum sodium in the prediction of survival of patients with cirrhosis awaiting liver transplantation. *Gut* **2007**, *56*, 1283–1290. [CrossRef]
17. Sakaida, I.; Terai, S.; Kurosaki, M.; Okada, M.; Hirano, T.; Fukuta, Y. Real-world effectiveness and safety of tolvaptan in liver cirrhosis patients with hepatic edema: Results from a post-marketing surveillance study (START study). *J. Gastroenterol.* **2020**, *55*, 800–810. [CrossRef]
18. Hanai, T.; Shiraki, M.; Nishimura, K.; Ohnishi, S.; Imai, K.; Suetsugu, A.; Takai, K.; Shimizu, M.; Moriwaki, H. Sarcopenia impairs prognosis of patients with liver cirrhosis. *Nutrition* **2015**, *31*, 193–199. [CrossRef]
19. Mandai, S.; Furukawa, S.; Kodaka, M.; Hata, Y.; Mori, T.; Nomura, N.; Ando, F.; Mori, Y.; Takahashi, D.; Yoshizaki, Y.; et al. Loop diuretics affect skeletal myoblast differentiation and exercise-induced muscle hypertrophy. *Sci. Rep.* **2017**, *7*, 46369. [CrossRef]
20. Uchida, Y.; Tsuji, S.; Uemura, H.; Kouyama, J.; Naiki, K.; Sugawara, K.; Nakao, M.; Inao, M.; Nakayama, N.; Imai, Y.; et al. Furosemide as a factor to deteriorate therapeutic efficacy of tolvaptan in patients with decompensated cirrhosis. *Hepatol. Res* **2020**, *50*, 1355–1364. [CrossRef]
21. Kogiso, T.; Sagawa, T.; Kodama, K.; Taniai, M.; Tokushige, K. Impact of continued administration of tolvaptan on cirrhotic patients with ascites. *BMC Pharmacol. Toxicol.* **2018**, *19*, 87. [CrossRef] [PubMed]

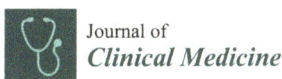

Journal of
Clinical Medicine

Review

Recent Advances in the Management of Acute Variceal Hemorrhage

Alberto Zanetto [1], **Sarah Shalaby** [1], **Paolo Feltracco** [2], **Martina Gambato** [1], **Giacomo Germani** [1], **Francesco Paolo Russo** [1], **Patrizia Burra** [1] and **Marco Senzolo** [1,*]

1   Gastroenterology and Multivisceral Transplant Unit, Department of Surgery, Oncology, and Gastroenterology, Padova University Hospital, Via Giustiniani 2, 35128 Padova, Italy; alberto.zanetto@yahoo.it (A.Z.); sarahshalaby18@gmail.com (S.S.); martina.gambato@gmail.com (M.G.); germani.giacomo@gmail.com (G.G.); francescopaolo.russo@unipd.it (F.P.R.); burra@unipd.it (P.B.)
2   Anesthesiology and Intensive Care Unit, Department of Medicine, Padova University Hospital, 35128 Padova, Italy; paolo.feltracco@unipd.it
*   Correspondence: marcosenzolo@hotmail.com

Abstract: Gastrointestinal bleeding is one of the most relevant causes of death in patients with cirrhosis and clinically significant portal hypertension, with gastroesophageal varices being the most frequent source of hemorrhage. Despite survival has improved thanks to the standardization on medical treatment aiming to decrease portal hypertension and prevent infections, mortality remains significant. In this review, our goal is to discuss the most recent advances in the management of *esophageal* variceal hemorrhage in cirrhosis with specific attention to the treatment algorithms involving the use of indirect measurement of portal pressure (HVPG) and transjugular intrahepatic portosystemic shunt (TIPS), which aim to further reduce mortality in high-risk patients after acute variceal hemorrhage and in the setting of secondary prophylaxis.

Keywords: cirrhosis; decompensation; bleeding; varices; survival; infection

Citation: Zanetto, A.; Shalaby, S.; Feltracco, P.; Gambato, M.; Germani, G.; Russo, F.P.; Burra, P.; Senzolo, M. Recent Advances in the Management of Acute Variceal Hemorrhage. *J. Clin. Med.* **2021**, *10*, 3818. https://doi.org/10.3390/jcm10173818

Academic Editors: Pierluigi Toniutto and Hidekazu Suzuki

Received: 30 July 2021
Accepted: 24 August 2021
Published: 25 August 2021

Publisher's Note: MDPI stays neutral with regard to jurisdictional claims in published maps and institutional affiliations.

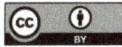
1. Introduction

Gastrointestinal (GI) bleeding is the second most frequent decompensating event in cirrhosis [1], with gastroesophageal varices representing the most frequent source of bleeding. Despite significant advances in the management of this complication, development of acute variceal hemorrhage (VH) is still associated with a six-week mortality risk of ~15–20% [2]. In patients who recover from VH, the risk of rebleeding is influenced by the treatment of underlying portal hypertension, with ~60% of untreated patients that will experience recurrent bleeding within on to two years, in contrast with only ~30% of those receiving therapies that lower portal pressure [3].

In this review, we discuss the management of patients with cirrhosis presenting with *esophageal* VH, including both treatment of the acute event (first section) and strategies to prevent recurrent hemorrhage (second section). The management of *gastric* variceal hemorrhage requires specific consideration and has been recently reviewed in depth elsewhere [4], therefore, it will not be included in the present review.

2. Control of Hemorrhage

The main goals of therapy in hospitalized patients with cirrhosis presenting with acute upper GI bleeding are (a) to control bleeding and (b) to prevent early rebleeding and death. Management can be divided into *general* measures, before the source of bleeding has been identified, and *specific* measures, once upper endoscopy has determined that hemorrhage is from esophageal varices.

85

2.1. General Measures

In combination with initial systemic stabilization (i.e., protection of circulatory and respiratory status) and start of intravenous proton pump inhibitors (PPIs), as in any patient hospitalized with upper GI bleeding, specific nuances in the management of patients with cirrhosis include a *restrictive* transfusion strategy and the use of prophylactic antibiotic therapy [5–8]. Additional measures include management of both coagulopathy and therapy with PPIs. For patients with alcohol-related liver disease, immediate and sustained cessation of alcohol consumption is particularly important to improve liver function and reduce risks of further bleeding, decompensation and mortality by reducing liver damage and portal pressure [9].

2.1.1. Blood Transfusion Strategy

The main driver for development of esophageal VH is clinically significant portal hypertension [10]. In a way, the acute loss of intravascular volume due to bleeding reduces splanchnic pressure and may lead to self-limitation or self-interruption of active hemorrhage. By contrast, a sudden restitution of intravascular volume is associated with a rebound increase in portal pressure, which in turn may lead to failure to control bleeding and/or early rebleeding [11]. In a seminal randomized control trial (RCT), a "restrictive" transfusion strategy (hemoglobin threshold for transfusion of 7 g/dL with target range of 7–9 g/dL) was associated with a significantly higher probability of survival compared with a "liberal" strategy (hemoglobin threshold for transfusion of 9 g/dL with target range of 9–11 g/dL) [12]. Therefore, current guidelines recommend initiating transfusions in cirrhosis when hemoglobin levels decrease to <7 g/dL, with a target level of 7–9 g/dL [5–8].

Restitution of intravascular volume should be managed with large peripheral lines (16–18 gauges), and blood loss has to be replaced by red blood packed cells [8]. Replacement of fluids and electrolytes is important to prevent pre-renal acute kidney injury, which is common in cirrhosis with GI bleeding and is associated with increased mortality [13]. Nephrotoxic drugs such as nonsteroidal anti-inflammatory drugs, non-selective beta-blockers (NSBBs), and other hypotensive drugs may be suspended during the acute course of VH [6]. As occurrence of acute decompensation may be associated with instability in the feeble hemostatic balance of decompensated cirrhosis, the need for invasive procedures should be evaluated carefully on an individual basis. As discussed below, clotting factors may be replaced only to correct an eventual dilutional coagulopathy, whereas there is no indication to prophylactically correct a prolonged prothrombin time or a low platelet count [5–8].

2.1.2. Antibiotic Prophylaxis

Bacterial infections are observed in up to 50% patients with cirrhosis hospitalized for GI bleeding, and are associated with strong risks of failure to control bleeding, early re-bleeding and mortality [14–16]. A recent meta-analysis including 12 studies comparing antibiotic prophylaxis vs. either placebo or no intervention demonstrated that the administration of prophylactic antibiotics was associated with reduced all-cause mortality (relative risk (RR): 0.79, 95% CI: 0.63–0.98), infection-driven mortality (RR: 0.43, 95% CI: 0.19–0.97), risk of bacterial infection (RR: 0.35, 95% CI: 0.26–0.47), rebleeding (RR: 0.53, 95% CI: 0.38–0.74), and length of stay (mean difference −1.9 days, 95% CI: −3.8–0.02) [17]. Therefore, a timely, short-term course of prophylactic antibiotics is an important step in the management of patients with cirrhosis and VH, and shall be instituted as early as possible upon admission, before upper endoscopy [5–8].

Whether severity of cirrhosis affects the importance of prophylaxis is unclear. In fact, while the role of prophylaxis is incontrovertible in patients with most advanced liver dysfunction (Child B and C), in those with less advanced liver disease conflicting data have been reported. In one retrospective analysis, Child A patients had lower risks of infection in the absence of prophylaxis (2%), and no difference in mortality was observed in treated vs. non treated patients [18]. The same study showed that the use of antibiotics was associated with a substantial reduction in mortality in Child C class [18]. However, prospective data are required to evaluate whether antibiotic prophylaxis can be avoided in Child A and current recommendation is to administer prophylaxis in all patients with cirrhosis presenting with VH, independent of child [5–8].

Intravenous ceftriaxone (1 g/24 h) for 7 days is the first choice in patients belonging to Child B and C classes, in those who were on quinolone prophylaxis, and in hospitals in which there is a high frequency of quinolone-resistant bacteria. Norfloxacin 400 mg twice daily may be used in the other patients. However, due to widespread quinolone resistance, ceftriaxone (a third-generation cephalosporin) has become the antibiotic of choice [5–7]. As approximately 30% of infection are from multidrug resistance antibiotics bacteria [19], evaluation of local resistance, if doable, may further improve definition of antibiotic regimen and should be considered [8]. Prophylactic antibiotics should be administered for a maximum of seven days, and their use should not be extended after discharge from the hospital [5–7]. In patients discharged before Day 7, transition to an oral antibiotic with the goal of completing seven days of treatment may be considered [8].

In a recent, nationwide study from Spain including 1656 patients with cirrhosis hospitalized for VH between 2013 and 2015, Martinez et al. investigated current epidemiology and trends of bacterial infections in these patients [20]. Interestingly, despite prophylaxis as currently recommended by international guidelines [5–7], 20% of patients developed bacterial infections, particularly respiratory tract infection. Development of infection was observed early (median time from admission 3 days) and was independently associated with Child C class (odds ratio (OR): 3.1; 95% CI: 1.4–6.7), Grade III–IV encephalopathy at admission (OR: 2.8; 95% CI: 1.8–4.4), orotracheal intubation for endoscopy (OR: 2.6; 95% CI: 1.8–3.8), and placement of nasogastric tube/balloon tamponade (OR: 1.7; 95% CI: 1.2–2.4 and 2.4; 95% CI: 1.2–4.9, respectively) [20]. Such procedures should, therefore, be minimized whenever possible, particularly in patients with additional risk factors, and active screening for respiratory infections shall be performed in case of early clinical deterioration. Whether patients at risk for respiratory infection would benefit from tailored regiments of antibiotic prophylaxis, particularly in settings with high risk of resistant strains bacteria, it remains to be evaluated in further studies.

2.1.3. Additional Measures
No Need for Correction of Coagulopathy

Hospitalized patients with decompensated cirrhosis have severe coagulopathy [21–23]. However, a prolonged prothrombin time does not reflect an increased bleeding tendency in these patients [21,23], and correction of INR by fresh frozen plasma should not be performed [5–8]. Not surprisingly, administration of recombinant FVII, which can correct prolongation of INR, was not associated with additional benefit compared with standard of care in an individual patient data meta-analysis of two RCTs [24]. Administration of plasma to correct coagulopathy in cirrhosis with bleeding is a very common practice [25]; however, this practice not only is ineffective, but is also likely harmful [26]. In a recent, multicenter cohort study administration of fresh frozen plasma in cirrhosis with VH was independently associated with increased risks of 42-day mortality (primary outcome, OR: 9.41, 95% CI: 3.71–23.90), failure to control bleeding at five days (OR: 3.87, 95% CI: 1.28–11.70) and length of stay (adjusted OR: 1.88, 95% CI: 1.03–3.42) (secondary outcomes) [27]. No specific data exist regarding the management of severe thrombocytopenia in the setting of VH, and therefore, no recommendation can be made. In patients without chronic liver disease, desmopressin increases levels of plasmatic Von Willebrand factor/procoagulant Factor VIII, and its use was associated with reduced bleeding time in an old study including compensated patients [28]. However, in a subsequent RCT no difference in control of VH was observed between patients randomized to terlipressin alone vs. patients treated with terlipressin plus desmopressin [29]. Therefore, desmopressin is not currently recommended.

Limited Usefulness of PPIs

As peptic ulcers are the source of bleeding in ~30% of patients with cirrhosis presenting with GI bleeding [30], intravenous PPIs should be initiated as soon as possible. However, when portal hypertensive bleeding is confirmed at endoscopy, discontinuation of PPIs may be considered as they have shown no efficacy in this clinical setting. Limited evidence suggested that a short-term use (10 days) of PPIs might reduce banding ulcer size [31], however, this was not associated with a significant reduction of bleeding risk. PPIs in decompensated cirrhosis are associated with significantly increased risks of hepatic encephalopathy, bacterial infection, and readmission at 30-days [32–34]. In a landmark analysis including 1198 patients from three RCTs evaluating the use of satavaptan in patients with cirrhosis and ascites, Dam et al. demonstrated that the use of PPIs was associated with a significantly increased risk of encephalopathy (OR: 1.88, 95% CI: 1.21–1.91) and spontaneous bacterial peritonitis (OR: 1.72, 95% CI: 1.10–2.69) during follow-up [33]. Recent data with extended period of follow-up confirmed that regular use of PPIs not only is associated with increased risk of spontaneous bacterial peritonitis, but also predicts liver-related mortality independent of MELD and stage of cirrhosis (OR: 2.01, 95% CI: 1.38–2.93) [34]. Therefore, their use should not be extended past discharge.

2.2. Specific Management of Acute Esophageal VH

Standard therapy for acute VH includes intravenous splanchnic vasoconstrictors and placement of rubber bands around esophageal varices, especially the one that is expected to be the source of bleeding [5–8]. Endotracheal intubation to protect the airway system may be considered in patients with massive bleeding prior to endoscopy. However, whether intubation is really protective or increases the risk of respiratory infections is unclear [20], therefore, it cannot be recommended for every patient.

2.2.1. Intravenous Splanchnic Vasoconstrictors

Three intravenous splanchnic vasoconstrictors are available: terlipressin, somatostatin or octreotide. These drugs exert their action by reducing splanchnic blood flow, therefore lowering portal pressure [35]. They are very effective and a recent meta-analysis clearly demonstrated that the use of vasoconstrictors is associated with a significantly higher probability of bleeding control and a lower seven-day mortality [36]. As a proof of concept, treatment with vasoconstrictors alone was previously found to control bleeding in >80% of patients [37]. It is most likely the widespread adoption of these drugs, together with the optimization of general medical care, that has significantly lowered the VH-related short-term mortality in the recent years [38].

A vasoconstrictor shall be initiated as soon as possible and early administration is associated with improved survival [5–8]. A placebo-controlled trial in which terlipressin was administered during the ambulance transfer showed that such early timing of administration was associated with increased probability to control of bleeding and survival in the treatment arm [39].

In clinical practice, the choice among these three intravenous vasoconstrictors is dictated by local availability and cost [40]. Recommended dose for terlipressin of 2 mg/4 h during the first 48 h, followed by 1 mg/4 h. If terlipressin is contraindicated, somatostatin is an alternative and should be administered as a continuous infusion of 250 mg/h (that can be increased up to 500 mg/h), with an initial bolus of 250 mg. The recommended dose of octreotide is a continuous infusion of 50 mg/h with an initial bolus of 50 mg [5–8].

Vasoconstrictors should be continued up to five days after the confirmation of VH because the risk of rebleeding during this time is particularly high [5–8]. However, as vasoconstrictors may be associated with potentially serious adverse events, the feasibility of a shorter administration (i.e., 24–48 h vs. 3–5 days) has been considered. In a recent meta-analysis, although the risk of 42-day mortality was not significantly different between one to three and five days, risk stratification was missing [41]. It may be that Child A patients could receive a shorter duration of therapy, whereas all others would require five days, but further studies are required to answer this question.

In summary, guidelines recommend that an intravenous splanchnic vasoconstrictor shall be initiated as soon as possible, prior to diagnostic endoscopy, and be administered for three to five days [5–8].

2.2.2. Endoscopic Therapy

Once hemodynamic stability has been reached, an upper GI endoscopy shall be performed to determine the cause of bleeding and to provide specific treatment [42]. Early data and one relatively recent retrospective study suggested that endoscopy within 12 h from the index event might be associated with reduced rates of recurrent bleeding and mortality [43]. On the other hand, in a larger multicenter study including 1373 patients with cirrhosis and VH, endoscopy within 24 h from admission was associated with lower mortality in patients with Child A or B cirrhosis (OR: 0.38, 95% CI: 0.16–0.86; $p = 0.020$) and in those with systolic blood pressure <90 mmHg (OR: 0.053, 95% CI: 0.006–0.51; $p = 0.011$) [44]. In contrast, performance of endoscopy within either 6 or 12 h was not associated with a further reduction in mortality compared with endoscopy within 24 h. Interestingly, the association between endoscopy within 24 h and reduced mortality was seen in Child A and B patients, but not in the overall group including also Child C [44].

This notwithstanding, current guidelines recommend that once hemodynamic stability has been achieved, endoscopy should be performed as early as possible, and within 12 h since presentation [5–8]. When VH is confirmed, either by the presence of a bleeding varix, a clot, or a "white nipple" over the varix, or when varices are the only abnormality observed that would explain the hemorrhage, all esophageal varices should be ligated, particularly the one that is considered the source of hemorrhage. Endoscopic variceal ligation (EVL) should be performed within the same endoscopy session. EVL is more effective than sclerotherapy, is associated with fewer adverse effects, and does not lead to further increase in portal hypertension [45]. Therefore, sclerotherapy should be restricted to the rare cases in whom ligation is not technically feasible. Hemostatic powder applied endoscopically may be considered as a rescue therapy, however, few data exist and its applicability remains to be determined [46,47].

In patients with uncontrolled bleeding, guidelines recommend placement of balloon tamponade (Sengastaken-Blackemore or Minnesota tubes) [5–8]. However, tamponade carries a high risk of complications, particularly respiratory infection [20], and shall be considered only as a temporary (maximum 24 h) bridge to TIPS [5]. Recent data suggest that placement of a self-expandable esophageal metal stent (placed orally or endoscopically) may be associated with greater bleeding control and lower adverse events compared to balloon [48]. As these stents may remain in place for up to 7 days, this would allow more time to plan for a definitive treatment. Per the last Baveno consensus, if available, the application of stents may be considered as a preferred alternative compared with balloons [5].

2.2.3. Transjugular Intrahepatic Portosystemic Shunt (TIPS)
Rescue TIPS (in Patients Who Fail Standard Therapy)

Despite combination therapy with prophylactic antibiotics, intravenous splanchnic vasoconstrictors, and EVL, 10–15% of patients will have either persistent bleeding or early rebleeding, which are associated with high risk of death [49]. Negative predictors for failure to control bleeding or early rebleeding include Child C class, portal vein thrombosis, severity of portal hypertension as defined by a hepatic venous pressure gradient (HVPG) >20 mmHg, and systolic blood pressure < 100 mmHg at admission [50,51].

In patients with mild-moderate rebleeding, a second session of endoscopy with ligation may be attempted. In patients with persistent or severe rebleeding (i.e., those with failure of endoscopic therapy), rescue TIPS is the therapy of choice [5–8]. In fact, by connecting the hypertensive portal venous system to the normotensive system of inferior vena cava, TIPS will quickly reduce portal pressure and resolve bleeding.

Given the lack of therapeutic alternatives, the only factor that would limit the use of rescue TIPS is futility. One issue to consider is patient's eligibility for transplantation. Additional factors include number and severity of organ failures. However, development of acute on-chronic liver failure (ACLF) per se is not an absolute contraindication for placement of rescue TIPS. In fact, in a recent multicenter study including 174 patients with either acute decompensation or ACLF and uncontrolled variceal bleeding, the insertion of rescue TIPS was an independent predictor of survival at 42 days [52]. There are multiple studies that looked for predictors of futility in patients undergoing rescue TIPS. In a recent, large multicenter cohort including 164 patients who received rescue TIPS, those with arterial lactate $\leq$ 2.5 mmol/L and MELD score $\leq$ 15 had 6-week survival > 85%, whereas those with baseline lactate level $\geq$ 12 mmol/L and/or MELD score $\geq$ 30 had >90% risk of death [53]. A recent, large observational study of rescue TIPS showed that stay in intensive care unit prior to TIPS, MELD, and Child-Pugh score were independently associated with mortality at six weeks, and the authors commented on the futility of rescue TIPS in patients with Pugh score > 13 [54].

Preemptive TIPS (In Patients at High-Risk of Failing Standard Therapy)

Patients with acute VH who are more likely to fail, despite initial control of hemorrhage by standard therapy, are those belonging to Child C class or those with HVPG > 20 mmHg [50,55]. It was, therefore, postulated that the placement of a TIPS before failure of standard therapy ("pre-emptive TIPS") could improve survival [56]. A first RCT in which 52 patients with HVPG > 20 mmHg was randomized to standard treatment vs. pre-emptive TIPS (uncovered) demonstrated significantly lower failure rates and all cause short-term mortality in the TIPS arm (12% vs. 50% and 17% vs. 38%, respectively) [57]. When covered TIPS became the standard-of-care, a second RCT confirmed an improved survival in patients randomized to TIPS vs. standard of care [58]. Both the one-year rate of failure to control bleeding/rebleeding and mortality were decreased by TIPS, the absolute reduction being 47% and 25%, respectively [58]. In this RCT, high-risk patients were defined as those with Child C cirrhosis and a Pugh score of 10–13, or those belonging to a Child B class with active bleeding at time of endoscopy.

Later on, however, large international observational cohorts confirmed the beneficial effect on survival of pre-emptive TIPS only in Child C patients (score 10–13), but not in those with Child B and active bleeding [59,60]. Therefore, the inclusion of Child B with active bleeding at endoscopy was questioned for potentially overrating the risk of mortality.

A recent RCT from China including 132 patients in Child B and C class and randomized 2:1 to pre-emptive TIPS vs. standard of care reported better transplant-free survival at six weeks and one year (OR: 0.50, 95% CI: 0·25–0·98; p = 0.04) and improved control of bleeding or rebleeding with early TIPS (OR: 0.26, 95% CI: 0.12–0.55; p < 0.0001) [61]. Importantly, the survival benefit was found in all subgroups, independent of either active bleeding or stage of cirrhosis, and no difference was found in the rate of hepatic encephalopathy. However, the reduction in mortality risk was relatively small (one-year survival 86% vs. 73% in pre-emptive TIPS vs. standard of care, respectively), which likely reflects the inclusion of patients at relatively lower risk of failure (57% of patients were Child B with no active bleeding and proportion of Child C was only 22%) [61]. It is also important to note that 75% of patients had HBV-related cirrhosis, which could have influenced the outcomes and may limit applicability of these results to Eastern countries. Furthermore, sclerotherapy was used in more than 5% of patients in standard of care group, which is not in line with current guidelines [5–7].

Another RCT from England in 58 patients with Child–Pugh score $\geq$ 8 showed no difference in survival (OR: 1.154, 95% CI: 0.3289–3.422; p = 0.79) and risk of rebleeding between pre-emptive TIPS and standard treatment, independent of severity of cirrhosis or active bleeding. However, the study was underpowered and only 23/29 patients (79%)

underwent preemptive TIPS, with only 13/23 within 72 h (therefore, not deemed early by definition) [62]. Remarkably, the one-year transplant-free survival in the control arm was higher than that in the 2010 RCT by Garcia-Pagan (76% vs. 61%) [58]. This may be related to the significant improvements in overall management of VH in cirrhosis, which would question the extrapolation of results from the 2010 study by Garcia-Pagan to present times [58]. On the other hand, an alternative explanation could be that patients included by Dunne et al. were not at high-risk of failure to control bleeding, which would not have allowed to assess the true benefits of pre-emptive TIPS [62].

Opposite to Dunne's findings, a large meta-analysis with individual data from 1327 patients included in seven studies, of whom 602 were Child B with active bleeding, found that placement of pre-emptive TIPS was associated with improved survival not only in the overall group (OR = 0.443, CI 95%: 0.323–0.607, $p < 0.001$), but also when Child B (OR = 0.524, CI 95%: 0.307–0.896, $p = 0.018$) and Child C (OR = 0.374, CI 95%: 0.253–0.553, $p < 0.001$) patients were analyzed separately [63]. This would support the use of pre-emptive TIPS in both Child C and Child B patients with active bleeding. However, results in Child B are less convincing/consistent compared with those obtained in Child C. Additional limitations are the inclusion or more observational studies than RCTs (four versus three), definition of high risk patients by only one specific criterion (therefore, not being able to assess if additional criteria might have better classified patients with VH at high risk), and the heterogeneity in both TIPS expertise and treatments in standard of care arms across different centers [63].

Therefore, a multicenter trial collecting large numbers of patients undergoing pre-emptive TIPS remains a research priority in this field. Importantly, such trial should assess not only which group(s) of patients are most likely to benefit from pre-emptive TIPS, but also whether there is a maximum threshold of severity of liver disease above which there is no improvement of survival.

While awaiting such trial, guidelines recommend to consider pre-emptive TIPS in patients with Child C cirrhosis (score 10–13) [5–8]. Patients with Child A cirrhosis and those with Child B cirrhosis without active bleeding should not be considered for pTIPS. Further data are required before to make a strong recommendation in patients with Child B and active bleeding at time of endoscopy.

As one major goal of pre-emptive TIPS is to prevent development of ACLF, one would think that pre-emptive TIPS should not be considered in patients who have already developed ACLF at time of admission/decision making. However, a recent study from a European collaborative group found that ACLF is an independent predictor of bleeding-related mortality, and that pre-emptive TIPS may improve outcomes in selected patients with ACLF [64]. Although prospective data are needed, these preliminary findings indicate that ACLF per se is not an absolute contraindication for pre-emptive TIPS, and instead eligibility should be a case-by-case decision according to number and severity of organ failures.

Despite RCTs and observational cohorts have demonstrated that pre-emptive TIPS is associated with a survival benefit, and the use of pre-emptive TIPS in these patients has been recommended since the Baveno V consensus (published 11 years ago) [65], a recent French survey revealed that only 7% of eligible patients finally received a pre-emptive TIPS [60]. Similarly, in another large observational cohort, a pre-emptive TIPS was placed in only 13% of high-risk patients [59]. This indicates a significant underutilization of pre-emptive TIPS in real-life practice, which is somewhat concerning considering its substantial effect on patient survival. Further efforts are required to lower the bar for a widespread adoption of pre-emptive TIPS in daily practice. These efforts include creation of dedicated networks through which selected patients may be referred early to tertiary care centers with specific expertise in invasive management of portal hypertension and its complications.

3. Prevention of Recurrent Hemorrhage

Per current guidelines, patients who had a TIPS placed after VH do not require further medical or endoscopic therapy for secondary prophylaxis, and should instead be referred for liver transplant evaluation in case they have additional complications of cirrhosis [5–8]. Patency of TIPS should be assessed at regular intervals by doppler ultrasound together with screening for hepatocellular carcinoma.

3.1. First Line Therapy

Combined therapy with NSBBs (propranolol or nadolol) plus EVL is the first line therapy in prevention of rebleeding [5–8]. This recommendation is based on multiple meta-analyses of RCTs performed to prevent rebleeding. One of these meta-analyses demonstrated that the added effect of NSBBs to EVL improved the efficacy of EVL alone and reduced mortality, whereas the added effect of EVL to NSBB was only associated with a non-significant decrease of rebleeding with no effect on survival [66]. A recent individual patient data meta-analysis evaluated data from three trials comparing NSBBs vs. combination therapy and from four trials analyzing EVL vs. combination therapy [67]. As these were individual data, the authors were able to perform risk stratification in Child A vs. Child B/C patients. Interestingly, in Child A (mostly compensated), combination therapy was associated with lower all-source rebleeding, without an effect on mortality. In Child B/C patients (mostly decompensated), combination therapy was associated with lower all-source rebleeding rates only in trials in which it was compared to EVL alone, indicating that NSBBs alone could be enough to prevent all-source rebleeding in these patients. Importantly, mortality was also lower in trials in which combination therapy was compared to EVL alone, suggesting that NSBBs not only are essential in preventing rebleeding, but also death [67].

These data, obtained from RCTs, are in contrast with a previous cohort study including patients with refractory ascites in which mortality was significantly higher in those receiving NSBBs [68]. However, study groups were different at baseline and patients were sicker in the NSBB group. Additionally, the determination of NSBBs was evaluated at diagnosis of refractory ascites with no information on their use thorough follow-up. Multiple trials in different groups of patients with decompensated cirrhosis have been conducted to confirm or refute these findings, and two meta-analyses have summarized these data both showing that the use of NSBBs is not associated with a higher mortality [69,70].

In studies that showed a detrimental effect of NSBBs [68,71], the arterial pressure in NSBBs users was lower than that in non-users, and a higher dose of propranolol was used, or a higher percentage of patients were treated with carvedilol. This indicates that patients in whom a negative inotropic effect or a vasodilatory effect from NSBBs/carvedilol were the ones that were negatively affected by beta-blockers [72]. In a way, this can be expected as this clinically-evident, likely dose-related deleterious hemodynamic effect of NSBBs would worsen the already vasodilated state of decompensated patients, leading to renal hypoperfusion, renal failure and death [73]. Indeed, in a propensity-matched analysis including only patients with refractory ascites, the use of propranolol was associated with an increased survival, except for the subgroup on a high dose (160 mg/day or more) [74].

Propranolol and nadolol should be used cautiously in patients with ascites and should be started at a lower dose than in patients without ascites, and the maximum dose should be capped also at a lower dose: propranolol should be capped to 160 mg/day (320 mg/day in patients without ascites) and nadolol to 80 mg/day (160 mg/day in patients without ascites) [7]. Importantly, the dose of NSBB should be reduced or drug should be discontinued in patients with refractory ascites who developed circulatory dysfunction defined by systolic blood pressure < 90 mm Hg, serum sodium < 130 meq/L, or acute kidney injury [7].

In summary, current guidelines recommend that first line therapy to prevent recurrent VH is the combination of NSBBs (propranolol or nadolol) plus EVL, independent of the presence or absence of ascites/refractory ascites or other complications of cirrhosis [5–8].

However, it is possible that refinements in risk stratification could lead to identification of "higher" risk patients in whom an aggressive approach, such as placement of TIPS, may be beneficial as first line therapy (i.e., before development of recurrent VH). This was recently evaluated by La Mura and Bosch in a retrospective study including 424 patients with cirrhosis candidates to secondary prophylaxis [75]. Inclusion criteria were diagnosis of cirrhosis, admission for VH within the previous seven days, baseline HVPG ≥ 12 mmHg, subsequent long-term treatment with propranolol or nadolol plus EVL, and a second HVPG assessment after one to three months of continued NSBBs. By combining clinical data (i.e., presence of ascites or encephalopathy) plus severity of portal hypertension (HVPG ≥ 16 mmHg), they identified two groups of patients at significantly different risks of rebleeding and mortality during follow-up. "Low" risk group included patients without ascites or encephalopathy and patients with VH plus ascites or encephalopathy but HVPG < 16 mmHg. "High" risk group included patients with VH plus one among the follows: ascites or HE, HVPG ≥ 16 mmHg, and lack of response to NSBBs as defined by an HVPG decrease by at least 20% of <12 mmHg. If confirmed by prospective series, this algorithm may improve risk stratification and lead to a more tailored management of patients with cirrhosis and history of VH. In fact, as shown in previous studies for acute VH [58] and "difficult ascites" [76], anticipating a decision for TIPS may be better compared with using it as rescue therapy.

In patients receiving secondary prophylaxis for VH, assessment of baseline HVPG and its response to NSBBs may provide useful information and guide therapy [77–79]. In this setting, the "goal-standard" is to measure HVPG at baseline and then re-assess HVPG after chronic administration of NSBBs (i.e., after four to six weeks) [80]. However, the measurement of "acute" HVPG response to intravenous propranolol may be a preferred alternative as it would be quicker and has an acceptable correlation with chronic response [77]. In one seminal RCT by Villanueva et al., an HVPG-guided therapy based on acute response to intravenous NSBBs significantly lowered the risk of portal hypertension related complications and mortality compared with standard of care [78]. In another retrospective study including both candidates for primary and secondary prophylaxis, acute response to intravenous propranolol was independently correlated with a 50% decrease in the probability of re-bleeding (23% at 2 years vs. 46% in non-responders; p = 0.032) and a better survival (95% vs. 65%; p = 0.003) [79]. Although further evidence is required to evaluate benefits and cost of such approach, current data suggest that HVPG-guided therapy in patients who are not deemed candidates for pre-emptive TIPS, could improve the management of secondary prophylaxis by reducing costs and adverse events due to ineffective therapy [77].

3.2. Second Line Therapy

Current guidelines recommend covered TIPS as second line therapy of choice in patients who experience rebleeding despite combination therapy with NSBB plus EVL [5–8].

Regarding prevention of recurrent VH by TIPS, RCTs comparing uncovered TIPS vs. NSBBs plus EVL (standard of care) agreed that TIPS is very effective in preventing rebleeding, but it is associated with higher risk of over encephalopathy and does not improve survival [81]. Comparable findings were confirmed by two RCTs in which covered TIPS was used [82,83]. Therefore, TIPS is considered the treatment of choice only in patients who fail first-line therapy (NSBBs plus EVL), in whom the risk of bleeding-related mortality is very high and exceeds those associated with TIPS [5–8].

Patients who experience the first episode of VH while on primary prophylaxis with NSBBs have a higher risk of rebleeding and mortality compared to those who experience VH not being on NSBBs, despite being treated with recommended combination therapy [84]. Although the best treatment strategy in these patients is unknown, they may benefit from a more aggressive strategy, and TIPS may be considered earlier rather than later in these patients. A second group of patients in whom to consider TIPS before failure of standard therapy are those who are or who become intolerant to NSBBs. In fact, as mentioned before,

NSBBs are the cornerstone of combined therapy, particularly in decompensated patients (Child B and C) [67].

In patients with cirrhosis and portal vein thrombosis who have recently bled, variceal obliteration with EVL takes longer and varices recur at a higher rate compared to patients without thrombosis [85]. Additionally, a small RCT showed that TIPS is more effective than EVL and NSBBs in preventing rebleeding in patients with cirrhosis and portal vein thrombosis, with a higher rate of thrombus resolution but without differences in mortality [61]. Patients with cirrhosis and portal vein thrombosis, which is the most common thrombotic complications in cirrhosis [86–88], may be a third group in which to consider TIPS earlier rather than later in the setting of secondary prophylaxis. This would be particularly important if the patient is awaiting liver transplantation, as the presence of thrombosis at time of transplantation is associated with a higher risk of post-transplant mortality [89].

A major clinical challenge in patients who receive TIPS for second-line prophylaxis of VH remains prediction of survival and prognosis (i.e., identification of patients with poor outcomes after TIPS in whom early evaluation for transplantation should be indicated). Recently, Bettinger et al. proposed to combine four simple variables (age, bilirubin, albumin and creatinine) in a new score named the "Freiburg index of post-TIPS survival" (FIPS score) [90]. In a very large cohort of patients who received TIPS for various indication, including second line prophylaxis of VH, the FIPS score was able to identify those at higher-risk for progression and death, and its prognostic discrimination was superior to other currently used score such as MELD, MELD-Na, and Child-Pugh [90].

4. Conclusions

Development of variceal hemorrhage in patients with cirrhosis poses a complex challenge requiring a multidisciplinary approach that is important to prevent rebleeding and improve survival. The management of variceal hemorrhage in these patients should take into consideration the severity of underlying portal hypertension and the presence (or absence) of other complications of cirrhosis, especially ascites. In patients presenting with variceal hemorrhage, the advances in the therapy of portal hypertension have resulted in lower rates of rebleeding and death, particularly for therapies associated with a decrease of portal pressure. Further improvement in risk stratification and in therapies of patients with cirrhosis and variceal hemorrhage are eagerly awaited.

Author Contributions: Conceptualization, A.Z. and M.S.; methodology, A.Z., S.S., P.F., M.G., G.G., F.P.R., P.B., M.S.; writing—original draft preparation, A.Z., S.S., P.F., M.G., G.G., F.P.R., P.B.; writing—review and editing, A.Z., M.S.; supervision, M.S. All authors have read and agreed to the published version of the manuscript.

Funding: This research received no external funding.

Institutional Review Board Statement: Not applicable.

Informed Consent Statement: Not applicable.

Data Availability Statement: Not applicable.

Conflicts of Interest: The authors declare no conflict of interest.

References

1. D'Amico, G.; Garcia-Tsao, G.; Pagliaro, L. Natural history and prognostic indicators of survival in cirrhosis: A systematic review of 118 studies. *J. Hepatol.* **2006**, *44*, 217–231. [CrossRef]
2. Bosch, J.; Garcia-Pagan, J.C. Prevention of variceal rebleeding. *Lancet* **2003**, *361*, 952–954. [CrossRef]
3. D'Amico, G.; Pagliaro, L.; Bosch, J. Pharmacological treatment of portal hypertension: An evidence-based approach. *Semin. Liver Dis.* **1999**, *19*, 475–505. [CrossRef]
4. Henry, Z.; Patel, K.; Patton, H.; Saad, W. AGA Clinical Practice Update on Management of Bleeding Gastric Varices: Expert Review. *Clin. Gastroenterol. Hepatol.* **2021**, *19*, 1098–1107.e1091. [CrossRef]
5. de Franchis, R.; Baveno, V.I.F. Expanding consensus in portal hypertension: Report of the Baveno VI Consensus Workshop: Stratifying risk and individualizing care for portal hypertension. *J. Hepatol.* **2015**, *63*, 743–752. [CrossRef] [PubMed]

6. European Association for the Study of the Liver. Electronic address eee, European Association for the Study of the L. EASL Clinical Practice Guidelines for the management of patients with decompensated cirrhosis. *J. Hepatol.* **2018**, *69*, 406–460. [CrossRef] [PubMed]
7. Garcia-Tsao, G.; Abraldes, J.G.; Berzigotti, A.; Bosch, J. Portal hypertensive bleeding in cirrhosis: Risk stratification, diagnosis, and management: 2016 practice guidance by the American Association for the study of liver diseases. *Hepatology* **2017**, *65*, 310–335. [CrossRef]
8. Bruno, R.; Cammà, C.; Caraceni, P.; D'Amico, G.; Grattagliano, I.; La Mura, V.; Riggio, O.; Schepis, F.; Senzolo, M.; Angeli, P.; et al. Portal Hypertension and Ascites: Patient- and Population-centered Clinical Practice Guidelines by the Italian Association for the Study of the Liver (AISF). *Dig. Liver Dis.* **2021**, 21. [CrossRef]
9. Burra, P.; Zanetto, A.; Germani, G. Liver Transplantation for Alcoholic Liver Disease and Hepatocellular Carcinoma. *Cancers* **2018**, *10*, 46. [CrossRef] [PubMed]
10. Zanetto, A.; Barbiero, G.; Battistel, M.; Sciarrone, S.S.; Shalaby, S.; Pellone, M.; Battistella, S.; Gambato, M.; Germani, G.; Russo, F.P.; et al. Management of portal hypertension severe complications. *Minerva Gastroenterol. (Torino)* **2021**, *67*, 26–37. [CrossRef]
11. Kravetz, D.; Bosch, J.; Arderiu, M.; Pilar Pizcueta, M.; Rodes, J. Hemodynamic effects of blood volume restitution following a hemorrhage in rats with portal hypertension due to cirrhosis of the liver: Influence of the extent of portal-systemic shunting. *Hepatology* **1989**, *9*, 808–814. [CrossRef]
12. Villanueva, C.; Colomo, A.; Bosch, A.; Concepcion, M.; Hernandez-Gea, V.; Aracil, C.; Graupera, I.; Poca, M.; Alvarez-Urturi, C.; Gordillo, J.; et al. Transfusion strategies for acute upper gastrointestinal bleeding. *N. Engl. J. Med.* **2013**, *368*, 11–21. [CrossRef]
13. Cardenas, A.; Gines, P.; Uriz, J.; Bessa, X.; Salmeron, J.M.; Mas, A.; Ortega, R.; Calahorra, B.; De Las Heras, D.; Bosch, J.; et al. Renal failure after upper gastrointestinal bleeding in cirrhosis: Incidence, clinical course, predictive factors, and short-term prognosis. *Hepatology* **2001**, *34*, 671–676. [CrossRef]
14. Ferrarese, A.; Zanetto, A.; Becchetti, C.; Sciarrone, S.S.; Shalaby, S.; Germani, G.; Gambato, M.; Russo, F.P.; Burra, P.; Senzolo, M. Management of bacterial infection in the liver transplant candidate. *World J. Hepatol.* **2018**, *10*, 222–230. [CrossRef]
15. Goulis, J.; Armonis, A.; Patch, D.; Sabin, C.; Greenslade, L.; Burroughs, A.K. Bacterial infection is independently associated with failure to control bleeding in cirrhotic patients with gastrointestinal hemorrhage. *Hepatology* **1998**, *27*, 1207–1212. [CrossRef]
16. Hou, M.C.; Lin, H.C.; Liu, T.T.; Kuo, B.I.; Lee, F.Y.; Chang, F.Y.; Lee, S.D. Antibiotic prophylaxis after endoscopic therapy prevents rebleeding in acute variceal hemorrhage: A randomized trial. *Hepatology* **2004**, *39*, 746–753. [CrossRef]
17. Chavez-Tapia, N.C.; Barrientos-Gutierrez, T.; Tellez-Avila, F.; Soares-Weiser, K.; Mendez-Sanchez, N.; Gluud, C.; Uribe, M. Meta-analysis: Antibiotic prophylaxis for cirrhotic patients with upper gastrointestinal bleeding—An updated Cochrane review. *Aliment. Pharmacol. Ther.* **2011**, *34*, 509–518. [CrossRef] [PubMed]
18. Tandon, P.; Abraldes, J.G.; Keough, A.; Bastiampillai, R.; Jayakumar, S.; Carbonneau, M.; Wong, E.; Kao, D.; Bain, V.G.; Ma, M. Risk of Bacterial Infection in Patients With Cirrhosis and Acute Variceal Hemorrhage, Based on Child-Pugh Class, and Effects of Antibiotics. *Clin. Gastroenterol. Hepatol.* **2015**, *13*, 1189–1196.e1182. [CrossRef]
19. Ferrarese, A.; Zanetto, A.; Germani, G.; Burra, P.; Senzolo, M. Rethinking the role of non-selective beta blockers in patients with cirrhosis and portal hypertension. *World J. Hepatol.* **2016**, *8*, 1012–1018. [CrossRef] [PubMed]
20. Martinez, J.; Hernandez-Gea, V.; Rodriguez-de-Santiago, E.; Tellez, L.; Procopet, B.; Giraldez, A.; Amitrano, L.; Villanueva, C.; Thabut, D.; Ibanez-Samaniego, L.; et al. Bacterial infections in patients with acute variceal bleeding in the era of antibiotic prophylaxis. *J. Hepatol.* **2021**, *75*, 342–350. [CrossRef] [PubMed]
21. Campello, E.; Zanetto, A.; Bulato, C.; Maggiolo, S.; Spiezia, L.; Russo, F.P.; Gavasso, S.; Mazzeo, P.; Tormene, D.; Burra, P.; et al. Coagulopathy is not predictive of bleeding in patients with acute decompensation of cirrhosis and acute-on-chronic liver failure. *Liver Int.* **2021**, 15001. [CrossRef]
22. Zanetto, A.; Rinder, H.M.; Campello, E.; Saggiorato, G.; Deng, Y.; Ciarleglio, M.; Wilson, F.P.; Senzolo, M.; Gavasso, S.; Bulato, C.; et al. Acute Kidney Injury in Decompensated Cirrhosis Is Associated With Both Hypo-coagulable and Hyper-coagulable Features. *Hepatology* **2020**, *72*, 1327–1340. [CrossRef]
23. Zanetto, A.; Rinder, H.M.; Senzolo, M.; Simioni, P.; Garcia-Tsao, G. Reduced Clot Stability by Thromboelastography as a Potential Indicator of Procedure-Related Bleeding in Decompensated Cirrhosis. *Hepatol. Commun.* **2021**, *5*, 272–282. [CrossRef]
24. Bendtsen, F.; D'Amico, G.; Rusch, E.; de Franchis, R.; Andersen, P.K.; Lebrec, D.; Thabut, D.; Bosch, J. Effect of recombinant Factor VIIa on outcome of acute variceal bleeding: An individual patient based meta-analysis of two controlled trials. *J. Hepatol.* **2014**, *61*, 252–259. [CrossRef] [PubMed]
25. Zanetto, A.; Senzolo, M.; Blasi, A. Perioperative management of antithrombotic treatment. *Best Pract. Res. Clin. Anaesthesiol.* **2020**, *34*, 35–50. [CrossRef] [PubMed]
26. Lisman, T.; Procopet, B. Fresh frozen plasma in treating acute variceal bleeding: Not effective and likely harmful. *Liver Int.* **2021**, *41*, 1710–1712. [CrossRef] [PubMed]
27. Mohanty, A.; Kapuria, D.; Canakis, A.; Lin, H.; Amat, M.J.; Rangel Paniz, G.; Placone, N.T.; Thomasson, R.; Roy, H.; Chak, E.; et al. Fresh frozen plasma transfusion in acute variceal haemorrhage: Results from a multicentre cohort study. *Liver Int.* **2021**, *41*, 1901–1908. [CrossRef]
28. Burroughs, A.K.; Matthews, K.; Qadiri, M.; Thomas, N.; Kernoff, P.; Tuddenham, E.; McIntyre, N. Desmopressin and bleeding time in patients with cirrhosis. *Br. Med. J. (Clin. Res. Ed.)* **1985**, *291*, 1377–1381. [CrossRef]

29. de Franchis, R.; Arcidiacono, P.G.; Carpinelli, L.; Andreoni, B.; Cestari, L.; Brunati, S.; Zambelli, A.; Battaglia, G.; Mannucci, P.M. Randomized controlled trial of desmopressin plus terlipressin vs. terlipressin alone for the treatment of acute variceal hemorrhage in cirrhotic patients: A multicenter, double-blind study. *New Italian Endoscopic Club. Hepatology* **1993**, *18*, 1102–1107. [CrossRef]

30. Hsu, Y.C.; Lin, J.T.; Chen, T.T.; Wu, M.S.; Wu, C.Y. Long-term risk of recurrent peptic ulcer bleeding in patients with liver cirrhosis: A 10-year nationwide cohort study. *Hepatology* **2012**, *56*, 698–705. [CrossRef]

31. Shaheen, N.J.; Stuart, E.; Schmitz, S.M.; Mitchell, K.L.; Fried, M.W.; Zacks, S.; Russo, M.W.; Galanko, J.; Shrestha, R. Pantoprazole reduces the size of postbanding ulcers after variceal band ligation: A randomized, controlled trial. *Hepatology* **2005**, *41*, 588–594. [CrossRef]

32. Bajaj, J.S.; Acharya, C.; Fagan, A.; White, M.B.; Gavis, E.; Heuman, D.M.; Hylemon, P.B.; Fuchs, M.; Puri, P.; Schubert, M.L.; et al. Proton Pump Inhibitor Initiation and Withdrawal affects Gut Microbiota and Readmission Risk in Cirrhosis. *Am. J. Gastroenterol.* **2018**, *113*, 1177–1186. [CrossRef]

33. Dam, G.; Vilstrup, H.; Watson, H.; Jepsen, P. Proton pump inhibitors as a risk factor for hepatic encephalopathy and spontaneous bacterial peritonitis in patients with cirrhosis with ascites. *Hepatology* **2016**, *64*, 1265–1272. [CrossRef]

34. Janka, T.; Tornai, T.; Borbely, B.; Tornai, D.; Altorjay, I.; Papp, M.; Vitalis, Z. Deleterious effect of proton pump inhibitors on the disease course of cirrhosis. *Eur. J. Gastroenterol. Hepatol.* **2020**, *32*, 257–264. [CrossRef] [PubMed]

35. Kulkarni, A.V.; Arab, J.P.; Premkumar, M.; Benitez, C.; Tirumalige Ravikumar, S.; Kumar, P.; Sharma, M.; Reddy, D.N.; Simonetto, D.A.; Rao, P.N. Terlipressin has stood the test of time: Clinical overview in 2020 and future perspectives. *Liver Int.* **2020**, *40*, 2888–2905. [CrossRef] [PubMed]

36. Wells, M.; Chande, N.; Adams, P.; Beaton, M.; Levstik, M.; Boyce, E.; Mrkobrada, M. Meta-analysis: Vasoactive medications for the management of acute variceal bleeds. *Aliment. Pharmacol. Ther.* **2012**, *35*, 1267–1278. [CrossRef] [PubMed]

37. D'Amico, G.; Pietrosi, G.; Tarantino, I.; Pagliaro, L. Emergency sclerotherapy versus vasoactive drugs for variceal bleeding in cirrhosis: A Cochrane meta-analysis. *Gastroenterology* **2003**, *124*, 1277–1291. [CrossRef]

38. Carbonell, N.; Pauwels, A.; Serfaty, L.; Fourdan, O.; Levy, V.G.; Poupon, R. Improved survival after variceal bleeding in patients with cirrhosis over the past two decades. *Hepatology* **2004**, *40*, 652–659. [CrossRef]

39. Levacher, S.; Letoumelin, P.; Pateron, D.; Blaise, M.; Lapandry, C.; Pourriat, J.L. Early administration of terlipressin plus glyceryl trinitrate to control active upper gastrointestinal bleeding in cirrhotic patients. *Lancet* **1995**, *346*, 865–868. [CrossRef]

40. Zanetto, A.; Garcia-Tsao, G. Gastroesophageal Variceal Bleeding Management. In *The Critically Ill Cirrhotic Patient*; Rahimi, R.S., Ed.; Springer: Cham, Switzerland, 2020. [CrossRef]

41. Yan, P.; Tian, X.; Li, J. Is additional 5-day vasoactive drug therapy necessary for acute variceal bleeding after successful endoscopic hemostasis? A systematic review and meta-analysis. *Medicine (Baltimore)* **2018**, *97*, e12826. [CrossRef] [PubMed]

42. Zanetto, A.; Garcia-Tsao, G. Management of acute variceal hemorrhage. *F1000Research* **2019**, *8*, 966. [CrossRef]

43. Chen, P.H.; Chen, W.C.; Hou, M.C.; Liu, T.T.; Chang, C.J.; Liao, W.C.; Su, C.W.; Wang, H.M.; Lin, H.C.; Lee, F.Y.; et al. Delayed endoscopy increases re-bleeding and mortality in patients with hematemesis and active esophageal variceal bleeding: A cohort study. *J. Hepatol.* **2012**, *57*, 1207–1213. [CrossRef]

44. Laursen, S.B.; Stanley, A.; Hernandez-Gea, V.; Procopet, B.; Giraldez, A.; Amitrano, L.; Villanueva, C.; Thabut, D.; Ibanez-Samaniego, L.; Silva-Junior, G.; et al. Optimal timing of endoscopy is associated with lower 42-day mortality in variceal bleeding. *J. Hepatol.* **2019**, *70*, e952. [CrossRef]

45. Laine, L.; el-Newihi, H.M.; Migikovsky, B.; Sloane, R.; Garcia, F. Endoscopic ligation compared with sclerotherapy for the treatment of bleeding esophageal varices. *Ann. Intern. Med.* **1993**, *119*, 1–7. [CrossRef]

46. Ibrahim, M.; El-Mikkawy, A.; Abdalla, H.; Mostafa, I.; Deviere, J. Management of acute variceal bleeding using hemostatic powder. *United Eur. Gastroenterol. J.* **2015**, *3*, 277–283. [CrossRef]

47. Ibrahim, M.; El-Mikkawy, A.; Abdel Hamid, M.; Abdalla, H.; Lemmers, A.; Mostafa, I.; Deviere, J. Early application of haemostatic powder added to standard management for oesophagogastric variceal bleeding: A randomised trial. *Gut* **2019**, *68*, 844–853. [CrossRef] [PubMed]

48. Escorsell, A.; Pavel, O.; Cardenas, A.; Morillas, R.; Llop, E.; Villanueva, C.; Garcia-Pagan, J.C.; Bosch, J.; Variceal Bleeding Study, G. Esophageal balloon tamponade versus esophageal stent in controlling acute refractory variceal bleeding: A multicenter randomized, controlled trial. *Hepatology* **2016**, *63*, 1957–1967. [CrossRef]

49. Garcia-Tsao, G.; Bosch, J. Management of varices and variceal hemorrhage in cirrhosis. *N. Engl. J. Med.* **2010**, *362*, 823–832. [CrossRef] [PubMed]

50. Abraldes, J.G.; Villanueva, C.; Banares, R.; Aracil, C.; Catalina, M.V.; Garci, A.P.J.C.; Bosch, J.; Spanish Cooperative Group for Portal, H.; Variceal, B. Hepatic venous pressure gradient and prognosis in patients with acute variceal bleeding treated with pharmacologic and endoscopic therapy. *J. Hepatol.* **2008**, *48*, 229–236. [CrossRef]

51. Amitrano, L.; Guardascione, M.A.; Manguso, F.; Bennato, R.; Bove, A.; DeNucci, C.; Lombardi, G.; Martino, R.; Menchise, A.; Orsini, L.; et al. The effectiveness of current acute variceal bleed treatments in unselected cirrhotic patients: Refining short-term prognosis and risk factors. *Am. J. Gastroenterol.* **2012**, *107*, 1872–1878. [CrossRef] [PubMed]

52. Kumar, R.; Kerbert, A.J.C.; Sheikh, M.F.; Roth, N.; Calvao, J.A.F.; Mesquita, M.D.; Barreira, A.I.; Gurm, H.S.; Ramsahye, K.; Mookerjee, R.P.; et al. Determinants of mortality in patients with cirrhosis and uncontrolled variceal bleeding. *J. Hepatol.* **2021**, *74*, 66–79. [CrossRef]

53. Walter, A.; Rudler, M.; Olivas, P.; Moga, L.; Trepo, E.; Robic, M.A.; Ollivier-Hourmand, I.; Baiges, A.; Sutter, O.; Bouzbib, C.; et al. Combination of Model for End-Stage Liver Disease and Lactate Predicts Death in Patients Treated With Salvage Transjugular Intrahepatic Portosystemic Shunt for Refractory Variceal Bleeding. *Hepatology* **2021**, 31913. [CrossRef]

54. Maimone, S.; Saffioti, F.; Filomia, R.; Alibrandi, A.; Isgro, G.; Calvaruso, V.; Xirouchakis, E.; Guerrini, G.P.; Burroughs, A.K.; Tsochatzis, E.; et al. Predictors of Re-bleeding and Mortality Among Patients with Refractory Variceal Bleeding Undergoing Salvage Transjugular Intrahepatic Portosystemic Shunt (TIPS). *Dig. Dis. Sci* **2019**, *64*, 1335–1345. [CrossRef] [PubMed]

55. Moitinho, E.; Escorsell, A.; Bandi, J.C.; Salmeron, J.M.; Garcia-Pagan, J.C.; Rodes, J.; Bosch, J. Prognostic value of early measurements of portal pressure in acute variceal bleeding. *Gastroenterology* **1999**, *117*, 626–631. [CrossRef]

56. Magaz, M.; Baiges, A.; Hernandez-Gea, V. Precision medicine in variceal bleeding: Are we there yet? *J. Hepatol.* **2020**, *72*, 774–784. [CrossRef] [PubMed]

57. Monescillo, A.; Martinez-Lagares, F.; Ruiz-del-Arbol, L.; Sierra, A.; Guevara, C.; Jimenez, E.; Marrero, J.M.; Buceta, E.; Sanchez, J.; Castellot, A.; et al. Influence of portal hypertension and its early decompression by TIPS placement on the outcome of variceal bleeding. *Hepatology* **2004**, *40*, 793–801. [CrossRef]

58. Garcia-Pagan, J.C.; Caca, K.; Bureau, C.; Laleman, W.; Appenrodt, B.; Luca, A.; Abraldes, J.G.; Nevens, F.; Vinel, J.P.; Mossner, J.; et al. Early use of TIPS in patients with cirrhosis and variceal bleeding. *N. Engl. J. Med.* **2010**, *362*, 2370–2379. [CrossRef]

59. Hernandez-Gea, V.; Procopet, B.; Giraldez, A.; Amitrano, L.; Villanueva, C.; Thabut, D.; Ibanez-Samaniego, L.; Silva-Junior, G.; Martinez, J.; Genesca, J.; et al. Preemptive-TIPS Improves Outcome in High-Risk Variceal Bleeding: An Observational Study. *Hepatology* **2019**, *69*, 282–293. [CrossRef] [PubMed]

60. Thabut, D.; Pauwels, A.; Carbonell, N.; Remy, A.J.; Nahon, P.; Causse, X.; Cervoni, J.P.; Cadranel, J.F.; Archambeaud, I.; Bramli, S.; et al. Cirrhotic patients with portal hypertension-related bleeding and an indication for early-TIPS: A large multicentre audit with real-life results. *J. Hepatol.* **2017**, *68*, 73–81. [CrossRef] [PubMed]

61. Lv, Y.; Qi, X.; He, C.; Wang, Z.; Yin, Z.; Niu, J.; Guo, W.; Bai, W.; Zhang, H.; Xie, H.; et al. Covered TIPS versus endoscopic band ligation plus propranolol for the prevention of variceal rebleeding in cirrhotic patients with portal vein thrombosis: A randomised controlled trial. *Gut* **2018**, *67*, 2156–2168. [CrossRef] [PubMed]

62. Dunne, P.D.J.; Sinha, R.; Stanley, A.J.; Lachlan, N.; Ireland, H.; Shams, A.; Kasthuri, R.; Forrest, E.H.; Hayes, P.C. Randomised clinical trial: Standard of care versus early-transjugular intrahepatic porto-systemic shunt (TIPSS) in patients with cirrhosis and oesophageal variceal bleeding. *Aliment. Pharmacol. Ther.* **2020**, *52*, 98–106. [CrossRef]

63. Nicoara-Farcau, O.; Han, G.; Rudler, M.; Angrisani, D.; Monescillo, A.; Torres, F.; Casanovas, G.; Bosch, J.; Lv, Y.; Thabut, D.; et al. Effects of Early Placement of Transjugular Portosystemic Shunts in Patients With High-Risk Acute Variceal Bleeding: A Meta-analysis of Individual Patient Data. *Gastroenterology* **2021**, *160*, 193–205.e110. [CrossRef]

64. Trebicka, J.; Gu, W.; Ibanez-Samaniego, L.; Hernandez-Gea, V.; Pitarch, C.; Garcia, E.; Procopet, B.; Giraldez, A.; Amitrano, L.; Villanueva, C.; et al. Rebleeding and mortality risk are increased by ACLF but reduced by pre-emptive TIPS. *J. Hepatol.* **2020**, *73*, 1082–1091. [CrossRef]

65. de Franchis, R.; Baveno, V.F. Revising consensus in portal hypertension: Report of the Baveno V consensus workshop on methodology of diagnosis and therapy in portal hypertension. *J. Hepatol.* **2010**, *53*, 762–768. [CrossRef] [PubMed]

66. Puente, A.; Hernandez-Gea, V.; Graupera, I.; Roque, M.; Colomo, A.; Poca, M.; Aracil, C.; Gich, I.; Guarner, C.; Villanueva, C. Drugs plus ligation to prevent rebleeding in cirrhosis: An updated systematic review. *Liver Int.* **2014**, *34*, 823–833. [CrossRef]

67. Albillos, A.; Zamora, J.; Martinez, J.; Arroyo, D.; Ahmad, I.; De-la-Pena, J.; Garcia-Pagan, J.C.; Lo, G.H.; Sarin, S.; Sharma, B.; et al. Stratifying risk in the prevention of recurrent variceal hemorrhage: Results of an individual patient meta-analysis. *Hepatology* **2017**, *66*, 1219–1231. [CrossRef] [PubMed]

68. Serste, T.; Melot, C.; Francoz, C.; Durand, F.; Rautou, P.E.; Valla, D.; Moreau, R.; Lebrec, D. Deleterious effects of beta-blockers on survival in patients with cirrhosis and refractory ascites. *Hepatology* **2010**, *52*, 1017–1022. [CrossRef]

69. Chirapongsathorn, S.; Valentin, N.; Alahdab, F.; Krittanawong, C.; Erwin, P.J.; Murad, M.H.; Kamath, P.S. Nonselective beta-Blockers and Survival in Patients With Cirrhosis and Ascites: A Systematic Review and Meta-analysis. *Clin. Gastroenterol. Hepatol.* **2016**, *14*, 1096–1104.e1099. [CrossRef]

70. Facciorusso, A.; Roy, S.; Livadas, S.; Fevrier-Paul, A.; Wekesa, C.; Kilic, I.D.; Chaurasia, A.K.; Sadeq, M.; Muscatiello, N. Nonselective Beta-Blockers Do Not Affect Survival in Cirrhotic Patients with Ascites. *Dig. Dis. Sci.* **2018**, *63*, 1737–1746. [CrossRef] [PubMed]

71. Mandorfer, M.; Bota, S.; Schwabl, P.; Bucsics, T.; Pfisterer, N.; Kruzik, M.; Hagmann, M.; Blacky, A.; Ferlitsch, A.; Sieghart, W.; et al. Nonselective beta blockers increase risk for hepatorenal syndrome and death in patients with cirrhosis and spontaneous bacterial peritonitis. *Gastroenterology* **2014**, *146*, 1680–1690.e1681. [CrossRef] [PubMed]

72. Garcia-Tsao, G. Beta blockers in cirrhosis: The window re-opens. *J. Hepatol.* **2016**, *64*, 532–534. [CrossRef] [PubMed]

73. Turco, L.; Garcia-Tsao, G.; Magnani, I.; Bianchini, M.; Costetti, M.; Caporali, C.; Colopi, S.; Simonini, E.; De Maria, N.; Banchelli, F.; et al. Cardiopulmonary hemodynamics and C-reactive protein as prognostic indicators in compensated and decompensated cirrhosis. *J. Hepatol.* **2018**, *68*, 949–958. [CrossRef] [PubMed]

74. Bang, U.C.; Benfield, T.; Hyldstrup, L.; Jensen, J.E.; Bendtsen, F. Effect of propranolol on survival in patients with decompensated cirrhosis: A nationwide study based Danish patient registers. *Liver Int.* **2016**, *36*, 1304–1312. [CrossRef]

75. La Mura, V.; Garcia-Guix, M.; Berzigotti, A.; Abraldes, J.G.; Garcia-Pagan, J.C.; Villanueva, C.; Bosch, J. A Prognostic Strategy Based on Stage of Cirrhosis and HVPG to Improve Risk Stratification After Variceal Bleeding. *Hepatology* **2020**, *72*, 1353–1365. [CrossRef] [PubMed]

76. Bureau, C.; Thabut, D.; Oberti, F.; Dharancy, S.; Carbonell, N.; Bouvier, A.; Mathurin, P.; Otal, P.; Cabarrou, P.; Peron, J.M.; et al. Transjugular Intrahepatic Portosystemic Shunts With Covered Stents Increase Transplant-Free Survival of Patients With Cirrhosis and Recurrent Ascites. *Gastroenterology* **2017**, *152*, 157–163. [CrossRef]

77. Garcia-Pagan, J.C.; Francoz, C.; Montagnese, S.; Senzolo, M.; Mookerjee, R.P. Management of the major complications of cirrhosis: Beyond guidelines. *J. Hepatol.* **2021**, *75* (Suppl. 1), S135–S146. [CrossRef]

78. Villanueva, C.; Graupera, I.; Aracil, C.; Alvarado, E.; Minana, J.; Puente, A.; Hernandez-Gea, V.; Ardevol, A.; Pavel, O.; Colomo, A.; et al. A randomized trial to assess whether portal pressure guided therapy to prevent variceal rebleeding improves survival in cirrhosis. *Hepatology* **2017**, *65*, 1693–1707. [CrossRef]

79. La Mura, V.; Abraldes, J.G.; Raffa, S.; Retto, O.; Berzigotti, A.; Garcia-Pagan, J.C.; Bosch, J. Prognostic value of acute hemodynamic response to i.v. propranolol in patients with cirrhosis and portal hypertension. *J. Hepatol.* **2009**, *51*, 279–287. [CrossRef] [PubMed]

80. Bosch, J.; Abraldes, J.G.; Berzigotti, A.; Garcia-Pagan, J.C. The clinical use of HVPG measurements in chronic liver disease. *Nat. Rev. Gastroenterol. Hepatol.* **2009**, *6*, 573–582. [CrossRef]

81. Zheng, M.; Chen, Y.; Bai, J.; Zeng, Q.; You, J.; Jin, R.; Zhou, X.; Shen, H.; Zheng, Y.; Du, Z. Transjugular intrahepatic portosystemic shunt versus endoscopic therapy in the secondary prophylaxis of variceal rebleeding in cirrhotic patients: Meta-analysis update. *J. Clin. Gastroenterol.* **2008**, *42*, 507–516. [CrossRef]

82. Holster, I.L.; Tjwa, E.T.; Moelker, A.; Wils, A.; Hansen, B.E.; Vermeijden, J.R.; Scholten, P.; van Hoek, B.; Nicolai, J.J.; Kuipers, E.J.; et al. Covered transjugular intrahepatic portosystemic shunt versus endoscopic therapy + beta-blocker for prevention of variceal rebleeding. *Hepatology* **2016**, *63*, 581–589. [CrossRef] [PubMed]

83. Sauerbruch, T.; Mengel, M.; Dollinger, M.; Zipprich, A.; Rossle, M.; Panther, E.; Wiest, R.; Caca, K.; Hoffmeister, A.; Lutz, H.; et al. Prevention of Rebleeding From Esophageal Varices in Patients With Cirrhosis Receiving Small-Diameter Stents Versus Hemodynamically Controlled Medical Therapy. *Gastroenterology* **2015**, *149*, 660–668.e661. [CrossRef]

84. de Souza, A.R.; La Mura, V.; Reverter, E.; Seijo, S.; Berzigotti, A.; Ashkenazi, E.; Garcia-Pagan, J.C.; Abraldes, J.G.; Bosch, J. Patients whose first episode of bleeding occurs while taking a beta-blocker have high long-term risks of rebleeding and death. *Clin. Gastroenterol. Hepatol.* **2012**, *10*, 670–676. [CrossRef]

85. Zanetto, A.; Garcia-Tsao, G. Some Answers and More Questions About Portal Vein Thrombosis in Patients With Decompensated Cirrhosis. *Clin. Gastroenterol. Hepatol.* **2020**, *18*, 2432–2434. [CrossRef] [PubMed]

86. Zanetto, A.; Senzolo, M.; Vitale, A.; Cillo, U.; Radu, C.; Sartorello, F.; Spiezia, L.; Campello, E.; Rodriguez-Castro, K.; Ferrarese, A.; et al. Thromboelastometry hypercoagulable profiles and portal vein thrombosis in cirrhotic patients with hepatocellular carcinoma. *Dig. Liver Dis.* **2017**, *49*, 440–445. [CrossRef] [PubMed]

87. Shalaby, S.; Simioni, P.; Campello, E.; Spiezia, L.; Gavasso, S.; Bizzaro, D.; Cardin, R.; D'Amico, F.; Gringeri, E.; Cillo, U.; et al. Endothelial Damage of the Portal Vein is Associated with Heparin-Like Effect in Advanced Stages of Cirrhosis. *Thromb Haemost* **2020**, *120*, 1173–1181. [CrossRef] [PubMed]

88. Russo, F.P.; Zanetto, A.; Campello, E.; Bulato, C.; Shalaby, S.; Spiezia, L.; Gavasso, S.; Franceschet, E.; Radu, C.; Senzolo, M.; et al. Reversal of hypercoagulability in patients with HCV-related cirrhosis after treatment with direct-acting antivirals. *Liver Int.* **2018**, *38*, 2210–2218. [CrossRef]

89. Zanetto, A.; Rodriguez-Kastro, K.I.; Germani, G.; Ferrarese, A.; Cillo, U.; Burra, P.; Senzolo, M. Mortality in liver transplant recipients with portal vein thrombosis—An updated meta-analysis. *Transpl. Int.* **2018**, *31*, 1318–1329. [CrossRef] [PubMed]

90. Bettinger, D.; Sturm, L.; Pfaff, L.; Hahn, F.; Kloeckner, R.; Volkwein, L.; Praktiknjo, M.; Lv, Y.; Han, G.; Huber, J.P.; et al. Refining prediction of survival after TIPS with the novel Freiburg index of post-TIPS survival. *J. Hepatol.* **2021**, *74*, 1362–1372. [CrossRef]

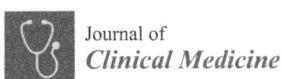

Review

New Therapies of Liver Diseases: Hepatic Encephalopathy

Chiara Mangini and Sara Montagnese *

Department of Medicine, University of Padova, 35128 Padova, Italy; chiara.manginij@gmail.com
* Correspondence: sara.montagnese@unipd.it; Tel.: +39-(0)49-8218675

Abstract: Hepatic encephalopathy (HE) is a common complication of advanced liver disease which has profound implications in terms of the patients' ability to fulfil their family and social roles, to drive and to provide for themselves. Recurrent and persistent HE is still a serious management challenge, translating into a significant burden for patients and their families, health services and society at large. The past few years have been characterized by significantly more attention towards HE and its implications; its definition has been refined and a small number of new drugs/alternative management strategies have become available, while others are underway. In this narrative review we summarize them in a pragmatic and hopefully useful fashion.

Keywords: cirrhosis; portal-systemic shunt; ammonia; vigilance

Citation: Mangini, C.; Montagnese, S. New Therapies of Liver Diseases: Hepatic Encephalopathy. *J. Clin. Med.* **2021**, *10*, 4050. https://doi.org/10.3390/jcm10184050

Academic Editor: Pierluigi Toniutto

Received: 16 July 2021
Accepted: 4 September 2021
Published: 7 September 2021

Publisher's Note: MDPI stays neutral with regard to jurisdictional claims in published maps and institutional affiliations.

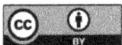

1. Introduction

Hepatic encephalopathy (HE) is a brain dysfunction caused by liver failure and/or portal-systemic shunt that results in a spectrum of neurological and psychiatric abnormalities ranging from subclinical alterations to coma [1].

Classification is based on the underlying condition leading to HE: "Type A" HE is due to acute liver failure, "Type B" HE is caused by portal-systemic shunt without significant liver disease and "Type C" HE by cirrhosis with or without portal-systemic shunt [1]. In terms of its severity, HE is qualified as covert (minor or no signs/symptoms but abnormalities on neuropsychological and/or neurophysiological tests) or overt (Grades II or over according to the West Haven criteria [1]). Finally, in terms of its time-course, overt HE is classified as episodic, recurrent (more than one episode over a period of six months) or persistent (no return to normal/baseline neuropsychiatric performance in between episodes) [1].

This narrative review will deal with the management of Type C HE, i.e., the one associated with cirrhosis with or without portal-systemic shunt [1]. Standard information on HE treatment (no formal literature search) plus 2018–2021 information on novel therapies is included. The 2018–2021 literature search was conducted on Pubmed using the terms hepatic encephalopathy plus: treatment, polyethylene glycol (PEG), branched-chain amino acids (BCAAs), L-ornithine L-aspartate (LOLA), nitrogen scavengers, Acetyl L-carnitine, albumin, probiotics, fecal microbiota transplantation (FMT), flumazenil, minocycline, ibuprofen, phosphodiesterase-5 inhibitors, indomethacin, benzodiazepine inverse agonists.

Prior to discussing available, recommended and more experimental (Table 1) treatment options, it is important to highlight how:

- The HE phenotype is nonspecific and differential diagnosis extremely important;
- Response to treatment can be utilized to confirm a working diagnosis of HE, especially in its mild forms;
- The lack thereof, should prompt fast differential diagnosis investigations, especially in severe forms;
- With the exception of direct modulation of vigilance/inflammation (*vide infra*), HE treatment is essentially synonymous of ammonia-lowering treatment. Hyperammonaemia is necessary but not sufficient for a working diagnosis of HE (i.e., there is no

99

HE without hyperammonaemia but the presence of hyperammonaemia does not necessarily translate into a HE phenotype, especially in young patients) [1].

2. General Management Principles

An episode of overt HE is generally managed by ensuring adequate airway protection for severe cases, correction of any identified precipitating factors and institution of ammonia-lowering treatment [1,2]. The most commonly utilized drugs for the subsequent commencement of secondary prophylaxis are non-absorbable disaccharides (i.e., lactulose or lactitol, which aim at reducing gut nitrogen load via their laxative and prebiotic effects, enhancing bacterial ammonia uptake and reducing ammonia production in the small intestine) and non-absorbable antibiotics (also affecting production/absorption of gut-derived neurotoxins, and reducing endotoxemia and inflammation), which are generally added after a second overt HE episode or, as a stand-alone, when non-absorbable disaccharides are not well tolerated [3,4]. Primary prophylaxis is not generally recommended, with the exception of the rapid removal of blood from the gastrointestinal tract after an upper gastrointestinal bleed, for example with lactulose [5] or mannitol [6]. By contrast, secondary prophylaxis is important, as once a patient has experienced an episode of overt HE, the likelihood of further episodes is high and a common cause of re-admission into hospital [7]. Secondary prophylaxis with a non-absorbable disaccharide (lactulose or lactitol) should be instituted [8,9]. If this is adequately titrated and the patient/caregivers instructed carefully, both constipation and diarrhoea/excessive flatulence and abdominal distension can be avoided. If overt HE becomes recurrent (i.e., more than one episode within six months [1]), rifaximin should be added to help maintain remission [1,10].

There are more uncertainties on the benefits of treatment of patients with mild forms of HE, especially as not all centres have the experience to diagnose them. Thus, treatment is not routinely recommended [1]. However, its initiation, especially if "ecological" (i.e., adding soluble fermentable fibre, probiotics such as yogurt, vegetables, cereal and milk-derived proteins to the habitual diet, plus getting used to in-between-meals snacks and a bedtime snack [11]), may both confirm the diagnosis and be beneficial. It is, therefore, reasonable, especially if the patients or their caregivers report symptoms compatible with mild HE, to institute it.

The management of patients with recurrent or persistent HE, which is more common in patients with large, spontaneous or surgical shunts [12] can be very difficult. Shunt closure/reduction can be considered in patients whose shunts are accessible. When related to TIPS, it can be treated and even prevented by reducing or occluding the stent [13–15]. Recurrent or persistent overt HE, and those forms of HE which are dominated by motor dysfunction (hepatic myelopathy) often require combination treatment, together with changes in the sources of dietary protein. Branched-chain amino acids (BCAAs), probiotics, L-ornithine L-aspartate (LOLA), non-ureic nitrogen scavengers and albumin have all been tested and can be used within this context [16]. Liver transplantation is the ultimate therapeutic option, and possibly the only real one for hepatic myelopathy [17]. It is crucial that all significant shunts are closed during transplantation, to avoid post-transplant Type B HE [1].

3. Therapies Other Than Non-Absorbable Disaccharides and Non-Absorbable Antibiotics

These are summarized in Table 1, at the end of this section.

3.1. Polyethylene Glycol (PEG)

The osmotic laxative PEG as a stand-alone [18] or in association with lactulose [19] has been associated with faster resolution of an episode of overt HE requiring hospitalization. Naso-gastric tubes have been used to administer PEG in patients with severe HE to avoid aspiration and guarantee adequate doses. Therefore, PEG applicability may be limited to patients in whom naso-gastric tube placement is safe and successful. A recent review and meta-analysis of four studies [20] showed that a single dose of PEG significantly improved clinical features of HE after 24 h and reduced the number of days for HE resolution compared to lactulose; however, no differences were observed in hospitalization length.

3.2. L-Ornithine L-Aspartate (LOLA)

LOLA is a substrate for the urea cycle and increases urea production in peri-portal hepatocytes. In addition, it activates glutamine synthetase in peri-venous hepatocytes and the skeletal muscle [21].

In a 2013 meta-analysis, LOLA was significantly more effective on HE than placebo/no-intervention [22]. Two comparative studies of LOLA and lactulose showed similar efficacy [23,24]. A double-blind randomised controlled trial (RCT) showed that LOLA was superior to placebo in the secondary prophylaxis of overt HE in 150 patients with cirrhosis [25]; improvement in psychometric test scores, critical flicker frequency and quality of life were documented, together with significant reductions in arterial ammonia levels. In one study, LOLA was shown to shorten a bout of overt HE requiring hospitalization when added to non-absorbable disaccharides and ceftriaxone [26]. The decrease in ammonia associated with LOLA seems to be temporary, and rebound hyperammonaemia has been observed on cessation [27]. Intravenous LOLA can be used to treat patients unresponsive to conventional therapy but further research is required in determining treatment dosage and duration. A Cochrane review [28] scored the available evidence in favour of LOLA as very low and qualified its benefits as uncertain, while a recent review and meta-analysis [29] suggests that LOLA is comparable to other ammonia-lowering agents in treating HE of varying severity.

3.3. Non Ureic Nitrogen Scavengers

Sodium benzoate provides an alternative pathway for nitrogen disposal and has been mostly used to treat patients with urea cycle defects. While the results of one, available RCT in patients with HE were encouraging [30], sodium benzoate has also been associated with increased ammonia levels in standard conditions and after a glutamine challenge [31]. A 2019 Cochrane systematic review did not find significant differences between sodium benzoate and non-absorbable disaccharides in terms of mortality, grade of HE or blood ammonia levels in patients with cirrhosis and an episode of overt HE [32]. Sodium benzoate may be particularly appropriate when HE and hyponatremia coexist [33].

Sodium phenylbutyrate may also reduce ammonia levels and improve neurological status/discharge survival in intensive care patients with overt HE [34]

Glycerol phenylbutyrate is mostly used in urea cycle disorders, as it favours nitrogen elimination by combining phenylacetic acid (a metabolite of phenylbutyric acid) with glutamine to form phenylacetyl-glutamine, which is then excreted in the urine. In a randomized, double-blind Phase IIb study of patients with cirrhosis who had had an episode of HE and were already on treatment with lactulose and rifaximin [35], glycerol phenylbutyrate significantly reduced ammonia levels and the likelihood of overt HE recurrence.

The rationale for treatment with **ornithine phenylacetate** relates to its capacity to stimulate glutamine synthetase in peripheral organs, by incorporating ammonia into the 'nontoxic' molecule phenylacetylglutamine, which is then excreted in the urine [36]. A randomized trial of 38 patients with cirrhosis enrolled within 24 h of an upper gastrointestinal bleed [37] showed that ornithine phenylacetate was well tolerated but did not significantly decrease ammonia. A subsequent RCT [38] of 231 patients did not document significant differences in time to clinical improvement compared to placebo.

3.4. Nutrition

Malnutrition, and sarcopenia in particular, are common in patients with cirrhosis and are associated with decreased survival [39]. Muscle loss impinges on nitrogen and ammonia metabolism and is associated with an increased risk of HE [40]. Thus, a low protein diet should be avoided in patients with HE [33,41,42], whose recommended daily energy and protein intake is not different from that of patients with cirrhosis and no HE (i.e., 35–40 kcal/kg ideal body weight and 1.2–1.5 g/kg ideal body weight, respectively). Nutritional therapy has been shown to improve psychometric performance and quality of life and to reduce the risk of overt HE compared with no intervention in patients with minimal HE in one RCT [43].

Small meals, evenly distributed throughout the day, and a late evening snack of complex carbohydrate [44] should be encouraged, as they decrease protein catabolism, and interrupt the long fast between dinner and breakfast. Personalized physical exercise should also be encouraged [45]. Despite solid rationale, there is limited evidence for the advantages of the replacing meat with vegetable/dairy protein. This is recommended only in the minority of patients who are truly intolerant of meat protein, and should be performed by experts and monitored closely to avoid reduction in caloric and protein intake [41].

A meta-analysis of four RCTs [46] showed that zinc supplementation improved some psychometric tests but did not reduce overt HE recurrence.

Diagnosed of suspected deficits in vitamins and micronutrients should be treated, as they may worsen mental function and confound HE diagnosis [33,41].

3.5. Albumin

Albumin may be effective in preventing overt HE in patients with decompensated cirrhosis, as demonstrated by a large retrospective study [47] and a recent meta-analysis [48]. In one RCT, high dose albumin was associated with decreased risk of high grade overt HE compared to standard of care in patients with cirrhosis and ascites [49].

3.6. Branched-Chain Amino Acids (BCAAs)

BCAAs availability is decreased in patients with cirrhosis, impinging on ammonia to glutamine conversion in the skeletal muscle. Thus, BCAA supplementation may enhance ammonia detoxification and reduce its concentrations. A Cochrane review [50] of 16 RCTs comparing BCAA (oral or intravenous) to placebo, no intervention, diet, neomycin or lactulose documented no beneficial effects of BCAAs on HE when trials including lactulose or neomycin were excluded, and no difference when BCAAs and lactulose or neomycin were compared. No effects on mortality, quality of life, or nutritional parameters was observed either. Recently, a multicenter prospective study evaluated long term oral BCAAs supplementation in decompensated cirrhosis [51]. In this study, MELD and Child-Pugh scores significantly improved in patients supplemented with BCAAs for more than six months; moreover, episodes of overt HE occurred less in the BCAA group compared to the control group. An increase in serum albumin in patients with a low albumin levels during BCAA supplementation was also observed. Furthermore, isoleucine long-term supplementation has been associated with increased brain perfusion and clinical improvement of overt HE compared to leucine [52]. BCAAs can be considered as a way to guarantee adequate protein intake in patients with recurrent/persistent HE on vegetable/diary diets [16]. However, palatability represents a significant issue [53].

3.7. Acetyl L-carnitine (ALC)

ALC contributes to blood and brain ammonia reduction and facilitates cellular energy production trough the uptake of acetyl-coenzyme A into the mitochondria, thereby preventing ammonia-induced neurotoxic damage in patients with HE [54].

A meta-analysis of seven RCTs (all single centre and of small to moderate size) [55] including 660 patients with varying degree of HE concluded that ALC reduced ammonia levels and improved one paper and pencil neuropsychological test. A 2019 Cochrane review of five single-centre small RCTs for a total of 398 patients [56] assessed the benefits/harms of ALC in patients with HE compared to intervention, placebo, or standard therapy. No summary information could be obtained on mortality, serious adverse events, or days of hospitalisation, nor were there any obvious differences in terms of fatigue, quality of life and minor adverse events. This may relate to limitations in the design and execution of the trials included. Blood ammonia lowering was documented in patients receiving acetyl-L-carnitine, although it was not associated with any obvious clinical benefit.

3.8. Probiotics

The rationale for the use of probiotics in treating HE relates to their capacity to modulate the gut microbiota composition and metabolic function, and to reduce inflammation. A recent review [57] compared the effects of probiotics or symbiotics (a combination of pre- and probiotics) with placebo/no intervention, or with any other treatment in patients with an episode or with persistent HE. A variety of probiotics and symbiotics were used and treatment duration ranged from three weeks to twelve months. Compared with placebo or no intervention, probiotics and symbiotics prevented overt HE recurrence [57]. However, this was not confirmed when probiotics were compared with lactulose, rifaximin or LOLA [57]. Based on a Cochrane review [58], the majority of trials were found to suffer from a high risk of both systematic and random error. A more recent meta-analysis [59] including 14 RCTs and 1132 patients found that probiotics decreased ammonia and endotoxin levels, improved minimal HE, and prevented overt HE. Of interest, the effects of fermentable fibre alone were comparable to those of a symbiotic on mental performance, ammonia levels and the gut flora in patients with minimal HE in one study [60].

3.9. Fecal Microbiota Transplantation (FMT)

The rationale for FMT for the treatment of HE is to modulate the composition and function of the gut microbiota. In one RCT, a small group of patients with recurrent HE where either treated with antibiotics and FMT or with standard of care: an improvement in short-term cognitive function and hospitalization was observed. Recently, this study was extended to assess the long-term impact of FMT on cognition, hospitalizations, and HE recurrence [61]: long-term safety and improvement in clinical and cognitive function parameters were confirmed in patients who received FMT with pre-treatment antibiotics compared with standard of care, especially regarding prevention of HE recurrence and hospitalizations. However, larger trials are needed. In addition, despite the promise of this initial experience, patients' and donors' selection, route and frequency of administration, follow-up and tolerability all need better definition.

3.10. Direct Vigilance Modulation

Finally, direct modulation of vigilance, possibly in combination with ammonia-lowering drugs, is worthy of study.

There is low quality evidence suggesting a short-term beneficial effect of **flumazenil** on HE in patients with cirrhosis, with no influence on all-cause mortality [62]. It is reasonable that this drug may produce a transient improvement in severe overt HE (allowing the administration of additional treatment by mouth) and also revert any known or unrecognized previous benzodiazepine intake.

Golexanolone is a novel GABA-A receptor-modulating steroid antagonist under development for the treatment of cognitive and vigilance disorders caused by allosteric over-activation of GABA-A receptors by neurosteroids. It has been shown to restore spatial learning and motor coordination in animal models of HE [63] and to mitigate the effects of intravenous allopregnanolone in healthy adults [64]. A multi-center pilot RCT assessed safety, pharmacokinetics and efficacy of golexanolone in a small group of patients with cirrhosis [65]. Treatment seemed to improve neuropsychiatric performance, as demonstrated by a significant decrease in slow electroencephalographic frequencies.

The effects of **caffeine** on induced hyperammonaemia (amino acid challenge) was investigated in a study involving both healthy volunteers and patients with cirrhosis [66]. In healthy volunteers, the increase in ammonia levels due to the amino acid challenge was contained by both the administration of LOLA and that of caffeine. The administration of caffeine also resulted in a reduction in subjective sleepiness and in the amplitude of the

EEG. Changes in ammonia levels, subjective sleepiness and the EEG were less obvious in patients. However, the timed administration of caffeine to top standard of care in patients with cirrhosis who also complain of sleepiness [67] may be both pleasant and useful.

3.11. Education

The provision of basic information on HE pathophysiology and simple hygienic and behavioural norms may have a significant impact on quality of life and HE recurrence in patients with cirrhosis. A 15 min educational session was administered to a small group of cirrhotic patients who had experienced at least one episode of overt HE [68]. This intervention was highly effective in increasing patients' understanding of treatment of the condition and, ultimately, reduced the risk of HE recurrence over a period of one year.

3.12. Miscellanea

Finally, minocycline [69], ibuprofen [70], indomethacin [71], phosphodiesterase-5 inhibitors (i.e., sildenafil) [72], benzodiazepine inverse agonists [73], AST-120 [74], a micro-spherical carbon with a selective adsorbent profile for small molecules such as ammonia, and liposome-supported peritoneal dialysis [75] are all being tested in animal models and/or early phase clinical studies. For some, anecdotal, direct clinical experience is also available, especially where the tested drug has alternative indications.

3.13. Local Experience

The authors of this review run a daily, dedicated HE clinic within a tertiary referral hepatology centre [76]. While they adhere, as they have in this manuscript, to published treatment guidelines, it is their impression that routine clinical HE reality is complex, and its management more varied and in many ways more interesting and more satisfactory than one would expect. We utilise treatment to facilitate differential diagnosis, as patients with cirrhosis have multiple and often coexisting risk factors for neuropsychiatric impairment [77]: if HE is treated adequately one can rule out alternative diagnoses and/or establish their relative contribution to overall neuropsychiatric status. We use dietary changes, under strict and frequent monitoring, for highly recurrent and persistent HE, sometimes very successfully. We often resolve iatrogenic HE by simply easing strict dietary prescriptions (sometimes self-imposed) that have resulted in malnutrition and sarcopenia. We do not miss an opportunity to test experimental HE treatment strategies if co-morbidities allow us to do so safely. For example, we all recall a patient with shunt-related, persistent HE whose neuropsychiatric status drastically improved when he was started on a brief course of a non-steroidal anti-inflammatory drug because of backache. We are fortunate enough to have the facilities [78] to test the effects of treatment over time in a comprehensive fashion, and to tailor treatment accordingly. We regret that this clinical experience, partly because of inherent difficulties in describing/summarising it and partly because of publication policies in relation to case reports/case series, remains largely unpublished and transferred to colleagues by traditional and somewhat haphazard teaching and collaboration strategies. Finally, we have sometimes been able to test treatment in controlled conditions, i.e., by inducing hyperammonaemia and then attempting to lower it in different ways [66]. We find this to be an under-utilised but potent tool to better understand the pathophysiology of HE [79], and thus, improve its management.

Table 1. Available treatments (other than general principles, non-absorbable disaccharides/antibiotics) with some commentary on the evidence for them and/or tips for use.

Treatment Category	Treatment	Evidence or Tips for Use
Laxative	Polyethylene glycol	In the acute setting, when administration is safe by mouth or by naso-gastric tube
	L-Ornithine L-Aspartate	
Non ureic nitrogen scavengers	Sodium benzoate	Particularly useful when hyponatremia is also present
Non ureic nitrogen scavengers	Sodium phenylbutyrate	
Non ureic nitrogen scavengers	Glycerol phenylbutyrate	
Non ureic nitrogen scavengers	Ornithine phenylacetate	
Nutritional measures	Vegetarian/dairy diets	In patients with highly recurrent/persistent HE or those who are truly intolerant to animal protein Under tight monitoring to avoid lowering overall calorie/protein intake
Nutritional measures	Food intake distribution over the 24 h	3 snacks to top up the 3 main meals can be suggested to malnourished/sarcopenic patients If not tolerated, please insist on the late-evening snack, which is the most important
Nutritional measures	Branched-chain amino acids	Useful also as a late-evening snack and in association with vegetarian/dairy diets, to ensure adequate protein intake
Nutritional measures	Prebiotics, probiotics and symbiotics	Ecological approaches, such as increased soluble fibre intake (albeit not necessarily easy to obtain) most likely useful and free of side effects
Albumin		In patients with ascites Possibly also acting as a nutritional measure
Acetyl L-carnitine		
Fecal Microbiota Transplantation		
Direct vigilance modulation	Golexanolone	
Direct vigilance modulation	Caffeine	With attention to timing (max effect for 60–90 min after intake)
Miscellanea	Minocycline, ibuprofen, indomethacin, phosphodiesterase-5 inhibitors, benzodiazepine inverse agonists, AST-120, liposome-supported peritoneal dialysis	Experimental
Education		Limited evidence but reasonable approach, especially if slim and structured, for both patients and caregivers
Tertiary referral centre experience		Needs to be better and more formally described, published where possible and disseminated in a structured fashion

Funding: S.M. is grateful to the University of Padova (Supporting TAlent in ReSearch @University of Padova 2019).

Conflicts of Interest: S.M.'s group has received research funding from AlfaSigma S.p.a., Norgine Ltd., Merz Pharmaceuticals GmbH, Umecrine Cognition AB and Versantis AG.

References

1. Vilstrup, H.; Amodio, P.; Bajaj, J.; Cordoba, J.; Ferenci, P.; Mullen, K.D.; Weissenborn, K.; Wong, P. Hepatic encephalopathy in chronic liver disease: 2014 Practice Guideline by the American Association for the Study of Liver Diseases and the European Association for the Study of the Liver. *Hepatology* **2014**, *60*, 715–735. [CrossRef] [PubMed]
2. Strauss, E.; Tramote, R.; Silva, E.P.; Caly, W.R.; Honain, N.Z.; Maffei, R.A. Doubleblind randomized clinical trial comparing neomycin and placebo in the treatment of exogenous hepatic encephalopathy. *Hepatogastroenterology* **1992**, *39*, 542–545.
3. Mullen, K.D.; Sanyal, A.J.; Bass, N.M.; Poordad, F.F.; Sheikh, M.Y.; Frederick, R.T.; Bortey, E.; Forbes, W.P. Rifaximin is safe and well tolerated for long-term maintenance of remission from overt hepatic encephalopathy. *Clin. Gastroenterol. Hepatol.* **2014**, *12*, 1390–1397.e2. [CrossRef]
4. Bajaj, J.S.; Barrett, A.C.; Bortey, E.; Paterson, C.; Forbes, W.P. Prolonged remission from hepatic encephalopathy with rifaximin: Results of a placebo crossover analysis. *Aliment. Pharmacol. Ther.* **2015**, *41*, 39–45. [CrossRef] [PubMed]
5. Sharma, P.; Agrawal, A.; Sharma, B.C.; Sarin, S.K. Prophylaxis of hepatic encephalopathy in acute variceal bleed: A randomized controlled trial of lactulose versus no lactulose. *J. Gastroenterol. Hepatol.* **2011**, *26*, 996–1003. [CrossRef] [PubMed]
6. Tromm, A.; Griga, T.; Greving, I.; Hilden, H.; Huppe, D.; Schwegler, U.; Micklefield, G.H.; May, B. Orthograde whole gut irrigation with mannite versus paromomycine + lactulose as prophylaxis of hepatic encephalopathy in patients with cirrhosis and upper gastrointestinal bleeding: Results of a controlled randomized trial. *Hepatogastroenterology* **2000**, *47*, 473–477.
7. Di Pascoli, M.; Ceranto, E.; De Nardi, P.; Donato, D.; Gatta, A.; Angeli, P. Hospitalizations due to cirrhosis: Clinical aspects in a large cohort of Italian patients and cost analysis report. *Dig. Dis.* **2017**, *35*, 433–438. [CrossRef]
8. Sharma, B.C.; Sharma, P.; Agrawal, A.; Sarin, S.K. Secondary prophylaxis of hepatic encephalopathy: An open-label randomized controlled trial of lactulose versus placebo. *Gastroenterology* **2009**, *137*, 885–891. [CrossRef]
9. Agrawal, A.; Sharma, B.C.; Sharma, P.; Sarin, S.K. Secondary prophylaxis of hepatic encephalopathy in cirrhosis: An open-label, randomized controlled trial of lactulose, probiotics, and no therapy. *Am. J. Gastroenterol.* **2012**, *107*, 1043–1050. [CrossRef]
10. Bass, N.M.; Mullen, K.D.; Sanyal, A.; Poordad, F.; Neff, G.; Leevy, C.B.; Sigal, S.; Sheikh, M.Y.; Beavers, K.; Frederick, T.; et al. Rifaximin treatment in hepatic encephalopathy. *N. Engl. J. Med.* **2010**, *362*, 1071–1081. [CrossRef]
11. Amodio, P. Hepatic encephalopathy: Diagnosis and management. *Liver Int.* **2018**, *38*, 966–975. [CrossRef] [PubMed]
12. Riggio, O.; Efrati, C.; Catalano, C.; Pediconi, F.; Mecarelli, O.; Accornero, N.; Nicolao, F.; Angeloni, S.; Masini, A.; Ridola, L.; et al. High prevalence of spontaneous portal-systemic shunts in persistent hepatic encephalopathy: A case-control study. *Hepatology* **2005**, *42*, 1158–1165. [CrossRef] [PubMed]
13. Kochar, N.; Tripathi, D.; Ireland, H.; Redhead, D.N.; Hayes, P.C. Transjugular intrahepatic portosystemic stent shunt (TIPSS) modification in the management of post-TIPSS refractory hepatic encephalopathy. *Gut* **2006**, *55*, 1617–1623. [CrossRef] [PubMed]
14. Riggio, O.; Angeloni, S.; Salvatori, F.M.; De Santis, A.; Cerini, F.; Farcomeni, A.; Attili, A.F.; Merli, M. Incidence, natural history, and risk factors of hepatic encephalopathy after transjugular intrahepatic portosystemic shunt with polytetrafluoroethylenecovered stent grafts. *Am. J. Gastroenterol.* **2008**, *3*, 2738–2746. [CrossRef] [PubMed]
15. Schepis, F.; Vizzutti, F.; Garcia-Tsao, G.; Marzocchi, G.; Rega, L.; De Maria, N.; Di Maira, T.; Gitto, S.; Caporali, C.; Colopi, S.; et al. Under-dilated TIPS Associate With Efficacy and Reduced Encephalopathy in a Prospective, Non-randomized Study of Patients With Cirrhosis. *Clin. Gastroenterol. Hepatol.* **2018**, *16*, 1153–1162.e7. [CrossRef]
16. Montagnese, S.; Russo, F.P.; Amodio, P.; Burra, P.; Gasbarrini, A.; Loguercio, C.; Marchesini, G.; Merli, M.; Ponziani, F.R.; Riggio, O.; et al. Hepatic encephalopathy 2018: A clinical practice guideline by the Italian Association for the Study of the Liver (AISF). *Dig. Liver Dis.* **2019**, *51*, 190–205. [CrossRef] [PubMed]
17. Weissenborn, K.; Tietge, U.J.; Bokemeyer, M.; Mohammadi, B.; Bode, U.; Manns, M.P.; Caselitz, M. Liver transplantation improves hepatic myelopathy: Evidence by three cases. *Gastroenterology* **2003**, *124*, 346–351. [CrossRef] [PubMed]
18. Rahimi, R.S.; Singal, A.G.; Cuthbert, J.A.; Rockey, D.C. Lactulose vs. polyethylene glycol 3350—Electrolyte solution for treatment of overt hepatic encephalopathy: The HELP randomized clinical trial. *JAMA Intern. Med.* **2014**, *174*, 1727–1733. [CrossRef]
19. Naderian, M.; Akbari, H.; Saeedi, M.; Sohrabpour, A.A. Polyethylene glycol and lactulose versus lactulose alone in the treatment of hepatic encephalopathy in patients with cirrhosis: A non-inferiority randomized controlled trial. *Middle East J. Dig. Dis.* **2017**, *9*, 12–29. [CrossRef]
20. Hoilat, G.J.; Ayas, M.F.; Hoilat, J.N.; Abu-Zaid, A.; Durer, C.; Durer, S.; Adhami, T.; John, S. Polyethylene glycol versus lactulose in the treatment of hepatic encephalopathy: A systematic review and meta-analysis. *BMJ Open Gastro.* **2021**, *8*, e000648. [CrossRef]
21. Rose, C.; Michalak, A.; Rao, K.V.; Quack, G.; Kircheis, G.; Butterworth, R.F. L-ornithine-L-aspartate lowers plasma and cerebrospinal fluid ammonia and prevents brain edema in rats with acute liver failure. *Hepatology* **1999**, *30*, 636–640. [CrossRef]
22. Bai, M.; Yang, Z.; Qi, X.; Fan, D.; Han, G. L-ornithine-L-aspartate for hepatic encephalopathy in patients with cirrhosis: A meta-analysis of randomized controlled trials. *J. Gastroenterol. Hepatol.* **2013**, *28*, 783–792. [CrossRef]
23. Poo, J.L.; Gongora, J.; Sanchez-Avila, F.; Aguilar-Castillo, S.; Garcia-Ramos, G.; Fernandez-Zertuche, M.; Rodríguez-Fragoso, L.; Uribe, M. Efficacy of oral L-ornithine-L-aspartate in cirrhotic patients with hyperammonemic hepatic encephalopathy. Results of a randomized, lactulose-controlled study. *Ann. Hepatol.* **2006**, *5*, 281–288. [CrossRef]
24. Mittal, V.V.; Sharma, B.C.; Sharma, P.; Sarin, S.K. A randomized controlled trial comparing lactulose, probiotics, and L-ornithine L-aspartate in treatment of minimal hepatic encephalopathy. *Eur. J. Gastroenterol. Hepatol.* **2011**, *23*, 725–732. [CrossRef] [PubMed]

25. Varakanahalli, S.; Sharma, B.C.; Srivastava, S.; Sachdeva, S.; Dahale, A.S. Secondary prophylaxis of hepatic encephalopathy in cirrhosis of liver: A double-blind randomized controlled trial of L-ornithine L-aspartate versus placebo. *Eur. J. Gastroenterol. Hepatol.* **2018**, *30*, 951–958. [CrossRef]

26. Sidhu, S.S.; Sharma, B.C.; Goyal, O.; Kishore, H.; Kaur, N. L-ornithine L-aspartate in bouts of overt hepatic encephalopathy. *Hepatology* **2018**, *67*, 700–710. [CrossRef]

27. Hadjihambi, A.; Arias, N.; Sheikh, M.; Jalan, R. Hepatic encephalopathy: A critical current review. *Hepatol. Int.* **2018**, *12* (Suppl. S1), 135–147. [CrossRef] [PubMed]

28. Goh, E.T.; Stokes, C.S.; Sidhu, S.S.; Vilstrup, H.; Gluud, L.L.; Morgan, M.Y. L-ornithine Laspartate for prevention and treatment of hepatic encephalopathy in people with cirrhosis. *Cochrane Database Syst. Rev.* **2018**, *5*, CD012410.

29. Butterworth, R.F.; McPhail, M.J.W. L-Ornithine L-Aspartate (LOLA) for Hepatic Encephalopathy in Cirrhosis: Results of Randomized Controlled Trials and Meta-Analyses. *Drugs* **2019**, *79*, S31–S37. [CrossRef]

30. Sushma, S.; Dasarathy, S.; Tandon, R.K.; Jain, S.; Gupta, S.; Bhist, M.S. Sodium benzoate inthe treatment of acute hepatic encephalopathy: A double-blind randomized trial. *Hepatology* **1992**, *16*, 138–144. [CrossRef]

31. Efrati, C.; Masini, A.; Merli, M.; Valeriano, V.; Riggio, O. Effect of sodium benzoate on blood ammonia response to oral glutamine challenge in cirrhotic patients: A note of caution. *Am. J. Gastroenterol.* **2000**, *95*, 3574–3578. [CrossRef] [PubMed]

32. Zacharias, H.D.; Zacharias, A.P.; Gluud, L.L.; Morgan, M.Y. Pharmacotherapies that specifically target ammonia for the prevention and treatment of hepatic encephalopathy in adults with cirrhosis. *Cochrane Database Syst. Rev.* **2019**, *6*, CD012334. [CrossRef]

33. Amodio, P.; Bemeur, C.; Butterworth, R.; Cordoba, J.; Kato, A.; Montagnese, S.; Uribe, M.; Vilstrup, H.; Morgan, M.Y. The nutritional management of hepatic encephalopathy in patients with cirrhosis: International Society for Hepatic Encephalopathy and Nitrogen Metabolism Consensus. *Hepatology* **2013**, *58*, 325–336. [CrossRef]

34. Weiss, N.; Tripon, S.; Lodey, M.; Guiller, E.; Junot, H.; Monneret, D.; Mayaux, J.; Brisson, H.; Mallet, M.; Rudler, M.; et al. Treating hepatic encephalopathy in cirrhotic patients admitted to ICU with sodium phenylbutyrate: A preliminary study. *Fundam. Clin. Pharmacol.* **2018**, *32*, 209–215. [CrossRef] [PubMed]

35. Rockey, D.C.; Vierling, J.M.; Mantry, P.; Ghabril, M.; Brown, R.S., Jr.; Alexeeva, O.; Zupanets, I.A.; Grinevich, V.; Baranovsky, A.; Dudar, L.; et al. Randomized, double-blind, controlled study of glycerol phenylbutyrate in hepatic encephalopathy. *Hepatology* **2014**, *59*, 1073–1083. [CrossRef]

36. Jover-Cobos, M.; Noiret, L.; Sharifi, Y.; Jalan, R. Ornithine phenylacetate revisited. *Metab. Brain Dis.* **2013**, *28*, 327–331. [CrossRef] [PubMed]

37. Ventura-Cots, M.; Concepcion, M.; Arranz, J.A.; Simon-Talero, M.; Torrens, M.; Blanco-Grau, A.; Fuentes, I.; Suñé, P.; Alvarado-Tapias, E.; Gely, C.; et al. Impact of ornithine phenylacetate (OCR-002) in lowering plasma ammonia after upper gastrointestinal bleeding in cirrhotic patients. *Therap. Adv. Gastroenterol.* **2016**, *9*, 823–835. [CrossRef] [PubMed]

38. Rahimi, R.S.; Safadi, R.; Thabut, D.; Bhamidimarri, K.R.; Pyrsopoulos, N.; Potthoff, A.; Bukofzer, S.; Bajaj, J.S. Efficacy and Safety of Ornithine Phenylacetate for Treating Overt Hepatic Encephalopathy in a Randomized Trial. *Clin. Gastroenterol. Hepatol.* **2020**, in press. [CrossRef] [PubMed]

39. Merli, M.; Riggio, O.; Dally, L. Does malnutrition affect survival in cirrhosis? PINC (Policentrica italiana nutrizione cirrosi). *Hepatology* **1996**, *23*, 1041–1046. [CrossRef]

40. Merli, M.; Giusto, M.; Lucidi, C.; Giannelli, V.; Pentassuglio, I.; Di Gregorio, V.; Lattanzi, B.; Riggio, O. Muscle depletion increases the risk of overt and minimal hepatic encephalopathy: Results of a prospective study. *Metab. Brain Dis.* **2013**, *28*, 281–284. [CrossRef]

41. European Association for the Study of the Liver. EASL Clinical Practice Guidelines on nutrition in chronic liver disease. *J. Hepatol.* **2019**, *70*, 172–193. [CrossRef]

42. Cordoba, J.; Lopez-Hellin, J.; Planas, M.; Sabin, P.; Sanpedro, F.; Castro, F.; Esteban, R.; Guardia, J. Normal protein diet for episodic hepatic encephalopathy: Results of a randomized study. *J. Hepatol.* **2004**, *41*, 38–43. [CrossRef] [PubMed]

43. Maharshi, S.; Sharma, B.C.; Sachdeva, S.; Srivastava, S.; Sharma, P. Efficacy of Nutritional Therapy for Patients With Cirrhosis and Minimal Hepatic Encephalopathy in a Randomized Trial. *Clin. Gastroenterol. Hepatol.* **2016**, *14*, 454–460. [CrossRef] [PubMed]

44. Tsien, C.D.; McCullough, A.J.; Dasarathy, S. Late evening snack: Exploiting a period of anabolic opportunity in cirrhosis. *J. Gastroenterol. Hepatol.* **2012**, *27*, 430–441. [CrossRef]

45. Tandon, P.; Ismond, K.P.; Riess, K.; Duarte-Rojo, A.; Al-Judaibi, B.; Dunn, M.A.; Holman, J.; Howes, N.; Haykowsky, M.J.F.; Josbeno, D.A.; et al. Exercise in cirrhosis: Translating evidence and experience to practice. *J. Hepatol.* **2018**, *69*, 1164–1177. [CrossRef]

46. Chavez-Tapia, N.C.; Cesar-Arce, A.; Barrientos-Gutierrez, T.; Villegas-Lopez, F.A.; Mendez-Sanchez, N.; Uribe, M. A systematic review and meta-analysis of the use of oral zinc in the treatment of hepatic encephalopathy. *Nutr. J.* **2013**, *12*, 74. [CrossRef]

47. Bai, Z.; Bernardi, M.; Yoshida, E.M.; Li, H.; Guo, X.; Méndez-Sánchez, N.; Li, Y.; Wang, R.; Deng, J.; Qi, X. Albumin infusion may decrease the incidence and severity of overt hepatic encephalopathy in liver cirrhosis. *Aging* **2019**, *8*, 8502–8525. [CrossRef] [PubMed]

48. Teh, K.B.; Loo, J.H.; Tam, Y.C.; Wong, Y.J. Efficacy and safety of albumin infusion for overt hepatic encephalopathy: A systematic review and meta-analysis. *Dig. Liver Dis.* **2021**, *53*, 817–823. [CrossRef]

49. Caraceni, P.; Pavesi, M.; Baldassarre, M.; Bernardi, M.; Arroyo, V. The use of human albumin in patients with cirrhosis: A European survey. *Expert Rev. Gastroenterol. Hepatol.* **2018**, *12*, 625–632. [CrossRef]

50. Gluud, L.L.; Dam, G.; Les, I.; Marchesini, G.; Borre, M.; Aagaard, N.K.; Vilstrup, H. Branched-chain amino acids for people with hepatic encephalopathy. *Cochrane Database Syst. Rev.* **2017**, *5*, CD001939. [CrossRef]
51. Park, J.G.; Tak, W.Y.; Park, S.Y.; Kweon, Y.O.; Chung, W.J.; Jang, B.K.; Bae, S.H.; Lee, H.J.; Jang, J.Y.; Suk, K.T.; et al. Effects of Branched-Chain Amino Acid (BCAA) Supplementation on the Progression of Advanced Liver Disease: A Korean Nationwide, Multicenter, Prospective, Observational, Cohort Study. *Nutrients* **2020**, *12*, 1429. [CrossRef] [PubMed]
52. Gomes Romeiro, F.; do Val Ietsugu, M.; de Campos Franzoni, L.; Augusti, L.; Alvarez, M.; Alves Amaral Santos, L.; Bazeia Lima, T.; Hiromoto Koga, K.; Marta Moriguchi, S.; Antonio Caramori, C.; et al. Which of the branched-chain amino acids increases cerebral blood flow in hepatic ncephalopathy? A double-blind randomized trial. *NeuroImage* **2018**, *19*, 302–310. [CrossRef]
53. Marchesini, G.; Bianchi, G.; Merli, M.; Amodio, P.; Panella, C.; Loguercio, C.; Rossi Fanelli, F.; Abbiati, R. Italian BCAA Study Group. Nutritional supplementation with branched-chain amino acids in advanced cirrhosis: A double-blind, randomized trial. *Gastroenterology* **2003**, *124*, 1792–1801. [CrossRef]
54. Malaguarnera, M. Acetyl-L-carnitine in hepatic encephalopathy. *Metab. Brain Dis.* **2013**, *28*, 193–199. [CrossRef] [PubMed]
55. Jiang, Q.; Jiang, G.; Shi, K.Q.; Cai, H.; Wang, Y.X.; Zheng, M.H. Oral acetyl-L-carnitine treatment in hepatic encephalopathy: View of evidence-based medicine. *Ann. Hepatol.* **2013**, *12*, 803–809. [CrossRef]
56. Martí-Carvajal, A.J.; Gluud, C.; Arevalo-Rodriguez, I.; Martí-Amarista, C.E. Acetyl-L-carnitine for patients with hepatic encephalopathy. *Cochrane Database Syst. Rev.* **2019**, *1*, CD011451. [CrossRef]
57. Viramontes Horner, D.; Avery, A.; Stow, R. The effects of probiotics and symbiotics on risk factors for hepatic encephalopathy: A systematic review. *J. Clin. Gastroenterol.* **2017**, *51*, 312–323. [CrossRef]
58. Dalal, R.; McGee, R.G.; Riordan, S.M.; Webster, A.C. Probiotics for people with hepatic encephalopathy. *Cochrane Database Syst. Rev.* **2017**, *2*, CD008716. [CrossRef]
59. Cao, Q.; Yu, C.B.; Yang, S.G.; Cao, H.C.; Chen, P.; Deng, M.; Li, L.J. Effect of probiotic treatment on cirrhotic patients with minimal hepatic encephalopathy: A meta-analysis. *Hepatob. Pancreat. Dis. Int.* **2018**, *17*, 9–16. [CrossRef]
60. Liu, Q.; Duan, Z.P.; Ha, D.K.; Bengmark, S.; Kurtovic, J.; Riordan, S.M. Synbiotic modulation of gut flora: Effect on minimal hepatic encephalopathy in patients with cirrhosis. *Hepatology* **2004**, *39*, 1441–1449. [CrossRef]
61. Bajaj, J.S.; Fagan, A.; Gavis, E.A.; Kassam, Z.; Sikaroodi, M.; Gillevet, P.M. Long-term Outcomes of Fecal Microbiota Transplantation in Patients With Cirrhosis. *Gastroenterology* **2019**, *156*, 1921–1923. [CrossRef] [PubMed]
62. Goh, E.T.; Andersen, M.L.; Morgan, M.Y.; Gluud, L.L. Flumazenil versus placebo or no intervention for people with cirrhosis and hepatic encephalopathy. *Cochrane Database Syst. Rev.* **2017**, *8*, CD002798. [PubMed]
63. Johansson, M.; Agusti, A.; Llansola, M.; Montoliu, C.; Strömberg, J.; Malinina, E.; Ragagnin, G.; Doverskog, M.; Bäckström, T.; Felipo, V. GR3027 antagonizes GABAA receptor-potentiating neurosteroids and restores spatial learning and motor coordination in rats with chronic hyperammonemia and hepatic encephalopathy. *Am. J. Physiol. Gastrointest. Liver Physiol.* **2015**, *309*, G400–G409. [CrossRef] [PubMed]
64. Johansson, M.; Strömberg, J.; Ragagnin, G.; Doverskog, M.; Bäckström, T. GABAA receptor modulating steroid antagonists (GAMSA) are functional in vivo. *J. Steroid Biochem. Mol. Biol.* **2016**, *160*, 98–105. [CrossRef]
65. Montagnese, S.; Lauridsen, M.; Vilstrup, H.; Zarantonello, L.; Lakner, G.; Fitilev, S.; Zupanets, I.; Kozlova, I.; Bunkova, E.; Tomasiewicz, K.; et al. A pilot study of golexanolone, a new GABA-A receptor-modulating steroid antagonist, in patients with covert hepatic encephalopathy. *J. Hepatol.* **2021**, *75*, 98–107. [CrossRef]
66. Garrido, M.; Skorucak, J.; Raduazzo, D.; Turco, M.; Spinelli, G.; Angeli, P.; Amodio, P.; Achermann, P.; Montagnese, S. Vigilance and wake EEG architecture in simulated hyperammonaemia: A pilot study on the effects of L-Ornithine-L-Aspartate (LOLA) and caffeine. *Metab. Brain Dis.* **2016**, *31*, 965–974. [CrossRef] [PubMed]
67. De Rui, M.; Schiff, S.; Aprile, D.; Angeli, P.; Bombonato, G.; Bolognesi, M.; Sacerdoti, D.; Gatta, A.; Merkel, C.; Amodio, P.; et al. Excessive daytime sleepiness and hepatic encephalopathy: It is worth asking. *Metab Brain. Dis.* **2013**, *28*, 245–248. [CrossRef]
68. Garrido, M.; Turco, M.; Formentin, C.; Corrias, M.; De Rui, M.; Montagnese, S.; Amodio, P. An educational tool for the prophylaxis of hepatic encephalopathy. *BMJ Open Gastro.* **2017**, *4*, e000161. [CrossRef]
69. Gamal, M.; Abdel Wahab, Z.; Eshra, M.; Rashed, L.; Sharawy, N. Comparative Neuroprotective effects of dexamethasone and minocycline during hepatic encephalopathy. *Neurol. Res. Int.* **2014**, *2014*, 254683. [CrossRef]
70. Cauli, O.; Rodrigo, R.; Piedrafita, B.; Boix, J.; Felipo, V. Inflammation and hepatic encephalopathy: Ibuprofen restores learning ability in rats with portacaval shunts. *Hepatology* **2007**, *46*, 514–519. [CrossRef]
71. Ahboucha, S.; Jiang, W.; Chatauret, N.; Mamer, O.; Baker, G.B.; Butterworth, R.F. Indomethacin improves locomotor deficit and reduces brain concentrations of neuroinhibitory steroids in rats following portacaval anastomosis. *Neurogastroenterol. Motil.* **2008**, *20*, 949–957. [CrossRef] [PubMed]
72. Agusti, A.; Hernandez-Rabaza, V.; Balzano, T.; Taoro-Gonzalez, L.; Ibanez-Grau, A.; Cabrera-Pastor, A.; Fustero, S.; Llansola, M.; Montoliu, C.; Felipo, V. Sildenafil reduces neuroinflammation in cerebellum, restores GABAergic tone, and improves motor in-coordination in rats with hepatic encephalopathy. *CNS Neurosci. Ther.* **2017**, *23*, 386–394. [CrossRef]
73. Steindl, P.; Puspok, A.; Druml, W.; Ferenci, P. Beneficial effect of pharmacological modulation of the GABAA-benzodiazepine receptor on hepatic encephalopathy in the rat: Comparison with uremic encephalopathy. *Hepatology* **1991**, *14*, 963–968. [CrossRef] [PubMed]
74. Bosoi, C.R.; Parent-Robitaille, C.; Anderson, K.; Tremblay, M.; Rose, C.F. AST-120 (spherical carbon adsorbent) lowers ammonia levels and attenuates brain edema in bile duct-ligated rats. *Hepatology* **2011**, *53*, 1995–2002. [CrossRef]

75. Matoori, S.; Forster, V.; Agostoni, V.; Bettschart-Wolfensberger, R.; Bektas, R.N.; Thöny, B.; Häberle, J.; Leroux, J.C.; Kabbaj, M. Preclinical evaluation of liposome-supported peritoneal dialysis for the treatment of hyperammonemic crises. *J. Control. Release* **2020**, *328*, 503–513. [CrossRef] [PubMed]

76. Formentin, C.; Zarantonello, L.; Mangini, C.; Frigo, A.C.; Montagnese, S.; Merkel, C. Clinical, neuropsychological and neurophysiological indices and predictors of hepatic encephalopathy (HE). *Liver Int.* **2021**, *41*, 1070–1082. [CrossRef] [PubMed]

77. Montagnese, S.; Schiff, S.; Amodio, P. Quick diagnosis of hepatic encephalopathy: Fact or fiction? *Hepatology* **2015**, *61*, 405–406. [CrossRef]

78. Montagnese, S.; De Rui, M.; Angeli, P.; Amodio, P. Neuropsychiatric performance in patients with cirrhosis: Who is "normal"? *J. Hepatol.* **2017**, *66*, 825–835. [CrossRef]

79. Bersagliere, A.; Raduazzo, I.D.; Nardi, M.; Schiff, S.; Gatta, A.; Amodio, P.; Achermann, P.; Montagnese, S. Induced hyperammonemia may compromise the ability to generate restful sleep in patients with cirrhosis. *Hepatology* **2012**, *55*, 869–878. [CrossRef]

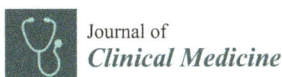

Journal of
Clinical Medicine

Review

Acute-on-Chronic Liver Failure in Cirrhosis

Carmine Gambino, Salvatore Piano * and Paolo Angeli

Unit of Internal Medicine and Hepatology (UIMH), Department of Medicine (DIMED), University of Padova, 35128 Padova, Italy; carmine.gabriele.gambino@gmail.com (C.G.); pangeli@unipd.it (P.A.)
* Correspondence: salvatorepiano@gmail.com

Abstract: Acute-on-chronic liver failure (ACLF) is a syndrome that develops in patients with acutely decompensated chronic liver disease. It is characterised by high 28-day mortality, the presence of one or more organ failures (OFs) and a variable but severe grade of systemic inflammation. Despite the peculiarity of each one, every definition proposed for ACLF recognizes it as a proper clinical entity. In this paper, we provide an overview of the diagnostic criteria proposed by the different scientific societies and the clinical characteristics of the syndrome. Established and experimental treatments are also described. Among the former, the most relevant are directed to support organ failures, treat precipitating factors and carry out early assessment for liver transplantation (LT). Further studies are needed to better clarify pathophysiology of the syndrome and discover new therapies.

Keywords: acute-on-chronic liver failure (ACLF); cirrhosis; liver transplantation (LT)

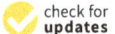
Citation: Gambino, C.; Piano, S.; Angeli, P. Acute-on-Chronic Liver Failure in Cirrhosis. *J. Clin. Med.* **2021**, *10*, 4406. https://doi.org/10.3390/jcm10194406

Academic Editors: Pierluigi Toniutto and Hiroki Nishikawa

Received: 31 August 2021
Accepted: 22 September 2021
Published: 26 September 2021

Publisher's Note: MDPI stays neutral with regard to jurisdictional claims in published maps and institutional affiliations.

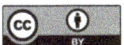
1. Definition of Acute-on-Chronic Liver Failure

Acute decompensation (AD) of cirrhosis refers to the development of ascites, gastrointestinal haemorrhage, hepatic encephalopathy or any combination of these, which leads to hospital admission [1]. Acute-on-chronic liver failure (ACLF) is a distinct syndrome that develops in patients with acutely decompensated chronic liver disease and is characterised by high 28-day mortality. Other major features of ACLF are the strong association with one or more precipitating factor(s), the development of single- or multiple organ failures (OFs) and a severe degree of systemic inflammation [2–4]. International scientific societies have proposed different definitions of ACLF in recent years; they differ from each other mainly in the type of precipitant (hepatic or extrahepatic), the stage of underlying liver disease (chronic hepatitis or cirrhosis) and the inclusion or not of extra-hepatic OFs. In spite of these differences, each of them recognizes ACLF as a definite clinical entity. Table 1 summarizes definitions, diagnostic criteria and stratification of ACLF used by the four major international consortia [2,5–9].

The definition proposed by the European Association for the Study of the Liver—Chronic Liver Failure (EASL-CLIF) Consortium is based on the results of the CANONIC study, a multi-center prospective investigation in which 1343 patients non-electively hospitalized for AD of cirrhosis were enrolled, irrespective of prior episode(s) of AD [2]. This definition considers both hepatic and extra-hepatic precipitants and both liver and extra-hepatic OFs. The diagnosis of OFs is based on a modified Sequential Organ Failure Assessment (SOFA) score, called CLIF-C organ failure (CLIF-C OF), which considers the function of six organ systems (liver, kidney, brain, coagulation, circulation and respiration) [2]. According to the number of OFs, patients with ACLF were stratified into three groups: (I) patients with a single kidney failure or another single OF if associated with brain or kidney disfunction (ACLF grade 1); (II) patients with two OFs (ACLF grade 2); (III) patients with three or more OFs (ACLF grade 3) [2]. We contributed to the development of this definition, which nowadays is the most studied. Thus, we currently use it in our center.

111

Table 1. Definitions, diagnostic criteria, and stratification of ACLF used by the four major international consortia *.

Characteristics	EASL-CLIF Consortium	NACSELD	COSSH	AARC
Population	Patients with AD of cirrhosis, independently from the absence/presence of previous AD	Patients with AD of cirrhosis, independently from the absence/presence of previous AD	Patients with AD of HBV-related chronic liver disease, with or without cirrhosis	Patients with CLD or compensated cirrhosis and acute liver insult that causes acute liver deterioration
Precipitating events	Intrahepatic (alcoholic hepatitis), extrahepatic (infection, gastrointestinal bleeding), or both	Intrahepatic, extrahepatic, or both	Intrahepatic (HBV flare), extrahepatic (bacterial infection) or both	Intrahepatic
Criteria of organ system failures used to define ACLF	Liver: Total bilirubin ≥ 12 mg/dL; Kidney: Creatinine ≥ 2 mg/dL or use of RRT; Coagulation: INR ≥ 2.5; Brain: HE Grade 3–4 in West Haven classification or use of mechanical ventilation because of HE; Circulation: Use of vasopressors including terlipressin; Lung: PaO$_2$/FiO$_2$ ≤ 200 or SpO$_2$/FiO$_2$ ≤ 214, or use of mechanical ventilation for reason other than HE	Kidney: Use of dialysis or other form of RRT; Brain: HE Grade 3–4 in West Haven classification; Circulation: MAP <60 mmHg or reduction of 40 mmHg in SBP from baseline, in spite of fluid resuscitation and adequate cardiac output; Lung: Use of mechanical ventilation	Same criteria as those used by the EASL-CLIF Consortium	Liver: Total bilirubin levels ≥ 5 mg/dL; Brain: clinical HE
Criteria for the presence of ACLF and ACLF stratification	ACLF is stratified into 3 grades of increasing severity: - ACLF grade 1 contains 3 subgroups of patients with: (1) single kidney failure (2) single liver, coagulation, circulatory or lung failure that is associated with either kidney dysfunction, brain dysfunction, [a] or both; (3) single brain failure and kidney dysfunction [a]; - ACLF grade 2: two OFs; - ACLF grade 3: three or more OFs.	Patients are stratified according to the number of organ failures (2, 3, or 4 organ failures)	ACLF is stratified into 3 grades of increasing severity. - ACLF grade 1 contains 4 subgroups of patients with: (1) single kidney failure; (2) single liver failure and either INR ≥ 1.5, kidney dysfunction, brain dysfunction, [a] or any combination of these; (3) single coagulation, circulatory or respiratory failure and either kidney dysfunction, brain dysfunction, [a] or both; (4) cerebral failure alone and kidney dysfunction; - ACLF grade 2: two OFs - ACLF grade 3: three or more OFs	Total bilirubin levels of 5 mg/dL or more and INR ≥ 1.5 or prothrombin activity <40% complicated within 4 weeks by clinical ascites, HE, or both. The severity of ACLF is assessed using the AARC score [#]: Grade 1 by scores 5–7, Grade 2 by scores 8–10 and Grade 3 for 11–15.
Short-term mortality rate of ACLF	By 28 days: Grade 1: 22% Grade 2: 32% Grade 3: 77%	By 30 days: 2 organ failures: 49% 3 organ failures: 64% 4 organ failures: 77%	By 28 days: Grade 1: 23% Grade 2: 61% Grade 3: 93%	By 30 days: Grade 1: 13% Grade 2: 45% Grade 3: 86%

EASL-CLIF, European Association for the Study of the Liver—Chronic Liver Failure; NACSELD, North American Consortium for the Study of End-stage Liver Disease; COSSH, Chinese Group on the Study of Severe Hepatitis B; AARC, APASL ACLF Research Consortium; APASL, Asian Pacific Association for the Study of the Liver; AD, acute decompensation; CLD, chronic liver disease ACLF, acute-on-chronic liver failure; RRT, renal replacement therapy; HE, hepatic encephalopathy; OFs, organ failures; INR, international normalised ratio; MAP, mean arterial pressure; SBP, systolic blood pressure. * Adapted from ref. [10]; [#] See ref. [9]. [a] Kidney dysfunction: serum creatinine from 1.5 mg/dL to 1.9 mg/dL. Brain dysfunction: grade 1 or grade 2 HE.

The definition proposed by the North American Consortium for the Study of End-stage Liver Disease (NACSELD) is based on an investigation involving 507 patients with AD of cirrhosis non electively hospitalised for infection [5]. Like the European one, the North American definition considers extra-hepatic OFs as part of the syndrome but does not include liver and coagulation. It defines ACLF by the presence of two or more OFs among kidney, brain, circulation and respiration and stratifies patients according to the number of organ failures [5]. The Chinese Group on the Study of Severe Hepatitis B (COSSH) developed a definition for hepatitis B virus (HBV)-related ACLF by using data from a large cohort of 1202 patients with HBV-related AD, with or without cirrhosis. The CLIF-C OF scoring system was used to define OFs; so, this definition and the consequent stratification of patients are quite similar to the European ones. The only difference is that, in the Chinese classification, a patient with single liver failure with INR ≥ 1.5 is considered as having ACLF grade 1 [6]. The Asian Pacific Association for the Study of the Liver (APASL) proposed a definition of ACLF in 2009 which was based on an expert opinion. This definition was updated by the APASL ACLF Research Consortium (AARC) in 2014 and then in 2019, using the results of the AARC database (5228 patients collected at that time) [7–9]. Unlike the above definitions, AARC investigators consider extra-hepatic OFs as manifestations but not as components of the syndrome, and extra-hepatic insults (for example, bacterial infections) as complications, but not triggers, of ACLF. So, ACLF is considered as an acute hepatic insult (for example, HBV reactivation or acute alcoholic hepatitis), manifested as jaundice (total bilirubin levels ≥ 5 mg/dL) and coagulation failure (INR ≥ 1.5 or prothrombin activity $< 40\%$) and complicated by clinical ascites, encephalopathy or both within 4 weeks in patients with chronic liver disease or compensated cirrhosis without prior decompensation and with no AD [9]. Thus, AARC investigators consider ACLF to be totally distinct from acutely decompensated cirrhosis. The severity of ACLF is assessed using a grading system based on the AARC score [9].

2. Clinical Features

ACLF has typical clinical features based on the definition used, on which its prevalence also depends. In the European cohort, the prevalence of the syndrome was 23% among patients with AD of cirrhosis at admission and 8.3% of patients developed it during hospitalization within a period of days (maximum of two weeks). In outpatients with cirrhosis, the incidence of the syndrome is about 40% at 10 years [11]. As confirmed by the PREDICT (PREDICTing Acute-on-Chronic Liver Failure) study, another large-scale European prospective investigation designed to identify predictors of this syndrome, patients with ACLF were younger, showed higher levels of white blood cells and C-reactive protein (CRP) and had a greater prevalence of bacterial infections, severe alcoholic hepatitis, variceal bleeding, drug-induced encephalopathy as precipitants, with respect to patients without ACLF [2,12,13]. Moreover, the PREDICT study demonstrated that the clinical course of AD that leads to ACLF is distinct from the other forms of AD of cirrhosis [12]. The 28-day mortality significantly rises with the increase in the number of OFs, ranging from 4.7% for patients without ACLF to 22%, 32% and 77% for patients with ACLF grade 1, 2 and 3, respectively [2].

In a validation study of NACSELD definition of ACLF, in which 2675 patients with AD of cirrhosis related or not to infection were included, the prevalence of ACLF was 10% and 30-day mortality rate was significantly different between patients with or without the syndrome (41% vs. 7%, respectively) [14]. In a recent study, the NACSELD criteria were demonstrated to be less sensitive compared to EASL-CLIF criteria in diagnosing ACLF [15].

When using NACSELD criteria, only about 40% of patients with a diagnosis of ACLF based on EASL-CLIF criteria were classified as affected by the syndrome, probably because the NACSELD definition considers only more severe patients and because it could be influenced by the medical strategies available in the different centers (renal replacement therapy (RRT), mechanical ventilation, use of vasopressors) [10,16].

In a cohort of patients with HBV-related AD of cirrhosis, the prevalence of ACLF was 30.2% according to the COSSH ACLF definition. As in the European cohort, patients with ACLF were younger, had a more severe grade of systemic inflammation (as demonstrated by higher levels of white blood cells and CRP) and more frequently had a bacterial infection (associated or not with HBV reactivation) as precipitant compared to those without ACLF, with a significantly higher short-term mortality (52.1% vs. 4.3%) [6]. Although EASL-CLIF and COSSH definitions of ACLF are very similar, clinical characteristics of patients are quite different, because of the higher prevalence of intra-hepatic precipitants in the Chinese cohort (most often HBV reactivation) with respect to the European cohort [16], with liver and coagulation failure being more frequent in the former and kidney and brain failure more frequent in the latter [4]. As expected, a flare of HBV infection was the most frequent trigger of ACLF in studies using AARC criteria [9,17]. In a study using AARC ACLF criteria which enrolled patients with HBV-related ACLF, about 32% had a bacterial or fungal infection as a complication. The 28-day mortality rate was 27.8% [18].

3. Pathophysiology

The pathophysiology of ACLF is yet to be fully understood. To date, ACLF is considered the extreme expression of systemic inflammation that drives AD of cirrhosis [19]. Systemic inflammation is characterised by activation of the immune system that leads to increased circulating levels of inflammatory mediators and, if severe, proliferation of neutrophils, monocytes and dendritic cells [20]. The mechanism of systemic inflammation depends on the precipitant of ACLF [3]. The recognition of pathogen-associated molecular patterns (PAMPs) activates the innate immune system by pattern-recognition receptors (PRR) in case of bacterial infection or translocation of viable bacteria and bacterial products through the intestinal wall [19,21]. Exceeding inflammation can cause direct tissue damage and necrotic cell death, resulting in the release of damage-associated molecular patterns (DAMPs) that perpetuate inflammation acting on PRR [21]. DAMPs are also released when an injury acts directly on the liver, as in case of alcoholic hepatitis or ischemia due to variceal haemorrhage [22,23]. This overactivation of the immune cells requires a large amount of energy sustained by reallocation of nutrients. This causes a reduced availability of substrates for other organ systems that leads to OFs by severe mitochondrial dysfunction and impaired energy production [19]. Moreover, recent findings suggest that systemic inflammation can explain and act with the traditionally accepted organ-specific mechanisms of AD (portal hypertension, hyperammonaemia, endogenous vasoconstrictors system and arterial blood volume) in determining OFs [19]. Blood metabolomics offers a new insight into the pathophysiology of systemic inflammation in patients with ACLF and could be an intriguing starting point to uncover new potential therapeutic targets [24]. Figure 1 summarizes the pathophysiology of ACLF.

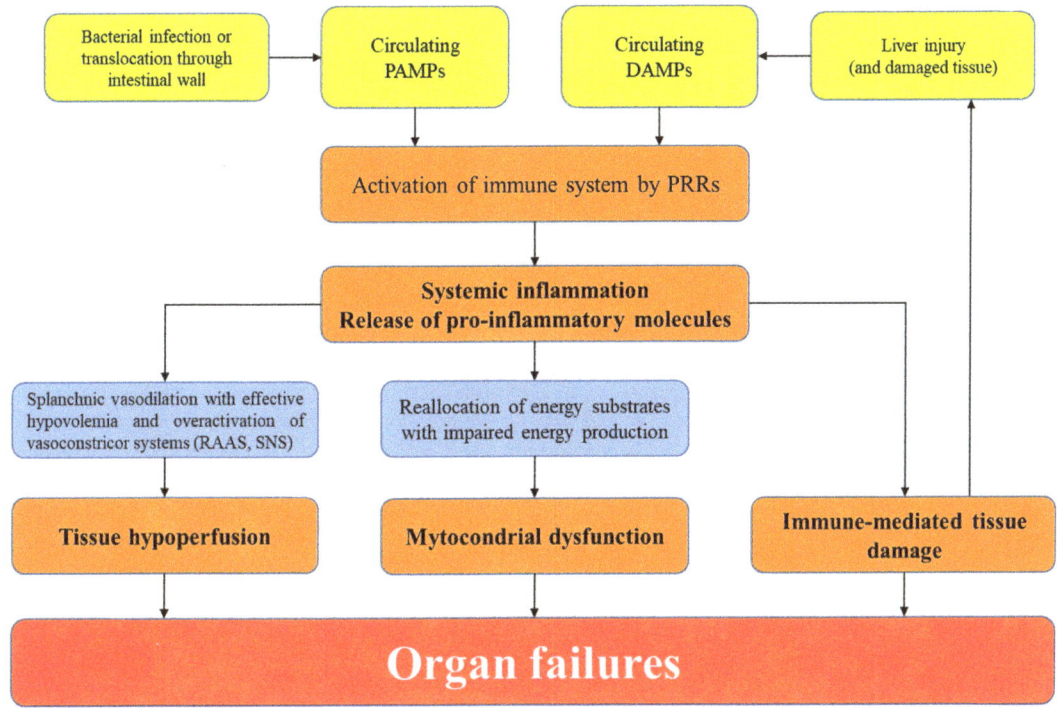

Figure 1. Pathophysiology of ACLF. PAMPs, pathogen-associated molecular patterns; DAMPs, damage-associated molecular patterns; PRR, pattern-recognition receptors; RAAS, renin-angiotensin-aldosterone system; SNS, sympathetic nervous system.

4. Prognostic Stratification

ACLF is a dynamic syndrome that can resolve, improve or worsen in a few days [25]. Outcomes for ACLF patients are strictly related both to severity of liver disease and to severity and number of OFs. Because ACLF patients may be considered for urgent Intensive Care Unit (ICU) referral and/or liver transplantation (LT), different consortia developed prognostic scores [16]. EASL-CLIF proposed the CLIF-C ACLF score, which demonstrated more accuracy in predicting death than MELD (Model for end-stage Liver Disease), MELD-Na (Model for end-stage Liver Disease-Sodium), Child-Pugh and CLIF-C OF scores [17]. CLIF-C ACLF score captures both intra- and extra-hepatic OFs but has a subjective element in the scoring of hepatic encephalopathy and a "ceiling effect" with INR, serum creatinine and bilirubin (for example, a patient with serum bilirubin 25 mg/dL has the same prognosis of a patient with serum bilirubin 12 mg/dL) [16]. The NACSELD organ failure score is simple to use but considers only the sickest patients. The AARC-ACLF score was found to be superior to MELD and CLIF-SOFA in predicting short-term mortality [26] but, as with CLIF-C ACLF score, has subjective elements and suffers from a "ceiling effect" for the considered laboratory values [16]. The COSSH-ACLF score showed higher predictive value for short-term mortality than other scores (MELD, MELD-Na, Child-Pugh, CLIF-C OF and CLIF-C ACLF) in patients with HBV-ACLF [6]. Recently, a simplified version of this score (COSSH-ACLF II) demonstrably improved prognostic accuracy and sensitivity for patients with HBV-ACLF. The COSSH-ACLF II score also allows easy division of patients into three different strata with significantly different 28-day mortality rates [27]. The COSSH-ACLF scores also include a subjective element in hepatic encephalopathy evaluation.

Prognosis is more accurately estimated when the scores are applied at 3 to 7 days than at time of diagnosis [25,28]. These findings are in keeping with the dynamic nature of

ACLF. Prognostic scores have also been applied to determine futility of treatments in ACLF patients [28,29]. Thus, it is necessary to overcome the above-mentioned limitations by creating models based only on objective, verifiable and continuous variables [16]. Finally, among OFs not actually included in the prognostic scores, relative adrenal insufficiency (RAI) has been shown to have a similar prognostic value for non-kidney OFs. RAI could be considered to better stratify patients with ACLF in clinical practice [30].

5. Management of ACLF

Principles of treatment of ACLF are summarized in Table 2.

5.1. Admission to Intensive Care Unit

The referral of patients with ACLF to ICU should be neither delayed nor denied only because of the underlying chronic liver disease or the possibility of poor prognosis in patients with OF(s) [31,32]. In fact, several findings suggest that acceptable survival rates can be achieved in patients with cirrhosis admitted to ICU [33]. In such a setting, CLIF-C OF and CLIF-C ACLF scores perform better than generally used and liver specific scores [31,34].

Table 2. Principles of treatment of ACLF [3]. ICA, International Club of Ascites; AKI, acute kidney injury; HRS, hepatorenal syndrome; RRT, renal replacement therapy; LT, liver transplantation; NSAID, non-steroidal anti-inflammatory drugs; MAP, mean arterial pressure; SBP, spontaneous bacterial peritonitis; LVP, large volume paracentesis; DVT deep-vein thrombosis; PaO_2 FiO_2 SpO_2 ACLF, acute-on-chronic liver failure.

Kidney	Circulation	Coagulation	Lung	Brain	Infections
Assess AKI severity using ICA Criteria * Taper/withdraw from diuretics and beta-blockers, withdraw from nephrotoxic drugs	Assess hemodynamic state early; consider a MAP ≥ 65 mmHg as target	Assess complete blood count and coagulation tests	Assess respiratory state by using also imaging techniques Calculate PaO_2/FiO_2 or SpO_2/FiO_2	Assess hepatic encephalopathy using West Haven criteria. Identify and treat the underlying cause	Perform a complete work up for infection at ACLF diagnosis
Administer albumin (1 g/kg for 48 h) if AKI stage > 1a * to volume expansion; if HRS-AKI, administer terlipressin by continuos infusion (2 mg/24 h) and albumin (20/40 g/day)	Administer crystalloids and 5% albumin as resuscitation fluids; norephinephrine as first line vasopressor	Administer platelets (if < 20.000 × 10^9/L) and fibrinogen (if <1 g/L) if invasive procedures	Administer oxygen and ventilation with lung protective strategy	Administer lactulose and enemas for hepatic encephalopathy.	Administer broad spectrum high-dose antibiotics at ACLF diagnosis and frequently re-assess therapy
Consider RRT as bridge to LT	Consider 20% albumin if AKI (see Kidney), SBP, LVP; consider terlipressin if additional agent needed	Consider prophylaxis for DVT in patients without severe coagulopathy	Consider intubation if risk of aspiration (West Haven grade III or IV hepatic encephalopathy)	Consider short-acting sedative agents if necessary	Consider antifungal agents if risk factors for fungal infections
Avoid NSAIDs	Avoid starches	Avoid fresh frozen plasma to correct INR if no bleeding	Avoid delay in intubation even if normal blood oxygen level	Avoid deep sedation and benzodiazepines	Avoid delay in antibiotics administration

* See ref. [34].

5.2. Treating Organ Failures

Acute kidney injury (AKI) should be treated with volume expansion with albumin and withdraw from diuretics and beta-blockers [35]. If there is no response after two days of volume expansion and hepatorenal syndrome (HRS)-AKI criteria are met [36], terlipressin given by continuous infusion should be started [37]. Response to terlipressin is inversely related to the number of OFs at baseline and to the creatinine value at the start of the treatment [38,39]. There are scarce data about the role of RRT in patients with ACLF. In a recent study in patients with type 1 HRS and no response to vasoconstrictors, RRT did not improve survival at 30 and 180 days [40]. To date, RRT should be considered as a bridge to LT in selected patients. A target of mean arterial pressure $\geq$ 65 mmHg should be reached within the first hours in patients with circulatory failure. Crystalloids and 5% albumin solution should be preferred over saline solutions as resuscitation fluids. Starches formulations should be avoided [4]. Norephinephrine is the first-line vasopressor agent [41]. Terlipressin demonstrated a better alternative in one study in patients with cirrhosis and septic shock [42]. Infusion of blood products should be considered only if clinically significant bleeding or invasive procedures in patients with coagulation failure. Respiratory failure should be treated with oxygen supplementation and ventilation, if needed. Intubation should be considered to prevent aspiration pneumonia in patients with severe hepatic encephalopathy by using short-acting sedative agents. Other measures include lactulose and enemas to clear the bowel and the treatment of the underlying cause [4,35].

6. Treating the Precipitating Event

6.1. Bacterial or Fungal Infection

The prevalence of infections in patients with ACLF, either as precipitants or complications of the syndrome, is about 50% and rises to 70% in patients with three or more OFs [43]. Bacterial infections are more frequent than fungal ones, being multidrug-resistant (MDR) pathogens involved in one-third of cases with different prevalence related to geographical region [43,44]. A complete work up for infection, including microbiological and imaging examinations, should be performed in all patients at diagnosis of ACLF before starting high-dose broad-spectrum antimicrobial therapy. The broad spectrum antibiotic treatment should be started as soon as possible. An effective antibiotic treatment is strongly associated with an improvement in survival in patients with ACLF [45,46]. Antifungal agents should be considered in patients with risk factors for fungal infections (e.g., nosocomial infections, previous antibiotic treatment, diabetes, AKI, recent endoscopy) [47,48].

6.2. Alcoholic Hepatitis

Corticosteroids are the first-line treatment for severe alcoholic hepatitis. The Lille score is used to identify response to treatment. The probability of response to corticosteroids is lower in patients with ACLF respect to those without (38% and 77%, respectively) and is negatively correlated with the number of OFs at diagnosis [49].

6.3. Acute Variceal Haemorrhage

Standard medical treatment for this life-threatening precipitant is made by a vasoconstrictor (terlipressin, somatostatin or analogues such as octreotide) and endoscopic therapy (preferably variceal ligation) plus a short-term antibiotic prophylaxis with ceftriaxone [50]. In a recent multicenter international study which enrolled patients with acute variceal bleeding and ACLF, the syndrome was identified as an independent risk factor for rebleeding and short-term mortality. Pre-emptive TIPS may improve survival in this cluster of patients, but further studies are needed before recommending its routinary use [51].

6.4. Hepatitis B Virus Reactivation

All patients with hepatitis B virus infection at presentation should be treated with a nucleoside or nucleotide analogue. Tenofovir, tenofovir alafenamide or entecavir should be used [9].

6.5. Liver Transplantation

Several studies showed that LT improved survival in patients with ACLF [52,53]. In a recent multi-center European investigation, one-year post-LT survival was >than 80% independently from ACLF grade [54]. Despite these findings, prioritization for LT of patients with ACLF remains complicated. Commonly used scores for listing patients with cirrhosis were demonstrated not to be accurate enough to predict survival in patients with OFs. Mortality of patients with ACLF of grade 3 and a MELD score < 25 was shown to be higher than in patients with a MELD score > 35 but without ACLF [52]. MELD-Na score underestimates mortality at 90-days in patients with ACLF, especially in those with MELD-Na < 30 [55]. Moreover, patients with ACLF grade 3 had a greater waitlist 14-day mortality than patients listed as status 1a, independent of MELD-Na score [56]. These findings emphasize the importance of early discussion for LT and consideration of priority for patients with ACLF, irrespective of traditional listing scores. Recently, a novel score which incorporates MELD score and ACLF grade demonstrably performs better than traditional scores by giving a higher impact to ACLF grade at lower MELD listing [57].

The Spanish Society of Liver Transplantation (SETH) proposed a consensus statement in which expedited organ allocation is recommended to allow ACLF patients to be transplanted [58]. SETH recommends the use of CLIF-C ACLF score instead of MELD to assess prognosis and suggests prioritisation of these patients because of their poor short-term prognosis [58]. NHS Blood and Transplant recently set the ACLF Liver Transplantation Tier (ACLFLTT) which gives a priority below that of super-urgent listed patients to those with cirrhosis and liver failure (as manifested by jaundice and coagulopathy) who stay on ICU for organ support and have risk of 28-day mortality of >50%. These patients usually fulfill EASL-CLIF criteria for ACLF of grade 2 or 3 [59].

An optimal selection of candidates for LT is equally important to avoid futile LT. Factors independently associated with poor post-LT survival were found to be lactate levels > 4 mmol/L, need for RRT at LT, older age of recipient, use of marginal organs and infections with MDROs while on the waiting list [52,54,60].

6.6. Extracorporeal Liver Support

Two large randomized clinical trials demonstrated no improvement in short-term survival in ACLF patients treated with albumin dialysis versus standard medical therapy [61,62]. Other two randomized trials are currently assessing plasma exchange (APACHE trial; ClinicalTrials.gov number, NCT03702920) and albumin exchange with endotoxin removal (DIALIVE trial, NCT03065699).

6.7. Granulocyte-Colony Stimulating Factor

Two small single-center studies reported improved survival and reduced rate of bacterial infections in ACLF patients treated with Granulocyte-Colony Stimulating Factor (G-CSF) [63,64]. This result was not confirmed by the recent large multicenter randomized trial (GRAFT study), which failed to demonstrate the superiority of G-CSF over standard medical treatment and reported serious drug-related adverse events [65].

6.8. Human Allogeneic Liver-Derived Progenitor Cells

Low doses of human allogeneic liver-derived progenitor cells (HALPC) appeared to be safe in a clinical phase II study which involved 24 patients [66]. Further studies are needed to confirm safety and assess efficacy of this medicinal product.

7. Conclusions

ACLF is a distinct syndrome without a universally accepted definition and is characterized by high short-term mortality due to OFs. Patients with ACLF should access ICU without delay if necessary. LT has good outcomes and should be considered irrespective of traditionally used scores for waiting list allocation. Prioritization of ACLF for LT should be improved using proper scores for ACLF patients. Further studies are needed in order to better clarify the pathophysiology of the syndrome and to develop treatments other than supportive measures for OFs.

Author Contributions: Writing—original draft, C.G., S.P. and P.A.; Writing—review & editing, C.G., S.P. and P.A. All authors have read and agreed to the published version of the manuscript.

Funding: This research received no external funding.

Conflicts of Interest: C.G.: None; S.P.: Mallinckrodt advisory board; P.A.: None.

References

1. D'Amico, G.; Garcia-Tsao, G.; Pagliaro, L. Natural history and prognostic indicators of survival in cirrhosis: A systematic review of 118 studies. *J. Hepatol.* **2006**, *44*, 217–231. [CrossRef]
2. Moreau, R.; Jalan, R.; Gines, P.; Pavesi, M.; Angeli, P.; Cordoba, J.; Durand, F.; Gustot, T.; Saliba, F.; Domenicali, M.; et al. Acute-on-chronic liver failure is a distinct syndrome that develops in patients with acute decompensation of cirrhosis. *Gastroenterology* **2013**, *144*, 1426–1437.e9. [CrossRef]
3. Arroyo, V.; Moreau, R.; Jalan, R. Acute-on-chronic liver failure. *N. Engl. J. Med.* **2020**, *382*, 2137–2145. [CrossRef] [PubMed]
4. Zaccherini, G.; Weiss, E.; Moreau, R. Acute-on-chronic liver failure: Definitions, pathophysiology and principles of treatment. *JHEP Rep.* **2020**, *3*, 100176. [CrossRef]
5. Bajaj, J.S.; O'Leary, J.G.; Reddy, K.R.; Wong, F.; Biggins, S.W.; Patton, H.; Fallon, M.B.; Garcia-Tsao, G.; Maliakkal, B.; Malik, R.; et al. Survival in infection-related acute-on-chronic liver failure is defined by extrahepatic organ failures. *Hepatology* **2014**, *60*, 250–256. [CrossRef] [PubMed]
6. Wu, T.; Li, J.; Shao, L.; Xin, J.; Jiang, L.; Zhou, Q.; Shi, D.; Jiang, J.; Sun, S.; Jin, L.; et al. Development of diagnostic criteria and a prognostic score for hepatitis B virus-related acute-on-chronic liver failure. *Gut* **2017**, *67*, 2181–2191. [CrossRef]
7. Sarin, S.K.; Kumar, A.; Almeida, J.A.; Chawla, Y.K.; Fan, S.T.; Garg, H.; De Silva, H.J.; Hamid, S.S.; Jalan, R.; Komolmit, P.; et al. Acute-on-chronic liver failure: Consensus recommendations of the Asian Pacific Association for the study of the liver (APASL). *Hepatol. Int.* **2009**, *3*, 269–282. [CrossRef] [PubMed]
8. Sarin, S.K.; Party, T.A.A.W.; Kedarisetty, C.K.; Abbas, Z.; Amarapurkar, D.; Bihari, C.; Chan, A.C.; Chawla, Y.K.; Dokmeci, A.K.; Garg, H.; et al. Acute-on-chronic liver failure: Consensus recommendations of the Asian Pacific Association for the Study of the Liver (APASL) 2014. *Hepatol. Int.* **2014**, *8*, 453–471. [CrossRef]
9. Sarin, S.K.; APASL ACLF Research Consortium (AARC) for APASL ACLF working Party; Choudhury, A.; Sharma, M.K.; Maiwall, R.; Al Mahtab, M.; Rahman, S.; Saigal, S.; Saraf, N.; Soin, A.S.; et al. Acute-on-chronic liver failure: Consensus recommendations of the Asian Pacific association for the study of the liver (APASL): An update. *Hepatol. Int.* **2019**, *13*, 353–390. [CrossRef]
10. Hernaez, R.; Kramer, J.R.; Liu, Y.; Tansel, A.; Natarajan, Y.; Hussain, K.B.; Ginès, P.; Solà, E.; Moreau, R.; Gerbes, A.; et al. Prevalence and short-term mortality of acute-on-chronic liver failure: A national cohort study from the USA. *J. Hepatol.* **2019**, *70*, 639–647. [CrossRef]
11. Piano, S.; Tonon, M.; Vettore, E.; Stanco, M.; Pilutti, C.; Romano, A.; Mareso, S.; Gambino, C.; Brocca, A.; Sticca, A.; et al. Incidence, predictors and outcomes of acute-on-chronic liver failure in outpatients with cirrhosis. *J. Hepatol.* **2017**, *67*, 1177–1184. [CrossRef] [PubMed]
12. Trebicka, J.; Fernández, J.; Papp, M.; Caraceni, P.; Laleman, W.; Gambino, C.; Giovo, I.; Uschner, F.E.; Jimenez, C.; Mookerjee, R.; et al. The PREDICT study uncovers three clinical courses of acutely decompensated cirrhosis that have distinct pathophysiology. *J. Hepatol.* **2020**, *73*, 842–854. [CrossRef] [PubMed]
13. Trebicka, J.; Fernandez, J.; Papp, M.; Caraceni, P.; Laleman, W.; Gambino, C.; Giovo, I.; Uschner, F.E.; Jansen, C.; Jimenez, C.; et al. PREDICT identifies precipitating events associated with the clinical course of acutely decompensated cirrhosis. *J. Hepatol.* **2020**, *74*, 1097–1108. [CrossRef]
14. O'Leary, J.G.; Reddy, K.R.; Garcia-Tsao, G.; Biggins, S.W.; Wong, F.; Fallon, M.B.; Subramanian, R.M.; Kamath, P.S.; Thuluvath, P.; Vargas, H.E.; et al. NACSELD acute-on-chronic liver failure (NACSELD-ACLF) score predicts 30-day survival in hospitalized patients with cirrhosis. *Hepatology* **2018**, *67*, 2367–2374. [CrossRef]
15. Li, F.; Thuluvath, P.J. EASL-CLIF criteria outperform NACSELD criteria for diagnosis and prognostication in ACLF. *J. Hepatol.* **2021**, in press. [CrossRef]
16. Moreau, R.; Gao, B.; Papp, M.; Bañares, R.; Kamath, P.S. Acute-on-chronic liver failure: A distinct clinical syndrome. *J. Hepatol.* **2021**, *75*, S27–S35. [CrossRef]
17. Jalan, R.; Saliba, F.; Pavesi, M.; Amoros, A.; Moreau, R.; Ginès, P.; Levesque, E.; Durand, F.; Angeli, P.; Caraceni, P.; et al. Development and validation of a prognostic score to predict mortality in patients with acute-on-chronic liver failure. *J. Hepatol.* **2014**, *61*, 1038–1047. [CrossRef]
18. Chen, T.; Yang, Z.; Choudhury, A.K.; Al Mahtab, M.; Li, J.; Chen, Y.; Tan, S.-S.; Han, T.; Hu, J.; Hamid, S.S.; et al. Complications constitute a major risk factor for mortality in hepatitis B virus-related acute-on-chronic liver failure patients: A multi-national study from the Asia–Pacific region. *Hepatol. Int.* **2019**, *13*, 695–705. [CrossRef]
19. Arroyo, V.; Angeli, P.; Moreau, R.; Jalan, R.; Clària, J.; Trebicka, J.; Fernández, J.; Gustot, T.; Caraceni, P.; Bernardi, M. The systemic inflammation hypothesis: Towards a new paradigm of acute decompensation and multiorgan failure in cirrhosis. *J. Hepatol.* **2020**, *74*, 670–685. [CrossRef]
20. Jalan, R.; D'Amico, G.; Trebicka, J.; Moreau, R.; Angeli, P.; Arroyo, V. New clinical and pathophysiological perspectives defining the trajectory of cirrhosis. *J. Hepatol.* **2021**, *75*, S14–S26. [CrossRef]
21. Angus, D.C.; van der Poll, T. Severe sepsis and septic shock. *N. Engl. J. Med.* **2013**, *369*, 840–851. [CrossRef]
22. Lucey, M.R.; Mathurin, P.; Morgan, T.R. Alcoholic hepatitis. *N. Engl. J. Med.* **2009**, *360*, 2758–2769. [CrossRef]
23. Cárdenas, A.; Ginès, P.; Uriz, J.; Bessa, X.; Salmerón, J.M.; Mas, A.; Ortega, R.; Calahorra, B.; Heras, D.D.L.; Bosch, J.; et al. Renal failure after upper gastrointestinal bleeding in cirrhosis: Incidence, clinical course, predictive factors, and short-term prognosis. *Hepatology* **2001**, *34*, 671–676. [CrossRef] [PubMed]

24. Moreau, R.; Clària, J.; Aguilar, F.; Fenaille, F.; Lozano, J.J.; Junot, C.; Colsch, B.; Caraceni, P.; Trebicka, J.; Pavesi, M.; et al. Blood metabolomics uncovers inflamma-tion-associated mitochondrial dysfunction as a potential mechanism underlying ACLF. *J Hepatol.* **2020**, *72*, 688–701. [CrossRef] [PubMed]

25. Gustot, T.; Fernandez, J.; Garcia, E.; Morando, F.; Caraceni, P.; Alessandria, C.; Laleman, W.; Trebicka, J.; Elkrief, L.; Hopf, C.; et al. Clinical Course of acute-on-chronic liver failure syndrome and effects on prognosis. *Hepatology* **2015**, *62*, 243–252. [CrossRef]

26. Choudhury, A.; Party, A.A.W.; Jindal, A.; Maiwall, R.; Sharma, M.K.; Sharma, B.C.; Pamecha, V.; Mahtab, M.; Rahman, S.; Chawla, Y.K.; et al. Liver failure determines the outcome in patients of acute-on-chronic liver failure (ACLF): Comparison of APASL ACLF research consortium (AARC) and CLIF-SOFA models. *Hepatol. Int.* **2017**, *11*, 461–471. [CrossRef]

27. Li, J.; Liang, X.; You, S.; Feng, T.; Zhou, X.; Zhu, B.; Luo, J.; Xin, J.; Jiang, J.; Shi, D.; et al. Development and validation of a new prognostic score for hepatitis B virus-related acute-on-chronic liver failure. *J. Hepatol.* **2021**, in press. [CrossRef] [PubMed]

28. Verma, N.; Dhiman, R.K.; Singh, V.; Duseja, A.; Taneja, S.; Choudhury, A.; Sharma, M.K.; Eapen, C.E.; Devarbhavi, H.; Al Mahtab, M.; et al. Comparative accuracy of prognostic models for short-term mortality in acute-on-chronic liver failure patients: CAP-ACLF. *Hepatol. Int.* **2021**, *15*, 753–765. [CrossRef] [PubMed]

29. Cao, Z.; Liu, Y.; Cai, M.; Xu, Y.; Xiang, X.; Zhao, G.; Cai, W.; Wang, H.; Wang, W.; Xie, Q. The Use of NACSELD and EASL-CLIF Classification systems of ACLF in the prediction of prognosis in hospitalized patients with cirrhosis. *Am. J. Gastroenterol.* **2020**, *115*, 2026–2035. [CrossRef]

30. Piano, S.; Favaretto, E.; Tonon, M.; Antonelli, G.; Brocca, A.; Sticca, A.; Mareso, S.; Gringeri, E.; Scaroni, C.; Plebani, M.; et al. Including relative adrenal insufficiency in definition and classification of acute-on-chronic liver failure. *Clin. Gastroenterol. Hepatol.* **2020**, *18*, 1188–1196.e3. [CrossRef]

31. Karvellas, C.J.; Garcia-Lopez, E.; Fernandez, J.; Saliba, F.; Sy, E.; Jalan, R.; Pavesi, M.; Gustot, T.; Ronco, J.; Arroyo, V.; et al. Dynamic prognostication in critically ill cirrhotic pa-tients with multiorgan failure in ICUs in Europe and North America: A multicenter analysis. *Crit. Care. Med.* **2018**, *46*, 1783–1791. [CrossRef] [PubMed]

32. Karvellas, C.; Bagshaw, S.M. Advances in management and prognostication in critically ill cirrhotic patients. *Curr. Opin. Crit. Care* **2014**, *20*, 210–217. [CrossRef] [PubMed]

33. Durand, F.; Roux, O.; Weiss, E.; Francoz, C. Acute-on-chronic liver failure: Where do we stand? *Liver Int.* **2021**, *41*, 128–136. [CrossRef] [PubMed]

34. Weil, D.; METAREACIR Group; Levesque, E.; McPhail, M.; Cavallazzi, R.; Theocharidou, E.; Cholongitas, E.; Galbois, A.; Pan, H.C.; Karvellas, C.J.; et al. Prognosis of cirrhotic patients admitted to intensive care unit: A meta-analysis. *Ann. Intensiv. Care* **2017**, *7*, 33. [CrossRef] [PubMed]

35. European Association for the Study of the Liver. EASL clinical practice guidelines for the management of patients with de-compensated cirrhosis. *J. Hepatol.* **2018**, *69*, 406–460. [CrossRef]

36. Angeli, P.; Ginès, P.; Wong, F.; Bernardi, M.; Boyer, T.D.; Gerbes, A.; Moreau, R.; Jalan, R.; Sarin, S.K.; Piano, S.; et al. Diagnosis and management of acute kidney injury in patients with cirrhosis: Revised consensus recommendations of the International Club of Ascites. *J. Hepatol.* **2015**, *62*, 968–974. [CrossRef]

37. Cavallin, M.; Kamath, P.S.; Merli, M.; Fasolato, S.; Toniutto, P.; Salerno, F.; Bernardi, M.; Romanelli, R.G.; Colletta, C.; Salinas, F.; et al. Terlipressin plus albumin versus midodrine and oc-treotide plus albumin in the treatment of hepatorenal syndrome: A randomized trial. *Hepatology* **2015**, *62*, 567–574. [CrossRef]

38. Piano, S.; Schmidt, H.H.; Ariza, X.; Amoros, A.; Romano, A.; Hüsing-Kabar, A.; Solà, E.; Gerbes, A.; Bernardi, M.; Alessandria, C.; et al. Association between grade of acute on chronic liver failure and response to terlipressin and albumin in patients with hepatorenal syndrome. *Clin. Gastroenterol. Hepatol.* **2018**, *16*, 1792–1800.e3. [CrossRef]

39. Boyer, T.D.; Sanyal, A.J.; Garcia-Tsao, G.; Blei, A.; Carl, D.; Bexon, A.S.; Terlipressin Study Group. Predictors of response to terlipressin plus albumin in hepatorenal syndrome (HRS) type 1: Relationship of serum creatinine to hemodynamics. *J Hepatol.* **2011**, *55*, 315–321. [CrossRef]

40. Zhang, Z.; Maddukuri, G.; Jaipaul, N.; Cai, C.X. Role of renal replacement therapy in patients with type 1 hepatorenal syndrome receiving combination treatment of vasoconstrictor plus albumin. *J. Crit. Care* **2015**, *30*, 969–974. [CrossRef]

41. Nadim, M.K.; Durand, F.; Kellum, J.A.; Levitsky, J.; O'Leary, J.G.; Karvellas, C.J.; Bajaj, J.S.; Davenport, A.; Jalan, R.; Angeli, P.; et al. Management of the critically ill patient with cirrhosis: A multidisciplinary perspective. *J. Hepatol.* **2015**, *64*, 717–735. [CrossRef]

42. Choudhury, A.; Kedarisetty, C.K.; Vashishtha, C.; Saini, D.; Kumar, S.; Maiwall, R.; Sharma, M.K.; Bhadoria, A.S.; Kumar, G.; Joshi, Y.K.; et al. A randomized trial comparing terlipressin and noradrenaline in patients with cirrhosis and septic shock. *Liver Int.* **2016**, *37*, 552–561. [CrossRef]

43. Fernández, J.; Acevedo, J.; Wiest, R.; Gustot, T.; Amoros, A.; Deulofeu, C.; Reverter, E.; Martínez, J.; Saliba, F.; Jalan, R.; et al. Bacterial and fungal infections in acute-on-chronic liver failure: Prevalence, characteristics and impact on prognosis. *Gut* **2017**, *67*, 1870–1880. [CrossRef]

44. Piano, S.; Singh, V.; Caraceni, P.; Maiwall, R.; Alessandria, C.; Fernandez, J.; Soares, E.C.; Kim, D.J.; Kim, S.E.; Marino, M.; et al. Epidemiology and effects of bacterial infections in patients with cirrhosis worldwide. *Gastroenterology* **2019**, *156*, 1368–1380.e10. [CrossRef]

45. Fernández, J.; Prado, V.; Trebicka, J.; Amoros, A.; Gustot, T.; Wiest, R.; Deulofeu, C.; Garcia, E.; Acevedo, J.; Fuhrmann, V.; et al. Multidrug-resistant bacterial infections in patients with decompensated cirrhosis and with acute-on-chronic liver failure in Europe. *J. Hepatol.* **2018**, *70*, 398–411. [CrossRef] [PubMed]

46. Wong, F.; Piano, S.; Singh, V.; Bartoletti, M.; Maiwall, R.; Alessandria, C.; Fernandez, J.; Soares, E.C.; Kim, D.J.; Kim, S.E.; et al. Clinical features and evolution of bacterial infection-related acute-on-chronic liver failure. *J. Hepatol.* **2020**, *74*, 330–339. [CrossRef] [PubMed]

47. Bajaj, J.S.; Reddy, R.K.; Tandon, P.; Wong, F.; Kamath, P.S.; Biggins, S.W.; Garcia-Tsao, G.; Fallon, M.; Maliakkal, B.; Lai, J.; et al. Prediction of fungal infection development and their impact on survival using the NACSELD cohort. *Am. J. Gastroenterol.* **2018**, *113*, 556–563. [CrossRef] [PubMed]

48. Bartoletti, M.; Rinaldi, M.; Pasquini, Z.; Scudeller, L.; Piano, S.; Giacobbe, D.R.; Maraolo, A.E.; Bussini, L.; Del Puente, F.; Incicco, S.; et al. Risk factors for Candidaemia in hospitalized patients with liver cirrhosis: A multicentre case–control–control study. *Clin. Microbiol. Infect.* **2020**, *27*, 276–282. [CrossRef]

49. Sersté, T.; Cornillie, A.; Njimi, H.; Pavesi, M.; Arroyo, V.; Putignano, A.; Weichselbaum, L.; Deltenre, P.; Degré, D.; Trépo, E.; et al. The prognostic value of acute-on-chronic liver failure during the course of severe alcoholic hepatitis. *J. Hepatol.* **2018**, *69*, 318–324. [CrossRef] [PubMed]

50. Garcia-Tsao, G.; Bosch, J. Management of varices and variceal hemorrhage in cirrhosis. *N. Engl. J. Med.* **2010**, *362*, 823–832. [CrossRef]

51. Trebicka, J.; Gu, W.; Ibáñez-Samaniego, L.; Hernández-Gea, V.; Pitarch, C.; Garcia, E.; Procopet, B.; Giráldez, Á.; Amitrano, L.; Villanueva, C.; et al. Rebleeding and mortality risk are increased by ACLF but reduced by pre-emptive TIPS. *J. Hepatol.* **2020**, *73*, 1082–1091. [CrossRef] [PubMed]

52. Sundaram, V.; Jalan, R.; Wu, T.; Volk, M.L.; Asrani, S.K.; Klein, A.S.; Wong, R.J. Factors associated with survival of patients with severe acute-on-chronic liver failure before and after liver transplantation. *Gastroenterology* **2019**, *156*, 1381–1391.e3. [CrossRef] [PubMed]

53. Artru, F.; Louvet, A.; Ruiz, I.; Levesque, E.; Labreuche, J.; Ursic-Bedoya, J.; Lassailly, G.; Dharancy, S.; Boleslawski, E.; Lebuffe, G.; et al. Liver transplantation in the most severely ill cirrhotic patients: A multicenter study in acute-on-chronic liver failure grade 3. *J. Hepatol.* **2017**, *67*, 708–715. [CrossRef] [PubMed]

54. Belli, L.S.; Duvoux, C.; Artzner, T.; Bernal, W.; Conti, S.; Cortesi, P.A.; Sacleux, S.-C.; Pageaux, G.-P.; Radenne, S.; Trebicka, J.; et al. Liver transplantation for patients with acute-on-chronic liver failure (ACLF) in Europe: Results of the ELITA/EF-CLIF collaborative study (ECLIS). *J. Hepatol.* **2021**, *75*, 610–622. [CrossRef] [PubMed]

55. Hernaez, R.; Liu, Y.; Kramer, J.R.; Rana, A.; El-Serag, H.B.; Kanwal, F. Model for end-stage liver disease-sodium underestimates 90-day mortality risk in patients with acute-on-chronic liver failure. *J. Hepatol.* **2020**, *73*, 1425–1433. [CrossRef]

56. Sundaram, V.; Shah, P.; Wong, R.J.; Karvellas, C.J.; Fortune, B.E.; Mahmud, N.; Kuo, A.; Jalan, R. Patients with acute on chronic liver failure grade 3 have greater 14-day waitlist mortality than status-1a patients. *Hepatology* **2019**, *70*, 334–345. [CrossRef]

57. Abdallah, M.A.; Kuo, Y.-F.; Asrani, S.; Wong, R.J.; Ahmed, A.; Kwo, P.; Terrault, N.; Kamath, P.S.; Jalan, R.; Singal, A.K. Validating a novel score based on interaction between ACLF grade and MELD score to predict waitlist mortality. *J. Hepatol.* **2020**, *74*, 1355–1361. [CrossRef]

58. Rodríguez-Perálvarez, M.; Gómez-Bravo, M.; Sánchez-Antolín, G.; De la Rosa, G.; Bilbao, I.; Colmenero, J. Expanding Indications of Liver Transplantation in Spain: Consensus Statement and Recommendations by the Spanish Society of Liver Transplantation. *Transplantation* **2020**, *105*, 602–607. [CrossRef]

59. Jalan, R.; Gustot, T.; Fernandez, J.; Bernal, W. 'Equity' and 'Justice' for patients with acute-on chronic liver failure: A call to action. *J. Hepatol.* **2021**. Online ahead of print. [CrossRef]

60. Artzner, T.; Michard, B.; Weiss, E.; Barbier, L.; Noorah, Z.; Merle, J.; Paugam-Burtz, C.; Francoz, C.; Durand, F.; Soubrane, O.; et al. Liver transplantation for critically ill cirrhotic patients: Stratifying utility based on pretransplant factors. *Arab. Archaeol. Epigr.* **2020**, *20*, 2437–2448. [CrossRef]

61. Bañares, R.; Nevens, F.; Larsen, F.S.; Jalan, R.; Albillos, A.; Dollinger, M.; Saliba, F.; Sauerbruch, T.; Klammt, S.; Ockenga, J.; et al. Extracorporeal albumin dialysis with the molecular adsorbent recirculating system in acute-on-chronic liver failure: The RELIEF trial. *Hepatology* **2012**, *57*, 1153–1162. [CrossRef] [PubMed]

62. Kribben, A.; Gerken, G.; Haag, S.; Herget–Rosenthal, S.; Treichel, U.; Betz, C.; Sarrazin, C.; Hoste, E.; Van Vlierberghe, H.; Escorsell, À.; et al. Effects of fractionated plasma separation and adsorption on survival in patients with acute-on-chronic liver failure. *Gastroenterology* **2012**, *142*, 782–789.e3. [CrossRef] [PubMed]

63. Garg, V.; Garg, H.; Khan, A.; Trehanpati, N.; Kumar, A.; Sharma, B.C.; Sakhuja, P.; Sarin, S.K. Granulocyte colony–stimulating factor mobilizes CD34+ cells and improves survival of patients with acute-on-chronic liver failure. *Gastroenterology* **2012**, *142*, 505–512.e1. [CrossRef] [PubMed]

64. Duan, X.-Z.; Liu, F.-F.; Tong, J.-J.; Yang, H.-Z.; Chen, J.; Liu, X.-Y.; Mao, Y.-L.; Xin, S.-J.; Hu, J.-H. Granulocyte-colony stimulating factor therapy improves survival in patients with hepatitis B virus-associated acute-on-chronic liver failure. *World J. Gastroenterol.* **2013**, *19*, 1104–1110. [CrossRef]

65. Engelmann, C.; Herber, A.; Franke, A.; Bruns, T.; Schiefke, I.; Zipprich, A.; Zeuzem, S.; Goeser, T.; Canbay, A.; Berg, C.; et al. Granulocyte-colony stimulating factor (G-CSF) to treat acuteon- chronic liver failure, a multicenter randomized trial (GRAFT study). *J. Hepatol.* **2021**, *5*. Online ahead of print.

66. Nevens, F.; Gustot, T.; Laterre, P.-F.; Lasser, L.L.; Haralampiev, L.E.; Vargas, V.; Lyubomirova, D.; Albillos, A.; Najimi, M.; Michel, S.; et al. A phase II study of human allogeneic liver-derived progenitor cell therapy for acute-on-chronic liver failure and acute decompensation. *JHEP Rep.* **2021**, *3*, 100291. [CrossRef] [PubMed]

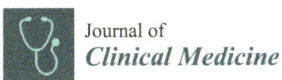
Journal of
Clinical Medicine

Review

HBV and HDV: New Treatments on the Horizon

Valentina Zuccaro [1,*], Erika Asperges [1], Marta Colaneri [1], Lea Nadia Marvulli [1,2] and Raffaele Bruno [1,2]

[1] U.O.C. Malattie Infettive I Fondazione IRCCS Policlinico San Matteo–Università di Pavia, 27100 Pavia, Italy; e.asperges@smatteo.pv.it (E.A.); marta.colaneri01@universitadipavia.it (M.C.); leanadia.marvulli01@universitadipavia.it (L.N.M.); raffaele.bruno@unipv.it (R.B.)

[2] Dipartimento di Scienze Clinico-Chirurgiche, Diagnostiche e Pediatriche–Università di Pavia, 27100 Pavia, Italy

* Correspondence: v.zuccaro@smatteo.pv.it; Tel.: +39-0382502660

Abstract: Despite the accumulating knowledge, chronic hepatitis B (CHB) and HDV infection represent a global health problem, and there are still several critical issues, which frequently remain uncovered. In this paper, we provided an overview of the current therapeutic options and summarized the investigational therapies in the pipeline. Furthermore, we discussed some critical issues such as a "functional cure" approach, the futility of long-term NA therapy and the relevance of understanding drug actions and safety of antivirals, especially in special populations.

Keywords: HBV; HDV; antivirals; functional cure; pharmacology

Citation: Zuccaro, V.; Asperges, E.; Colaneri, M.; Marvulli, L.N.; Bruno, R. HBV and HDV: New Treatments on the Horizon. *J. Clin. Med.* **2021**, *10*, 4054. https://doi.org/10.3390/jcm10184054

Academic Editors: Pierluigi Toniutto and Tatsuo Kanda

Received: 8 August 2021
Accepted: 6 September 2021
Published: 8 September 2021

Publisher's Note: MDPI stays neutral with regard to jurisdictional claims in published maps and institutional affiliations.

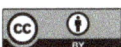
1. Introduction

Viral hepatitis has been recognized as a health and development priority only recently [1]. Most countries have implemented neonatal vaccination programs against hepatitis B virus (HBV) and reached a reduction in HBV prevalence among children; despite this, the burden this infection places, especially on the adult population, is still huge. In 2015, an estimated 257 million people were living with chronic HBV infection (CHB) worldwide, and its complications (especially long-term consequences, i.e., cirrhosis and hepatocellular carcinoma) were responsible for the 66% of the deaths caused by viral hepatitis; future perspectives are worrying, with 17 million deaths attributable to CHB in 2030 [2,3]. It is estimated that 5% of HBV-infected persons are also coinfected with hepatitis Delta virus (HDV) and have a more severe liver disease; however, there is substantial uncertainty, as in many countries, HDV infection is not tested [2].

Currently, the recommended treatment of choice for CHB regardless of the severity of the liver disease is the long-term administration of a nucleos(t)ide analog (NA) with a high barrier to resistance, such as entecavir, tenofovir disoproxil fumarate and telbivudine; alternatively, for patients with mild to moderate CHB, a 48 week-therapy with peginterferon alfa (PegIFNa) can be considered [4]. The main endpoint of all current treatment strategies is suppression of HBV DNA levels, as it is strongly associated with disease progression; however, this does not translate to an effective and complete cure of the HBV infection. Among the several barriers to cure, the most worrying one is the covalently closed circular DNA (cccDNA), which allows the virus to permanently persist in hepatocytes and against which NAs have little effect [5]. Moreover, NAs rarely achieve the so-called "functional cure", which was defined by clinical guidelines as seroclearance of hepatitis B surface antigen (HBsAg) with or without anti-HBs. Therefore, treatment is often lifelong and often leading to the selection of resistant mutants or causing side effects [4,6]. As for HDV infection, the ideal goal of treatment is the clearance of HBsAg plus a sustained HDV virological response at least 6 months after stopping the treatment, and the attainment of both the aforementioned aims is truly challenging. Pertaining to chronic HDV infection (CHD), the treatment of choice is a one year-course of PegIFNa, usually leading to a reduction of the HDV RNA viral load, but this may prove useless if not associated with

123

a clearance of the HBsAg [7]. When compared to other viral chronic hepatitis, there are certainly fewer data on the PegIFNa efficacy for chronic hepatitis D. To date, the largest available trial includes a total of 38 participants. Treatment success was achieved in only eight patients (21%) after 24 weeks of follow-up (all patients were maintained on PegINFa for 48 weeks) [8]. A higher virological response rate (43%) after a 12-month-follow-up was instead found in a subsequent trial. Nevertheless, it was carried out in a restricted group of 14 patients [9]. The European Association for the Study of the Liver (EASL) guidelines suggest tenofovir or entecavir treatment for those patients not eligible for interferon-based therapy with detectable HBV DNA levels in order to block residual HBV replication, mainly in patients with decompensated liver disease [4]. Unsurprisingly, rather than an ineffective drug with a well-known toxicity, we support the search for new molecules.

Although there are multiple comprehensive literature reviews on chronic hepatitis B and D treatments, there are still several critical issues, which frequently remain uncovered.

As CHB is associated with aging population, individuals often have co-morbid health concerns. Although current and investigational therapies do not carry high risks of toxicities, attention should be paid to subsets of the population called special populations, such as HIV coinfected patients, children, pregnant women, immunosuppressed patients, and patients undergoing chemotherapy and dialysis. Moreover, the futility of long-term NA therapy has become a very interesting topic, and the approach of finite NA treatment is not completely uniform.

The purpose of our study is not only to overview the different therapeutic options for chronic hepatitis B and D but to focus on those critical issues especially.

2. Overview of the Drug Pipeline

To succeed in the cure of the chronic infection, the prevailing theory at the moment is that the combination of two different strategies is required [3,10]. On the one hand, the recent progress in understanding the structure and life cycle of the virus allowed the development of novel antivirals directly targeting multiple steps in the virus replication, preventing the synthesis of new cccDNA. On the other hand, immunomodulators are also needed to subvert the state of tolerance found in the chronic phase of the disease and consequently promote the death of infected hepatocytes and neutralization of circulating virions [5]. According to the latest update, more than 50 compounds are currently being tested for CHB, and the majority of the studies are in a preclinical phase [11].

Adding to an existing class of drugs, new nucleotides analogs in development include besifovir, metacavir and two prodrugs of tenofovir (tenofovir exalidex, tenofovir disoproxil orotate). However, it is now widely recognized that an efficacious therapy should target more than one step of the virus replication cycle. For this reason, other drugs currently in development include attachment/entry inhibitors, such as bulevirtide.

Myrcludex-B (Myr), also known as bulevirtide, acts upon the sodium taurocholate cotransporting polypeptide (NTCP), a receptor of both HBV and HDV. Therefore, this new drug might block HBV and HDV entry, and it was approved in the European Union in July 2020 as the first effective drug for the treatment of chronic HDV in patients with compensated liver disease [11,12]. In a phase 2a trial, patients were treated with Myr for 72 weeks, and a follow-up was planned 6 months after the end of treatment. The estimation of efficacy parameters was planned to be performed after 24 and 48 weeks of therapy and after the end of follow-up. The results, though, were published as interim findings at week 24 and showed that all patients with measurable HDV RNA experienced a decline of HDV RNA under Myr monotherapy, while, remarkably, the combination of Myr with PegIFNα-2a profoundly enhanced this antiviral effect, achieving a decline >1 log in HDV RNA in all the subjects. Finally, ALT levels significantly declined in six of the eight patients of the Myr cohort [13]. Regarding the reduction of >0.5 log HBsAg, which we already described as an alternative therapeutic target, none of the patients achieved this endpoint. Similarly, Wedemeyer et al. showed a HDV RNA declined by 2 log and a normalization of ALT levels in patients treated with Myr and tenofovir, but regrettably, HDV RNA replication relapsed after the end of treatment in most of the patients and HBsAg remained unaffected [14]. Moreover, recent studies showed that the effect on HBsAg seemed to be more pronounced in the HDV patients receiving lower doses of Myr in combination with IFNa, rather than higher. The reason for this observation is not currently known.

Lonafarnib (LNF) is a farnesyl transferase inhibitor, which blocks assembly and secretion of virions in the cell (IC50: 36 nM) through the hepatitis delta antigen prenylation. LNF has been more extensively studied because of its potential activity in cancer patients and its proven efficacy in Hutchinson–Gilford progeria syndrome. In a phase 2a study, 14 patients were randomly assigned to receive LNF 100 mg or 200 mg twice daily for 28 days with greater decline in HDV RNA [15]. In a subsequent study, Yurdaydin et al. explored different potential LNF regimens: different doses of LNF, LNF plus ritonavir (RTV), LNF plus PEG-INF. A better antiviral response was achieved with the addition of RTV supporting the key role of the cytochrome P450 3A4 inhibitor and the need of exploration of boosting combinations [7].

Recently, nucleic acid polymers (NAPs), such REP 2139, have also been widely studied, showing promising results, as after a follow-up of 1 year, 7 and 5 of the 12 evaluated patients were HDV RNA and HBsAg negative, respectively. Asymptomatic and transient elevation of liver enzymes have been also reported [16]. Similarly, PEG-IFN-lambda was associated with improved or similar rates of virologic response with fewer adverse events than IFNa. The primary end point was once again a reduction of >2 log or negative HDV RNA at the end of 48-week-treatment and following a 24-week observation period [17]. We underline here that therapeutic targets remain generally similar in the older and newer studies assessing the efficacy of HBV or HDV treatment. In any case, depending on the treatment aim (HBV DNA or HBsAg decline, HDV-RNA long-term suppression, ALT normalization, etc.) and the degree of hepatic impairment, these novel regimens might potentially be successful, and with additional strategies, such as drug combinations, they might work even better.

Other molecules working with different mechanisms include:

- siRNAs (small interfering RNA that interfere with viral mRNA to prevent synthesis of viral antigens): GalNAc-siRNA, VIR-2218, DCR-HBVS, JNJ-3989, ARB-1467. Mostly now in phase 1 or 2 studies.
- Antisense nucleotides: GSK3389404, RO7062931, GSK3228836. In phase 2 studies.
- RNase H targeting (prevents degradation of pre-genomic RNA and synthesis of DNA): a-hydrocytropolones, N-hydroxyisoquinolinediones, N-hydroxylpyridinediones. These are the chemical class of molecules now under investigation, no single molecule has been developed yet.
- Capsid inhibitors (interfere with the formation of the HBC core protein): GLS4, JNJ 56136379, JNJ 56136379 (alone or in combination with JNJ 73763989), ABI-H0731, ABI-H2158, QL-007, RO7049389, EDP-514, AB-423, and JNJ-6379. Mainly in phase II, some in phase I or in vitro studies, alone or in combination with nucleotide inhibitors. A study of a capsid inhibitor in combination with Toll-like receptor 7 agonist is also in program (RO7049389 + RO7020531).
- HBsAg release inhibitors (prevent the assembly and secretion of HBV subviral particles: REP 2139 (also in combination with REP 2165), REP-2055, REP 301, REP 301-LTF, REP 401, REP 102. Some of these have been studied in combination with Peg-IFN and TDF. Now in phase II.
- cccDNA formation inhibitors: ccc_R08. Now in animal studies [5].

In the immunotherapy side of HBV treatment, mechanisms and molecules under study include:

- Toll-like receptor agonists (activation of innate immune system with production of IFN): GS-9620, GS9688, TQ-A3334, RO6864017. As explained above, there is also RO7020531 in combination with a capsid inhibitor (RO7049389 + RO7020531). They are mostly in phase II.

- Retinoic acid-inducible gene-1 agonist (lead to production of IFN and other cytokines that activate antiviral immunity): Inarigivir, SB-9200.
- Agonists of IFN genes stimulators (IFN production). Now in animal studies.
- Checkpoint inhibitors (restore T-cell functionality): CTLA-4, CD244/2B4, Tim-3, LAG-3, HLX10, cemiplimab, nivolumab in combination with a therapeutic vaccine.
- Therapeutic vaccines: ABX-203, INO-1800 (with or without INO-9112), HB-110 (with adefovir), GS-4774, TG-1050, JNJ-64300535, FP-02.2, DV-601, HBV0003, T101, GC1102. Mostly in phase I.
- Apoptosis inducers: APG-1387
- Ciclophilin inhibitor: CRV-31
- Transfer of genetically engineered T cells or CAR (chimeric antigen receptor) T cells [5].

3. Pharmacology and Safety of Current and Investigational Therapies of Hepatitis B and D

3.1. Myrcludex B (Myr)

Myr targets the hepatocytes exclusively, and this might allow subcutaneous administration of low drug doses [18]. Phase III clinical trials have established a subcutaneous injection of 10 mg as the optimal dose to reach more than 80% saturation of the NTCP receptor for at least 15 h [19]. The raised concern that NTCP blockage might cause an elevated plasma bile acid levels-related adverse reaction [20] is now insubstantial because, while the inhibition of HBV/HDV infection is reached with an inhibitory concentration (IC) 50 of 80 pM [21], the increase in bile acid transportation is impaired with an IC 50 of 47 nM, therefore significantly higher. Hence, Myr effectively inhibits HBV/HDV infection at concentrations where the NTCP-mediated transport of substrates is not yet affected. However, whether NTCP inhibition can also affect drug exposure is unknown. Conversely, plasma bile acid levels might work as the drug's marker. A study by Blank et al. recently investigated the pharmacokinetic data of Myr, and its effects on TDF 300 mg in 12 healthy volunteers after administration of a 10 mg SC dose. The authors noted that the steady-state AUC and the Cmax were significantly higher compared with those following the first dose, thus indicating an accumulation [19]. A further major consideration for clinical practice concerns the drug's excretion, and renal excretion resulted as a negligible route of elimination of Myr [22].

A critical issue is definitely the combination of antiviral therapies for hepatitis B infection. The reason behind it is precisely to achieve the HBsAg loss, acting at different stages of the disease, and simultaneously decrease HBV attachment and entry, ccc DNA formation, nucleocapsid and core assembly. For example, although Myr blocks viral entry, HDV and HBV can still propagate undisturbed through cell division, which is, conversely, efficiently restricted by IFN. IFN-α inhibits HBV transcription and replication in cell culture and in humanized mice by targeting the epigenetic regulation of the nuclear cccDNA minichromosome [23,24]. In the published first results of a phase 2 trial, a benefit of the antiviral combination of PegIFNα-2a and myrcludex was definitely observed [13]. However, follow-up showed a viral rebound after treatment cessation. Myr may thus be combined with current HBV drugs to improve HBV or HBV-HDV infected patient outcome; however, despite a decrease in HDV-RNA in a dose-dependent manner, only 10% of patients treated with Myr showed a definite virological response (defined as a 2 log10 reduction in HDV-RNA). The optimal duration of treatment to clear HDV RNA permanently is still unknown, since studies of 2 to 3-year duration are being planned, while the suggestion of potential benefit of a higher dose of Myr has been investigated by Loglio et al. [25].

3.2. Lonafarnib

Lonafarnib (LNF) is a farnesyl transferase inhibitor, which blocks assembly and secretion of virions in the cell (IC50: 36 nM) through the hepatitis delta antigen prenylation [15,26]. LNF has dose and time-dependent pharmacokinetics with an insignificant renal excretion [27]. Moreover, this drug notoriously has some adverse events, mostly in the multiple-dose rather than once-daily administration, mainly reported as minor gastrointestinal disorders, which significantly decreased with food intake [28]. Although the recommended dose is 200 mg bid [29], a recent PK and PD study showed that a high LNF dose of 610 mg bid would achieve 99% efficacy. However, such a high dose might cause several adverse effects [30]. Therefore, the authors provided an already explored suggestion regarding the use of a ritonavir booster to potentially optimize both the LNF tolerability and its antiviral effect [31]. The true ramifications of this option will need to be extensively investigated. Finally, the work of Lempp and colleagues indicates that, besides the suppression of viral secretion, LFN led to an intracellular accumulation of a hepatitis delta antigen [26].

3.3. JNJ-56136379

JNJ-5613379 (JNJ-6379) is an oral drug, which has at least two mechanisms of action on HBV infection. First, it interferes with the HBV capsid assembly, and second, it prevents cccDNA formation during de novo infection. Recently, Vandenbossche et al. demonstrated a dose-proportional increase in plasma concentration and AUC of the drug administered to healthy subjects [32]. However, this is true for dosages up to 300 mg, while with a double dose of 600 mg, the clearance decreased, determining a less than dose-proportional increase in the drug. Moreover, the drug showed a very long half-life of 120–140 h. Significantly, the drug clearance also decreased with lower weight [32]. No clear information regarding the metabolism of this drug is currently available. However, since a renal excretion of 18% has been recently reported, a certain share of hepatic metabolism probably exists. How this might potentially result in a drug–drug interaction (DDI) is still unclear [33]. Importantly, no severe adverse reactions were reported in the first in vivo single and multiple dose trial in healthy volunteers, and there was no dose limiting toxicity [34]. Only one patient experienced an elevation of ALT and AST during the treatment, but it was not possible to link it with any certainty to therapy [35]. A phase 2, randomized, open label study is currently ongoing to evaluate efficacy, pharmacokinetics, safety and tolerability of response-guided treatment with this drug combined with NA and Pegylated Interferon Alpha-2 [36].

3.4. ABI-H0731

ABI-H0731 is an orally administered, HBV core protein inhibitor, which also blocks several other steps in the HBV life cycle, including the HBV DNA synthesis and cccDNA formation. For this very reason, core inhibitors might have a more profound inhibitory effect on overall HBV replication than nucleoside analogs alone [37,38]. In a recent randomized, placebo-controlled, first-in-human study by Man-Fung Yuen et al., ABI-H0731 pharmacokinetics were assessed in healthy volunteers and HBV chronic patients. Overall, the authors' aim was to identify a safe and effective dosing schedule for phase 2 clinical studies [39]. Interestingly, this study showed that ABI-H0731 has dose-proportional pharmacokinetics, since steady-state Cmax, Cmin, and AUC increased when a higher dose of the drug was administered. The drug was rapidly absorbed, with mean time to maximum plasma concentration (Tmax) values of 2×50–4×17 h, and inter-individuals' variability in pharmacokinetic parameters was low. Furthermore, a moderate-fat meal intake has a significant impact on absorption, causing an approximately 45% increase in AUC. These findings are supportive of once-daily dosing of this drug. Nevertheless, it is interesting to note that chronic HBV patients experienced a higher exposure to the same dosages of ABI-H0731 than healthy individuals, suggesting a currently unexplored hepatic metabolism of the drug and hanging question marks over cirrhotic patients on the one hand, and potential drug–drug interactions on the other. Regarding the efficacy of ABI-H0731 in chronic HBV, when administered as monotherapy for 28 days (and 28 days of follow-up), the drug exhibited a dose-related antiviral activity, with mean maximal HBV DNA decline from baseline of 1×7 log10 IU/mL at 100 mg to 2×8 log10 IU/mL at 300 mg after 28 days, for both HBeAg positive and negative participants. To further confirm that a combination therapy is preferable, a more profound HBV DNA decline of treatment was seen when patients were treated with both an NA and ABI-H0731, compared with the placebo [40]. Therefore, the combination might not only maximize the antiviral potency but also avoid treatment-emergent resistance. Regarding the safety data, while a macular/maculopapular rash should be considered during the treatment, since some moderate cases occurred, the treatment was well tolerated overall [39].

3.5. REP-2139

REP-2139 is a nucleic acid polymer (NAP), which acts as a secretion inhibitor. The currently available studies investigated its role as monotherapy and in combination with NA or IFNa for 24–48 weeks, either IV or SC [16,41]. The suggested role of this compound is the removal of HBsAg from the blood, unmasking the anti-HBs response, and finally allowing the HBV clearance. Moreover, leading to a favorable immunological activation in the absence of HBsAg, this drug would potentially enhance the effect of IFNa and TDF [16,41]. Even considering all chance-related uncertainties, and due to the lack of pharmacokinetic data on REP-2139, its relative resemblance to other compounds under current use for different conditions, such as mipomersen for homozygous familial hypercholestcrolemia, might lead us to consider similarities in terms of absorption, distribution, metabolism and elimination. Hence, it showed a dose-dependent maximum plasma concentration at the end of a 2-h IV infusion or SC administration, while the time of peak concentrations (t max) were typically observed 3–4 h after SC dosing and the half-time was quite long, with post-distribution-phase plasma concentrations well predicting tissue concentrations and pharmacological activity [16]. Regarding REP-2139, some data on safety are currently available. Administration-related side effects, including fever and chills, were commonly experienced but generally did not require specific therapy. As in all oligonucleotides, an improved tolerability was then attributed to the neutralization of the chelation of calcium or magnesium. Importantly, significant elevation flares of ALT and AST (>10X ULN) were frequently observed during REP-2139-Ca monotherapy in HBV/HDV patients, treated either with monotherapy or combination therapy [42]. This phenomenon, though, was self-limited and so did not require any dose adjustment and/or interruption of treatment (Table 1).

Table 1. Summary of pharmacology and safety of current and investigational therapies of hepatitis B and D.

Myrcludex B (Myr)	• Injections by SC route • Recommended dose is 10 mg qd • Insignificant renal excretion
Lonafarnib (LNF)	• Oral drug • Recommended dose is 200 mg bid • Insignificant renal excretion • Gastrointestinal disorders, which significantly decrease with food intake
JNJ-6379	• Oral drug • Long half-life of 120–140 • Renal excretion and hepatic metabolism may exist (potential DDI)
ABI-H0731	• Oral drug • A moderate-fat meal intake has a significant impact on absorption, supportive of once-daily dosing • Hepatic metabolism (potential DDI)
REP-2139	• Injections IV or SC • Side effects reported, including fever and chills

4. Evaluating the Response to the Hepatitis D Treatment

The only recognized available and effective drug against HDV is interferon alfa (IFNa), and it is recommended for patients with detectable HDV RNA and active liver disease (elevated serum aminotransferase and/or chronic hepatitis on liver biopsy) [43]. The treatment of chronic hepatitis D remains unsatisfactory and the eradication of HDV and HBV and prevention of the long-term sequelae of chronic hepatitis, such as cirrhosis, liver decompensation, and HCC are still not commonly achieved. Since the primary endpoint of treatment is suppression of HDV RNA, the standard of therapeutic success was defined as negative HDV RNA at 6 months (24 weeks) or more after treatment, known as a sustained virological response (SVR) [9,44]. Detectable HDV RNA at 6 months of treatment might be a predictor for a failed virological response [45]. Although achieving a negative HDV viremia is still considered a hallmark of treatment efficacy, several studies have shown that the only robust endpoint might differently be the clearance of the HBsAg [46,47]. It finally seems that the ideal goal of HDV treatment should be both the clearance of HBsAg and the sustained HDV virological response at least 6 months after stopping the treatment, and the attainment of both the aforementioned aims is truly challenging [48]. Moreover, together with a negative HDV viremia, a successful treatment is also associated with amelioration of necroinflammatory activity, defined as a sustained biochemical response (normalization of ALT and/or AST levels at six months or more after treatment) or histological response (improvement of inflammatory activity confirmed by liver biopsy). These goals are commonly considered as secondary outcomes measures in the available trials [45]. Taking these into account, Yurdaydin et al. recently proposed the evaluation of HDV treatment success based on the improvement of liver function rather than the virologic response. Relying on this unorthodox method, a decline of two or more logs of HDV RNA even without achieving a negative HDV RNA test might be sufficient, if ALT are normalized [7].

Therapeutic targets remain generally similar in the older and newer studies assessing the efficacy of HDV treatment. In any case, depending on the treatment aim (HDV-RNA long-term suppression, ALT normalization, etc.) and the degree of hepatic impairment, these novel regimens might potentially be successful, even more if additional strategies, as the combination of drugs, are implemented. Our expert opinion is that the primary goal would be, first of all, the functional cure of HBV.

5. Finite Nucleos(t)ide Analog Therapy

Long-term therapy with NA is effective in achieving viral suppression; however, this is not indicative of HBV eradication [49]. As highlighted by Papatheodoridi et al., several reasons have driven the emergent proposal to stop long-term NA therapy: the futility of continuing a therapy that does not offer any further benefit; the unknown safety of a lifetime NA therapy; the cumulative cost; the undoubted risk to occur through a decline of treatment adherence [50]. Despite the lack of a well-defined endpoint for HBV treatments, international guidelines unanimously consider HBsAg loss as the most important one [6]. However, Dusheiko et al. reported that HBsAg loss rates were <1% per year during NA treatment [6,51]. With this in mind, over the past 5–10 years, the finite NA treatment became a very interesting topic [6], and since 2016, the international guidelines have begun accepting finite NA therapy as an option in a specific subset of patients.

Although the approach of finite NA treatment is not completely uniform, there is a consistent agreement among different guidelines: finite NA therapy was suggested in not-cirrhotic patients with undetectable levels of HBV DNA(on three separate occasions, 6 months apart) after 12–18 months from HBeAb seroconversion (consolidation therapy) [52]. The Asian guidelines, in contrast to EASL and AASLD, consider finite NA treatment also in patients with cirrhosis [4,53–55]. After discontinuation, virological relapse is quite common; however, not all patients necessarily have a biochemical relapse, which means that not all patients require retreatment [53]. Although several studies have focused on identifying factors that might predict relapse after treatment discontinuation, at present, there is no reliable marker able to predict such a response [53]. Liu Y et al.

performed a meta-analysis to evaluate those factors and data showed that older age, high levels of quantitative HBsAg (>1000 IU/mL) at baseline and at the end of treatment, and shorter duration of consolidation therapy result as factors predictive of relapse after NA discontinuation in HBeAg-negative CHB patients [56]. Certain viral markers have gained interest, such as the hepatitis B core-related antigen (HBcrAg), which seemed to serve as a useful marker on patients who are planning finite NA therapy. In particular, a decrease in HBcrAg levels was reported during NA therapy; Matsumoto et al. reported an experience from CHB patients treated with lamivudine where HbcrAg levels > 4.9 log U/mL at the time of NA discontinuation were correlated to clinical relapse. In contrast, HbcrAg levels < 3.4 log U/mL were the only independent predictive factor without relapse after NA cessation [57].

Moreover, immunological studies have highlighted the role of the host immune response as a pathobiological basis to facilitate HBsAg decline towards HBsAg loss [58]. Considering that, investigators have progressed to exploring immune biomarkers [53], such as soluble isoform of growth stimulation expressed gene 2 (ST2), which belongs to the Toll-like/interleukin-1 receptor superfamily. Xie et al. showed that ST2 was correlated with HBsAg, HBV DNA, ALT and anti-HBc levels. Although baseline levels of ST2 were not associated to clinical relapse, after 12 weeks after NA cessation, the level of ST2 was able to predict the clinical relapse [59].

5.1. When and Whom to Stop Long-Term NA Therapy?

After reviewing the current literature, we suggest that NAs should be discontinued:

- After HBsAg loss; [4]
- In patients with HBV DNA undetectability after 12–18 months from HBeAb seroconversion (consolidation therapy): [4];
- In HBsAg-positive patients without liver cirrhosis who achieved stable HBV DNA undetectability on three separate occasions, 6 months apart after treatment for 2–3 years [4,6].

Conversely, NAs discontinuation should be avoided in:

- Cirrhotic patients;
- Patients who are not motivated to adhere to close monitoring;
- Patients with HIV or HDV coinfection [6].

As already pointed above, predictors of post-NA relapse are lacking; however, Papatheodorid et al. showed an overview of biomarkers able to identify non-cirrhotic CHB patients who can safely discontinue NAs before HBsAg loss; HBsAg serum levels at NA discontinuation seem to be able to predict the clinical relapse, as already emerged from the meta-analysis of Liu Y et al. [53,56] (Table 2).

Table 2. Patients that should stop long-term NA therapy and when.

NAs Should Be Discontinued	NAs Discontinuation Should Be Avoided
• HBsAg loss	• Cirrhotic patients
• After 12–18 months from HBeAb seroconversion with HBV DNA undetectability	• Patients who are not motivated to adhere to close monitoring
• HBV DNA undetectability on three separate occasions, 6 months apart after treatment for 2–3 years	• Patients with HIV or HDV coinfection

5.2. Management of Patients after NA Cessation

Concerning the management of patients after NAs cessation, liver function tests (serum ALT/AST, bilirubin and prothrombin time) should be monitored at week 6, week 12, week 18, week 24, and 3 monthly thereafter for the first 2 years. Weekly or biweekly tests are recommended in the case of elevation of ALT or AST > 5X ULN.

HBV DNA and HBsAg should be monitored every 3 months in the first year or in case of virologic relapse or clinical relapse and every 6–12 months afterward [6,58].

6. Special Populations

Current guidelines for special populations in HBV-infected patients include HIV-HBV coinfected patients, children, pregnant women, immunosuppressed patients and patients undergoing chemotherapy and dialysis. In most cases, practice points are well defined: HIV patients should follow a TAF/TAF based regimen; safety and efficacy profiles for interferon, TDF and entecavir in children are similar to adults, allowing for easy treatment when warranted; HBsAg-positive patients undergoing immunosuppressive therapy should undergo prophylaxis according to their reactivation risk; renal failure/dialysis patients should be administered entecavir or TAF as treatment/prophylaxis. Studies regarding new drugs, are, however, still missing. A search on clinicaltrial.gov reveals that active studies regarding bulevirtide either exclude special populations or do not plan sub-analysis for them. Similarly, Pubmed searches for "bulevirtide + HIV", "bulevirtide + pregnancy", "bulevirtide + children" and similar or related keywords yields no results. Lonafarnib has been more extensively studied (though evidence is still scarce) because of its potential activity in cancer patients and its proven efficacy in Hutchinson–Gilford progeria syndrome. Studies on solid tumors and hematological patients include the following pathologies: myelodysplastic syndrome, chronic myelomonocytic and myelogenous leukemia, lymphoma, breast, central nervous system, gastrointestinal, genitourinary, head and neck, lung and liver cancer and soft tissue sarcomas. Most of these studies are still ongoing with no published results; however, some phase II studies that used standard lonafarnib dosage (100 to 200 mg twice daily) reported mainly grade 1 and 2 side effects, with no excess of hematological side effects when compared to standard therapy [60–65]. A case report in three chronic myelomonocytic leukemia patients describes hyperleukocytosis associated with respiratory distress that has not been observed in other patients [27,66–71]. Thus, we can conclude that in terms of side effects, cancer patients and patients undergoing chemotherapy require no special attention. A few studies also examined potential drug–drug interactions, finding no interactions with gemcitabine, imatinib, paclitaxel. Concerning children, a phase I study on pediatric cancer patients determined an optimal body surface area-dependent dose (yielding good serum levels with grade 1 or 2 side effects) similar to adults, and higher doses resulted in the same side effects. It also noted that myelosuppression occurred only with higher doses, as it happened in adults [72]. This might also make this drug ideal for immunosuppressed patients. Studies on Hutchinson–Gilford progeria syndrome were obviously directed at children, and showed pharmacological properties and side effects profiles similar to the ones observed in adults [73,74]. Obviously, children with Hutchinson–Gilford progeria syndrome represent a nearly unique category given the rarity of the disease, and this, plus the minuscule number of participants involved in these studies, do not guarantee reliability of the findings on pharmacodynamics-kinetics and uncommon side effects. Other drugs in the pipeline for HBV treatment are still too new in their development phases to have data about special populations.

7. Conclusions

In this paper, we provided an overview of the different therapeutic options for chronic hepatitis B and D. As discussed above, despite the accumulating knowledge, although HBV and HDV infections represent a global health problem, unmet clinical needs still remain. Firstly, the chance of a cure with the currently available antiviral drugs is very low. Secondly, as infections are associated with an aging population, individuals often have co-morbid health concerns. Although current and investigational therapies do not carry high risks of toxicities, attention should be paid in a subset of the population called a special population, such as HIV coinfected patients, children, pregnant women, immunosuppressed patients, and patients undergoing chemotherapy and dialysis.

In view of this, a basic understanding of actions and safety of current and investigational therapies should be useful to guide clinicians toward the correct therapeutic choice. Further studies will focus on the development of combination strategies targeting

J. Clin. Med. **2021**, *10*, 4054

different signaling pathways towards a functional cure, most probably with a combination of multiple drugs.

Author Contributions: E.A.: data curation, writing—review and editing; M.C.: data curation, writing—review and editing; L.N.M.: data curation, writing—review and editing; V.Z.: writing—original draft preparation, conceptualization, methodology; R.B.: conceptualization, validation, writing—review and editing. All authors have read and agreed to the published version of the manuscript.

Funding: No funding to declare.

Institutional Review Board Statement: Not applicable.

Informed Consent Statement: Not applicable.

Conflicts of Interest: The authors declare no conflict of interest.

References

1. World Health Organization. *Global Health Sector Strategy on Viral Hepatitis 2016–2021*; World Health Organization: Geneva, Switzerland, 2016.
2. World Health Organization. *Global Hepatitis Report*; World Health Organization: Geneva, Switzerland, 2017.
3. Nguyen, M.H.; Wong, G.; Gane, E.; Kao, J.-H.; Dusheiko, G. Hepatitis B virus: Advances in prevention, diagnosis, and therapy. *Clin. Microbiol. Rev.* **2020**, *33*, e00046-19. [CrossRef] [PubMed]
4. Lampertico, P.; Agarwal, K.; Berg, T.; Buti, M.; Janssen, H.L.A.; Papatheordoridis, G.; Zoulim, F. EASL 2017 Clinical practice guidelines on the management of Hepatitis B virus infection. *J. Hepatol.* **2017**, *67*, 370–398. [CrossRef] [PubMed]
5. Alexopoulou, A.; Vasilieva, L.; Karayiannis, P. New approaches to the treatment of chronic Hepatitis B. *J. Clin. Med.* **2020**, *9*, 3187. [CrossRef]
6. Hall, S.; Howell, J.; Visvanathan, K.; Thompson, A. The Yin and the Yang of treatment for chronic Hepatitis B—When to start, when to stop nucleos(t)ide analogue therapy. *Viruses* **2020**, *12*, 934. [CrossRef]
7. Yurdaydin, C.; Abbas, Z.; Buti, M.; Cornberg, M.; Esteban, R.; Etzion, O.; Gane, E.J.; Gish, R.G.; Glenn, J.S.; Hamid, S.; et al. Treating chronic hepatitis delta: The need for surrogate markers of treatment efficacy. *J. Hepatol.* **2019**, *70*, 1008–1015. [CrossRef] [PubMed]
8. Niro, G.A.; Ciancio, A.; Battista Gaeta, G.; Smedile, A.; Marrone, A.; Olivero, A.; Stanzione, M.; David, E.; Brancaccio, G.; Fontana, R.; et al. Pegylated interferon alpha-2b as monotherapy or in combination with ribavirin in chronic hepatitis delta. *Hepatology* **2006**, *44*, 713–720. [CrossRef] [PubMed]
9. Castelnau, C.; Le Gal, F.; Ripault, M.-P.; Gordien, E.; Martinot-Peignoux, M.; Boyer, N.; Pham, B.-N.; Maylin, S.; Bedossa, P.; Dény, P.; et al. Efficacy of peginterferon alpha-2b in chronic hepatitis delta: Relevance of quantitative RT-PCR for follow-up. *Hepatology* **2006**, *44*, 728–735. [CrossRef] [PubMed]
10. Kim, W.R. Emerging therapies toward a functional cure for Hepatitis B virus infection. *Gastroenterol. Hepatol.* **2018**, *14*, 439–442.
11. Kang, C.; Syed, Y.Y. Bulevirtide: First approval. *Drugs* **2020**, *80*, 1601–1605. [CrossRef]
12. European Medicines Agency. *Hepcludex*; European Medicines Agency: Brussels, Belgium, 2021.
13. Bogomolov, P.; Alexandrov, A.; Voronkova, N.; Macievich, M.; Kokina, K.; Petrachenkova, M.; Lehr, T.; Lempp, F.A.; Wedemeyer, H.; Haag, M.; et al. Treatment of chronic Hepatitis D with the entry inhibitor myrcludex B: First results of a phase Ib/IIa study. *J. Hepatol.* **2016**, *65*, 490–498. [CrossRef]
14. Wedemeyer, H.; Schöneweis, K.; Bogomolov, P.; Voronka, N.; Chulanov, V.; Stepanova, T.; Bremer, B.; Lehmann, P.; Raupach, R.; Allweis, L.; et al. Final results of a multicenter, open-label phase 2b clinical trial to assess safety and efficacy of Myrcludex B in combination with Tenofovir in patients with chronic HBV/HDV co-infection. *J. Hepatol.* **2018**, *68*, S3. [CrossRef]
15. Koh, C.; Canini, L.; Dahari, H.; Zhano, X.; Uprichard, S.L.; Haynes-Williams, V.; Winters, M.A.; Subramanya, G.; Cooper, S.L.; Pinto, P.; et al. Oral prenylation inhibition with lonafarnib in chronic hepatitis D infection: A proof-of-concept randomised, double-blind, placebo-controlled phase 2A trial. *Lancet Infect. Dis.* **2015**, *15*, 1167–1174. [CrossRef]
16. Bazinet, M.; Pântea, V.; Cebotarescu, V.; Cojuhari, L.; Jimberi, P.; Albrecht, J.; Schmid, P.; Le Gal, F.; Gordien, E.; Krawczyk, A.; et al. Safety and efficacy of REP 2139 and pegylated interferon alfa-2a for treatment-naive patients with chronic hepatitis B virus and hepatitis D virus co-infection (REP 301 and REP 301-LTF): A non-randomised, open-label, phase 2 trial. *Lancet Gastroenterol. Hepatol.* **2017**, *2*, 877–889. [CrossRef]
17. Etzion, O.; Hamid, S.S.; Lurie, Y.; Gane, E.; Bader, N.; Yardeni, D.; Nevo-Shor, A.; Channa, S.; Mawani, M.; Parkash, O.; et al. PS-052-End of study results from LIMT HDV study: 36% durable virologic response at 24 weeks post-treatment with pegylated interferon lambda monotherapy in patients with chronic hepatitis delta virus infection. *J. Hepatol.* **2019**, *70*, e32. [CrossRef]
18. Schieck, A.; Schulze, A.; Gähler, C.; Müller, T.; Haberkorn, U.; Alexandrov, A.; Urban, S.; Mier, W. Hepatitis B virus hepatotropism is mediated by specific receptor recognition in the liver and not restricted to susceptible hosts. *Hepatology* **2013**, *58*, 43–53. [CrossRef]

19. Blank, A.; Eidam, A.; Haag, M.; Hohmann, N.; Burhenne, J.; Schwab, M.; van de Graaf, S.; Meyer, M.R.; Meier, K.; Weiss, J.; et al. The NTCP-inhibitor Myrcludex B: Effects on bile acid disposition and tenofovir pharmacokinetics. *Clin. Pharmacol. Ther.* **2018**, *103*, 341–348. [CrossRef] [PubMed]

20. Haag, M.; Hofmann, U.; Mürdter, T.E.; Heinkele, G.; Leuthold, P.; Blank, A.; Haefeli, W.E.; Alexandrov, A.; Urban, S.; Schwab, M. Quantitative bile acid profiling by liquid chromatography quadrupole time-of-flight mass spectrometry: Monitoring hepatitis B therapy by a novel Na+-taurocholate cotransporting polypeptide inhibitor. *Anal. Bioanal. Chem.* **2015**, *407*, 6815–6825. [CrossRef]

21. Schulze, A.; Schieck, A.; Ni, Y.; Mier, W.; Urban, S. Fine mapping of pre-S sequence requirements for Hepatitis B virus large envelope protein-mediated receptor interaction. *J. Virol.* **2010**, *84*, 1989–2000. [CrossRef]

22. Smolders, E.J.; Burger, D.M.; Feld, J.J.; Kiser, J.J. Review article: Clinical pharmacology of current and investigational hepatitis B virus therapies. *Aliment. Pharmacol. Ther.* **2020**, *51*, 231–243. [CrossRef]

23. Belloni, L.; Allweiss, L.; Guerrieri, F.; Pediconi, N.; Volz, T.; Pollicino, T.; Petersen, J.; Raimondo, G.; Dandri, M.; Levrero, M. IFN-α inhibits HBV transcription and replication in cell culture and in humanized mice by targeting the epigenetic regulation of the nuclear cccDNA minichromosome. *J. Clin. Investig.* **2012**, *122*, 529–537. [CrossRef]

24. Zhang, Z.; Walther, T.; Lempp, F.A.; Ni, Y.; Urban, S. Synergistic Suppression of HDV Persistence In Vitro by Cotreatment with Investigational Drugs Targeting both Extracellular and Cell Division Mediated Spreading Pathways. In Proceedings of the Liver Meeting® 2019–AASLD, Boston, MA, USA, 8–12 November 2019.

25. Loglio, A.; Ferenci, P.; Uceda Renteria, S.C.; Tham, C.Y.L.; van Bömmel, F.; Borghi, M.; Holzmann, H.; Perbellini, R.; Trombetta, E.; Giovanelli, S.; et al. Excellent safety and effectiveness of high-dose myrcludex-B monotherapy administered for 48 weeks in HDV-related compensated cirrhosis: A case report of 3 patients. *J. Hepatol.* **2019**, *71*, 834–839. [CrossRef]

26. Lempp, F.A.; Schlund, F.; Rieble, L.; Nussbaum, L.; Link, C.; Zhang, Z.; Ni, Y.; Urban, S. Recapitulation of HDV infection in a fully permissive hepatoma cell line allows efficient drug evaluation. *Nat. Commun.* **2019**, *10*, 2265. [CrossRef]

27. Castaneda, C.; Meadows, K.L.; Truax, R.; Morse, M.A.; Kaufmann, S.H.; Petros, W.P.; Zhu, Y.; Statkevich, P.; Cutler, D.L.; Hurwitz, H.I. Phase I and pharmacokinetic study of lonafarnib, SCH 66336, using a 2-week on, 2-week off schedule in patients with advanced solid tumors. *Cancer Chemother. Pharmacol.* **2011**, *67*, 455–463. [CrossRef] [PubMed]

28. Zhu, Y.; Statkevich, P.; Cutler, D.L. Effect of food on the pharmacokinetics of lonafarnib (SCH 66336) following single and multiple doses. *Int. J. Clin. Pharmacol. Ther.* **2007**, *45*, 539–547. [CrossRef] [PubMed]

29. Chow, L.Q.M.; Eckhardt, S.G.; O'Bryant, C.L.; Schultz, M.K.; Morrow, M.; Grolnic, S.; Basche, M.; Gore, L. A phase I safety, pharmacological, and biological study of the farnesyl protein transferase inhibitor, lonafarnib (SCH 663366), in combination with cisplatin and gemcitabine in patients with advanced solid tumors. *Cancer Chemother. Pharmacol.* **2008**, *62*, 631–646. [CrossRef]

30. Canini, L.; Koh, C.; Cotler, S.J.; Uprichard, S.L.; Winters, M.A.; Han, M.A.T.; Kleiner, D.E.; Idilman, R.; Yurdaydin, C.; Glenn, J.S.; et al. Pharmacokinetics and pharmacodynamics modeling of lonafarnib in patients with chronic hepatitis delta virus infection. *Hepatol. Commun.* **2017**, *1*, 288–292. [CrossRef] [PubMed]

31. Treatment of Chronic Delta Hepatitis with Lonafarnib and Ritonavir. ClinicalTrials.gov Identifier: NCT02511431. Available online: ClinicalTrials.gov (accessed on 5 September 2021).

32. Vandenbossche, J.; Zoulim, F.; Lenz, O.; Talloen, W.; Moscalu, I.; Rosmawati, M.; Streinu-Cercel, A.; Chuang, W.-L.; Bourgeois, S.; Yang, S.-S.; et al. Safety, Antiviral Activity, and Pharmacokinetics of a Novel Hepatitis B Virus Capsid Assembly Modulator, JNJ-56136379, in Asian and Caucasian Patients with Chronic Hepatitis B (FRI-217). In Proceedings of the International Liver Congress EASL-European Association for the Study of the Liver 2019, Vienna, Austria, 10–14 April 2019.

33. Yogaratnam, J.Z.; Vandenbossche, J.; Lenz, O.; Gogate, J.; Verpoorten, N.; Biewenga, J.; Snoeys, J.; Blatt, L.; Fry, J. Safety, Tolerability and Pharmacokinetics of Single Ascending Doses of JNJ-56136379, a Novel HBV Capsid Assembly Modulator, in Japanese Adult Healthy Volunteers. In Proceedings of the APASL-27th Annual Conference of the Asian Pacific Association for the Study of the Liver, New Delhi, India, 14–18 March 2018.

34. Lenz, O.; Verbinnen, T.; Hodari, M.; Talloen, W.; Vandenbossche, J.; Shukla, U.; Berby, F.; Scholtes, C.; Blue, D.; Yogaratnam, J.; et al. FRI-189-HBcrAg decline in JNJ-56136379-treated chronic hepatitis B patients: Results of a phase 1 study. *J. Hepatol.* **2019**, *70*, e473–e474. [CrossRef]

35. Zoulim, F.; Yogaratnam, J.Z.; Vandenbossche, J.; Moscalu, I.; Streinu-Cercel, A.; Lenz, O.; Bourgeois, S.; Talloen, M.; Crespo, J.; Pascasio, J.M.; et al. Safety, Pharmacokinetics and Antiviral Activity of Novel HBV Capsid Assembly Modulator, JNJ-56136379, in Patients with Chronic Hepatitis B. In Proceedings of the Liver Meeting (AASLD), San Francisco, CA, USA, 9–13 November 2018.

36. ClinicalTrials.gov. *A Study of JNJ-73763989 + JNJ-56136379 + Nucleos(t)ide Analog (NA) Regimen with or without Pegylated Interferon Alpha-2a (PegIFN-α2a) in Treatment-Naive Participants with Hepatitis B e Antigen (HBeAg) Positive Chronic Hepatitis B Virus (HBV) Infection and Normal Alanine Aminotransferase (ALT)*; National Medicine Library of USA: Bethesda, MA, USA, 2019.

37. Huang, Q.; Mercier, A.; Zhou, Y.; Zong, Y.; Guo, L.; Mercier, A.; Zhou, Y.; Tang, A.; Henne, K.; Colonno, R. Preclinical characterization of potent core protein assembly modifiers for the treatment of chronic hepatitis B. *Antimicrob. Agents Chemother.* **2020**, *64*, e01463-20. [CrossRef]

38. Huang, Q.; Turner, W.W.; Haydar, S.; Li, L.; Rai, R.; Cai, D.; Yan, R.; Zhou, Y.; Zhou, X.; Zong, Y.; et al. Preclinical Profile of Potent Second Generation CpAMs Capable of Inhibiting the Generation of HBsAg, HBeAg, pgRNA and cccDNA in HBV-Infected Cells. In Proceedings of the Liver Meeting, Washington, DC, USA, 20–24 October 2017.

39. Yuen, M.-F.; Agarwal, K.; Gane, E.J.; Schwabe, C.; Ahn, S.-H.; Kim, D.-J.; Lim, Y.-S.; Cheng, W.; Sievert, W.; Visvanathan, K.; et al. Safety, pharmacokinetics, and antiviral effects of ABI-H0731, a hepatitis B virus core inhibitor: A randomised, placebo-controlled phase 1 trial. *Lancet Gastroenterol. Hepatol.* **2020**, *5*, 152–166. [CrossRef]
40. Xiaoli, M.A.; Lalezari, J.; Nguyen, T.; Bae, H.; Schiff, E.R.; Fung, S.; Yuen, M.-F.; Hassanein, T.; Hann, H.-W.; Elkhashab, M.; et al. Interim Safety and Efficacy Results of the ABI-H0731 Phase 2a Program Exploring the Combination of ABI-H0731 with Nuc Therapy in Treatment-Naïve and Treatment-Suppressed Chronic Hepatitis B Patients. In Proceedings of the International Liver Congress EASL-European Association for the Study of the Liver, Vienna, Austria, 10–14 April 2019.
41. Al-Mahtab, M.; Bazinet, M.; Vaillant, A. Safety and efficacy of nucleic acid polymers in monotherapy and combined with immunotherapy in treatment-naive bangladeshi patients with HBeAg + chronic Hepatitis B infection. *PLoS ONE* **2016**, *11*, e0156667. [CrossRef] [PubMed]
42. Bazinet, M.; Pântea, V.; Placinta, G.; Moscalu, I.; Cebotarescu, V.; Cojuhari, L.; Jimbei, P.; Iarovoi, L.; Smesnoi, V.; Mustetea, T.; et al. Safety and efficacy of 48 weeks REP 2139 or REP 2165, tenofovir disoproxil, and pegylated interferon alfa-2a in patients with chronic HBV infection naïve to nucleos(t)ide therapy. *Gastroenterology* **2020**, *158*, 2180–2194. [CrossRef] [PubMed]
43. Farci, P.; Mandas, A.; Coiana, A.; Lai, M.E.; Desmet, V.; Van Eyken, P.; Gibo, Y.; Caruso, L.; Scaccabarozzi, S.; Criscuolo, D.; et al. Treatment of chronic Hepatitis D with interferon alfa-2a. *N. Engl. J. Med.* **1994**, *330*, 88–94. [CrossRef] [PubMed]
44. Erhardt, A.; Gerlich, W.; Starke, C.; Wend, U.; Donner, A.; Sagir, A.; Heintges, T.; Haussinger, D. Treatment of chronic hepatitis delta with pegylated interferon-α2b. *Liver Int.* **2006**, *26*, 805–810. [CrossRef] [PubMed]
45. Abbas, Z.; Khan, M.A.; Salih, M.; Jafri, W. Interferon alpha for chronic hepatitis D. *Cochr. Database Syst. Rev.* **2011**, *2011*, CD006002. [CrossRef] [PubMed]
46. Triantos, C.; Kalafateli, M.; Nikolopoulou, V.; Burroughs, A. Meta-analysis: Antiviral treatment for hepatitis D. *Aliment. Pharmacol. Ther.* **2012**, *35*, 663–673. [CrossRef]
47. Ouzan, D.; Pénaranda, G.; Joly, H.; Halfon, P. Optimized HBsAg titer monitoring improves interferon therapy in patients with chronic hepatitis delta. *J. Hepatol.* **2013**, *58*, 1258–1259. [CrossRef]
48. Niro, G.A.; Smedile, A.; Fontana, R.; Olivero, A.; Ciancio, A.; Valvano, M.R.; Pittaluga, F.; Coppola, N.; Wedemeyer, H.; Zachou, K.; et al. HBsAg kinetics in chronic hepatitis D during interferon therapy: On-treatment prediction of response. *Aliment. Pharmacol. Ther.* **2016**, *44*, 620–628. [CrossRef]
49. Sbarigia, U.; Vincken, T.; Wigfield, P.; Hashim, M.; Heeg, B.; Postma, M. A comparative network meta-analysis of standard of care treatments in treatment-naïve chronic hepatitis B patients. *J. Comp. Eff. Res.* **2020**, *9*, 1051–1065. [CrossRef]
50. Papatheodoridi, M.; Papatheodoridis, G. Can we stop nucleoside analogues before HB sAg loss? *J. Viral Hepat.* **2019**, *26*, 936–941. [CrossRef]
51. Dusheiko, G. Will we need novel combinations to cure HBV infection? *Liver Int.* **2020**, *40*, 35–42. [CrossRef]
52. Wang, C.H.; Chang, K.K.; Lin, R.C.; Kuo, M.J.; Yang, C.C.; Tseng, Y.T. Consolidation period of 18 months no better at promoting off-treatment durability in HBeAg-positive chronic hepatitis B patients with tenofovir disoproxil fumarate treatment than a 12-month period: A prospective randomized cohort study. *Medicine* **2020**, *99*, e19907. [CrossRef]
53. Papatheodoridi, M.; Papatheodoridis, G. Emerging diagnostic tools to decide when to discontinue nucleos(t)ide analogues in chronic Hepatitis, B. *Cells* **2020**, *9*, 493. [CrossRef] [PubMed]
54. Terrault, N.A.; Lok, A.S.F.; McMahon, B.J.; Chang, K.M.; Hwang, J.P.; Jonas, M.M.; Brown, R.S., Jr.; Bzowej, N.H.; Wong, J.B. Update on prevention, diagnosis, and treatment of chronic Hepatitis B: AASLD 2018 Hepatitis B guidance. *Clin. Liver Dis.* **2018**, *12*, 33–34. [CrossRef] [PubMed]
55. Sarin, S.K.; Kumar, M.; Lau, G.K.; Abbas, Z.; Chan, H.L.; Chen, C.J.; Chen, D.S.; Chen, H.L.; Chen, P.J.; Chien, R.N.; et al. Asian-Pacific clinical practice guidelines on the management of Hepatitis B: A 2015 update. *Hepatol. Int.* **2016**, *10*, 1–98. [CrossRef] [PubMed]
56. Liu, Y.; Jia, M.; Wu, S.; Jiang, W.; Feng, Y. Predictors of relapse after cessation of nucleos(t)ide analog treatment in HBeAg-negative chronic hepatitis B patients: A meta-analysis. *Int. J. Infect. Dis.* **2019**, *86*, 201–207. [CrossRef] [PubMed]
57. Matsumoto, A.; Tanaka, E.; Minami, M.; Okanoue, T.; Yatsuhashi, H.; Nagaoka, S.; Suzuki, F.; Kobayashi, M.; Chayama, K.; Imamura, M.; et al. Low serum level of hepatitis B core-related antigen indicates unlikely reactivation of hepatitis after cessation of lamivudine therapy. *Hepatol. Res.* **2007**, *37*, 661–666. [CrossRef] [PubMed]
58. Liaw, Y.-F. Finite nucleos(t)ide analog therapy in HBeAg-negative chronic Hepatitis B: An emerging paradigm shift. *Hepatol. Int.* **2019**, *13*, 665–673. [CrossRef]
59. Xie, L.; Liao, G.; Chen, H.; Xia, M.; Huang, X.; Fan, R.; Peng, J.; Zhang, X.; Liu, H. Elevated expression of serum soluble ST2 in clinical relapse after stopping long-term Nucleos(t)ide analogue therapy for chronic Hepatitis B. *BMC Infect. Dis.* **2019**, *19*, 640. [CrossRef]
60. Hanrahan, E.O.; Kies, M.S.; Glisson, B.S.; Khuri, F.R.; Feng, L.; Tran, H.T.; Ginsberg, L.E.; Truong, M.T.; Hong, W.K.; Kim, E.S. A Phase II study of lonafarnib (SCH66336) in patients with chemorefractory, Advanced squamous cell carcinoma of the head and neck. *Am. J. Clin. Oncol.* **2009**, *32*, 274–279. [CrossRef] [PubMed]
61. Meier, W.; du Bois, A.; Rau, J.; Gropp-Meier, M.; Baumann, K.; Huober, J.; Wollschlaeger, K.; Kreienberg, R.; Canzler, U.; Schmalfeldt, B.; et al. Randomized phase II trial of carboplatin and paclitaxel with or without lonafarnib in first-line treatment of epithelial ovarian cancer stage IIB–IV. *Gynecol. Oncol.* **2012**, *126*, 236–240. [CrossRef]

62. Kim, E.S.; Kies, M.S.; Fossella, F.V.; Glisson, B.S.; Zaknoen, S.; Statkevich, P.; Munden, R.F.; Summey, C.; Pisters, K.M.; Papadimitrakopoulou, V.; et al. Phase II study of the farnesyltransferase inhibitor lonafarnib with paclitaxel in patients with taxane-refractory/resistant nonsmall cell lung carcinoma. *Cancer* **2005**, *104*, 561–569. [CrossRef]

63. Feldman, E.J.; Cortes, J.; DeAngelo, D.J.; Holyoake, T.; Simonsson, B.; O'Brien, S.G.; Reiffers, J.; Turner, A.R.; Roboz, G.J.; Lipton, J.H.; et al. On the use of lonafarnib in myelodysplastic syndrome and chronic myelomonocytic leukemia. *Leukemia* **2008**, *22*, 1707–1711. [CrossRef]

64. Sharma, S.; Kemeny, N.; Kelsen, D.P.; Ilson, D.; O'Reilly, E.; Zaknoen, S.; Baum, C.; Statkevich, P.; Hollywood, E.; Zhu, Y. A phase II trial of farnesyl protein transferase inhibitor SCH 66336, given by twice-daily oral administration, in patients with metastatic colorectal cancer refractory to 5-fluorouracil and irinotecan. *Ann. Oncol.* **2002**, *13*, 1067–1071. [CrossRef] [PubMed]

65. Winquist, E.; Moore, M.J.; Chi, K.N.; Ernst, D.S.; Hirte, H.; North, S.; Powers, J.; Walsh, W.; Boucher, T.; Patton, R.; et al. A multinomial phase II study of lonafarnib (SCH 66336) in patients with refractory urothelial cancer. *Urol. Oncol. Semin. Orig. Investig.* **2005**, *23*, 143–149. [CrossRef] [PubMed]

66. Buresh, A.; Perentesis, J.; Rimsza, L.; Kurtin, S.; Heaton, R.; Sugrue, M.; List, A. Hyperleukocytosis complicating lonafarnib treatment in patients with chronic myelomonocytic leukemia. *Leukemia* **2005**, *19*, 308–310. [CrossRef]

67. Eskens, F.A.; Awada, A.; Cutler, D.L.; de Jonge, M.J.; Luyten, G.P.; Faber, M.N.; Statkevich, P.; Sparreboom, A.; Verweij, J.; Hanauske, A.R.; et al. Phase I and pharmacokinetic study of the oral farnesyl transferase inhibitor SCH 66336 given twice daily to patients with advanced solid tumors. *J. Clin. Oncol.* **2001**, *19*, 1167–1175. [CrossRef]

68. Awada, A.; Eskens, F.A.; Piccart, M.; Cutler, D.L.; van der Gaast, A.; Bleiberg, H.; Wanders, J.; Faber, M.N.; Statkevich, P.; Fumoleau, P.; et al. Phase I and pharmacological study of the oral farnesyltransferase inhibitor SCH 66336 given once daily to patients with advanced solid tumours. *Eur. J. Cancer* **2002**, *38*, 2272–2278. [CrossRef]

69. Wong, N.S.; Meadows, K.L.; Rosen, L.S.; Adjei, A.A.; Kaufmann, S.H.; Morse, M.A.; Petros, W.P.; Zhu, Y.; Statkevich, P.; Cutler, D.L.; et al. A phase I multicenter study of continuous oral administration of lonafarnib (SCH 66336) and intravenous gemcitabine in patients with advanced cancer. *Cancer Investig.* **2011**, *29*, 617–625. [CrossRef] [PubMed]

70. Cortes, J.; Jabbour, E.; Daley, G.Q.; O'Brien, S.; Verstovsek, S.; Ferrajoli, A.; Koller, C.; Zhu, Y.; Statkevich, P.; Kantarjian, H. Phase 1 study of lonafarnib (SCH 66336) and imatinib mesylate in patients with chronic myeloid leukemia who have failed prior single-agent therapy with imatinib. *Cancer* **2007**, *110*, 1295–1302. [CrossRef] [PubMed]

71. Khuri, F.R.; Glisson, B.S.; Kim, E.S.; Statkevich, P.; Thall, P.F.; Meyers, M.L.; Herbst, R.S.; Munden, R.F.; Tendler, C.; Zhu, Y.; et al. Phase I study of the farnesyltransferase inhibitor lonafarnib with paclitaxel in solid tumors. *Clin. Cancer Res.* **2004**, *10*, 2968–2976. [CrossRef] [PubMed]

72. Kieran, M.W.; Packer, R.J.; Onar, A.; Blaney, S.M.; Phillips, P.; Pollack, I.F.; Geyer, J.R.; Gururangan, S.; Banerjee, A.; Goldman, S.; et al. Phase I and pharmacokinetic study of the oral farnesyltransferase inhibitor lonafarnib administered twice daily to pediatric patients with advanced central nervous system tumors using a modified continuous reassessment method: A pediatric brain tumor consortium study. *J. Clin. Oncol.* **2007**, *25*, 3137–3143. [PubMed]

73. Gordon, L.B.; Kleinman, M.E.; Miller, D.T.; Neuberg, D.S.; Giobbie-Hurder, A.; Gerhard-Herman, M.; Smoot, L.B.; Gordon, C.M.; Cleveland, R.; Snyder, B.D.; et al. Clinical trial of a farnesyltransferase inhibitor in children with Hutchinson-Gilford progeria syndrome. *Proc. Natl. Acad. Sci. USA* **2012**, *109*, 16666–16671. [CrossRef] [PubMed]

74. Gordon, L.B.; Massaro, J.; D'Agostino Sr, R.B.; Campbell, S.E.; Brazier, J.; Brown, W.T.; Kleinman, M.E.; Kieran, M.W.; Progeria Clinical Trials Collaborative. Impact of farnesylation inhibitors on survival in hutchinson-gilford progeria syndrome. *Circulation* **2014**, *130*, 27–34. [CrossRef] [PubMed]

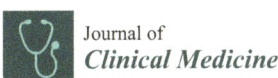

Journal of
Clinical Medicine

Review

Emerging Therapies for Advanced Cholangiocarcinoma: An Updated Literature Review

Anthony Vignone [1,*,†], **Francesca Biancaniello** [1,*,†], **Marco Casadio** [1], **Ludovica Pesci** [1], **Vincenzo Cardinale** [2],
Lorenzo Ridola [1] and **Domenico Alvaro** [1]

1   Department of Translational and Precision Medicine, Sapienza University of Rome, Viale dell'Università 37, 00185 Rome, Italy; marco.casadio@uniroma1.it (M.C.); ludovica.pesci@uniroma1.it (L.P.); lorenzo.ridola@uniroma1.it (L.R.); domenico.alvaro@uniroma1.it (D.A.)

2   Department of Medical-Surgical and Biotechnologies Sciences, Polo Pontino, Sapienza University of Rome, Corso della Repubblica 79, 04100 Latina, Italy; vincenzo.cardinale@uniroma1.it

*   Correspondence: anthony.vignone@uniroma1.it (A.V.); francesca.biancaniello@uniroma1.it (F.B.)

†   These authors contributed equally to this paper.

Abstract: Cholangiocarcinoma is a group of malignancies with poor prognosis. Treatments for the management of advanced-stage cholangiocarcinoma are limited, and the 5-year survival rate is estimated to be approximately 5–15%, considering all tumor stages. There is a significant unmet need for effective new treatment approaches. The present review is provided with the aim of summarizing the current evidence and future perspectives concerning new therapeutic strategies for cholangiocarcinoma. The role of targeted therapies and immunotherapies is currently investigational in cholangiocarcinoma. These therapeutic options might improve survival outcomes, as shown by the promising results of several clinical trials illustrated in the present review. The co-presence of driver mutations and markers of susceptibility to immunotherapy may lead to rational combination strategies and clinical trial development. A better understanding of immunologically based therapeutic weapons is needed, which will lead to a form of a precision medicine strategy capable of alleviating the clinical aggressiveness and to improve the prognosis of cholangiocarcinoma.

Keywords: cholangiocarcinoma; targeted therapy; immunotherapy

Citation: Vignone, A.; Biancaniello, F.; Casadio, M.; Pesci, L.; Cardinale, V.; Ridola, L.; Alvaro, D. Emerging Therapies for Advanced Cholangiocarcinoma: An Updated Literature Review. *J. Clin. Med.* **2021**, *10*, 4901. https://doi.org/10.3390/jcm10214901

Academic Editor: Pierluigi Toniutto

Received: 28 September 2021
Accepted: 22 October 2021
Published: 24 October 2021

Publisher's Note: MDPI stays neutral with regard to jurisdictional claims in published maps and institutional affiliations.

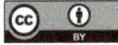
1. Introduction

Cholangiocarcinoma (CCA) is a rare malignant tumor that develops from the epithelium of the bile ducts or peribiliary glands (PBGs). Although CCA is considered a rare tumor in Western countries, it represents 3% of all gastrointestinal malignant tumors worldwide and the second most common primary liver cancer [1]. In Eastern countries, the incidence is higher than in Western ones, where it is estimated to be lower than 4 cases/100,000 people/year [2]. Northeast Thailand has the highest CCA rate in the world (90 cases/100,000 people/year) [3]. The highest incidence rate is in the seventh decade, with a slight prevalence in males. Due to classification coding (four different ICD-10 sub-codes) and variable terminology, CCA burden has been underestimated. CCA is the first cause of metastasis of unknown origin, and this further highlights how we still do not know the real burden of CCA [4]. While a reduction of the mortality rate from other cancers, including breast, lung, and colon cancer, has been observed in 1990–2009 (USA data), the mortality rate for liver and bile ducts tumors increased by more than 40% and 60% in females and males, respectively. While the mortality rate from hepatocellular carcinoma (HCC) has become more uniform across Europe, intrahepatic CCA mortality has substantially increased [5].

Anatomically, three types of cholangiocarcinoma can be distinguished: intrahepatic (iCCA), perihilar (pCCA) and distal (dCCA). Histologically, these are different kinds of tumors, considering cholangiocarcinogenesis as a process that starts from several cells of

137

origin. In particular, pCCA and dCCA are mainly mucinous adenocarcinomas, while iCCA is highly heterogeneous, since it could resemble conventional mucinous adenocarcinomas (large-duct type iCCA), similar to p/dCCA, or transformed interlobular bile ducts (small-duct type iCCA).

Currently, surgical resection with negative margins represents the best potentially curative therapy of CCA. Therapeutic options for the management of advanced-stage CCA are limited, and the 5-year survival rate is estimated to be approximately 5–15%, considering all tumor stages [6]. Cisplatin plus gemcitabine (GEMCIS) represents the first-line treatment for these patients, as established by the phase II BT22 trial and the phase III ABC-02 trial [7,8].

Few studies have enrolled specifically iCCA patients or have reported the anatomic subtypes of CCA (iCCA, pCCA, and dCCA). Many studies reviewed here concerned biliary tract cancers (BTCs), enrolling together CCA and gallbladder cancer (GBC) patients. Neglecting CCA heterogeneity in the study design, in terms of anatomical, histological, and molecular subtypes, might represent a strong limitation in patients' allocation to clinical trials. Moreover, given the possibilities shown by the development of targeted therapies, molecular profiling and efficient biomarkers would be needed to select the best therapeutic option for each patient [9].

The present review aims at summarizing the current evidence and future perspectives with regards to new therapeutic strategies for advanced CCA. Most drugs summarized in the following paragraphs are already used in the management of some oncological diseases, such as PD-L1 inhibitors (Pembrolizumab) that represent the first-line monotherapy for advanced non-small cell lung cancer (NSCLC) with a programmed death ligand 1 tumor proportion score of 50% or greater and without EGFR/ALK aberrations, based on the results of the phase III trial KEYNOTE 024 [10].

2. Targeted Therapy

2.1. FGFR2 Inhibitors

Approximately 15–20% of iCCAs have been observed to have FGRF2 translocations [11] (fusion or rearrangements), implicated in promoting cell proliferation and angiogenesis. These mutations are almost absent in extrahepatic cholangiocarcinomas. On this basis, several FGFR 1–3 inhibitors have been tested in advanced cholangiocarcinomas patients, showing good antitumor activity and safety. Particularly, the European Medicines Agency (EMA) approved in April 2021 the use of Pemigatinib for previously treated advanced cholangiocarcinomas showing FGFR2 fusion or rearrangement. Furthermore, a phase III study (FIGHT-302) [12] is currently ongoing to test the efficacy of Pemigatinib as a first-line treatment versus chemotherapy in patients with advanced cholangiocarcinoma with FGFR2 mutations (Table 1). The efficacy of Infigratinib (BGJ398), a reversible selective FGFR 1–3 inhibitor, is also under evaluation (NCT03773302) as a first-line treatment for patients with locally advanced or metastatic cholangiocarcinoma harboring FGFR2 mutations (Table 1).

However, point mutations of the FGFR 2 domain have been found capable of conferring resistance to FGFR inhibitors in previously treated patients [13]. In this category of patients, Futibatinib, a selective and irreversible FGFR inhibitor, has shown inhibitory activity and partial response, and a phase III study (Table 1) is underway to test its efficacy as a first-line treatment in patients with advanced CCA (FOENIX-CCA3 and NCT04093362). Another reversible ATP competitive inhibitor, Erdafitinib, showed promising result in a phase I–II study [14].

Table 1. Phase III targeted-therapy trials for BTC.

NCT	Phase	Condition or Disease	N. Patients	Regimen	Line of Therapy	Results
NCT02989857 ClarIDHy	III	Advanced and Metastatic CCA	187	Ivosidenib	II	OS: 8–10 months Median PFS: 2–7 months
NCT01149122	III	Advanced BTC	103	GEMOX + Erlotinib	I	ORR: 48% Median PFS: 7.3 months OS: 10.7 months
NCT03093870	II/III	BTC	151	Varlitinib + Capecitabine	I	ORR: 9.4% Median PFS: 2.8 months
NCT03345303	III	iCCA	50	Bortezomib	II	-
NCT03656536 Fight302	III	Advanced, CCA	432	Pemigatinib	I	ORR: 35.5% Median PFS: 6.93 months
NCT03773302	III	Advanced CCA	384	Infigratinib	I	-
NCT04093362	III	Advanced CCA	216	Futibatinib	I	-

2.2. Metabolic Regulator (IDH Inhibitors)

Reprogramming of cancer cells' metabolism has been defined as one of the hallmarks of cancer [15] and represents a possible target for precision medicine. Genomic and transcriptomic studies [16] have demonstrated that isocitrate dehydrogenase 1 and 2 (IDH1, IDH2) mutations occur in 13–25% of iCCA. These enzymes are involved in tricarboxylic acid cycle (TCA), β-oxidation of unsaturated fatty acids, response to oxidative stress, and expression of chromatin remodelers. In IDH1/2-mutated cells, the oncometabolite D-2-dihydroxyglutarate (2-HG) accumulates, leading to metabolic and epigenetic changes, enhanced proliferation, and susceptibility to DNA damage. This pathway may be hampered by inhibitors of IDH1 (AG120) and IDH2 (AG221), such as ivosidenib and enasidinib (NCT02273739), with encouraging results in randomized control trials (RCTs). Patients with IDH1-mutated iCCA who had progressed on previous therapy [17] showed a significant response to ivosidenib when compared to placebo-administered patients in the ClarIDHy phase III double-blind clinical trial (Table 1), in terms of both progression-free survival (2–7 vs. 1–4 months) and overall survival (10–8 vs. 9–7 months). Based on these results, ivosidenib has been recently approved by the FDA for locally advanced and metastatic cholangiocarcinoma with IDH1 mutations. IDH1 inhibitors are currently under investigation also in combination with other treatments. A phase Ib/II basket trial is evaluating Olutasidenib (FT-2102) alone, in combination with azacitidine, nivolumab, or gemcitabine and cisplatin in 200 patients with different solid tumors harboring the same IDH1 mutations (NCT03684811).

2.3. Tyrosine Kinase Inhibitors

Mutations of epidermal growth factor receptors play a pivotal role in different cancers [18], and several drugs are already approved for specific subsets of malignancies, i.e., EGFR-mutated non-small cell lung cancer [19] and colorectal cancer [20]. Nevertheless, convincing evidence of their efficacy in CCA is still lacking.

In the PiCCA phase II randomized clinical trial [21], panitumumab, a monoclonal anti-EGFR1 antibody, was administered in combination with gemcitabine and cisplatin in KRAS-wild-type patients versus gemcitabine and cisplatin alone, but it failed to improve ORR, PFS, and OS. Similar results were obtained in a phase II study in chemotherapy-naive patients with advanced BTC, treated with panitumumab and GEMOX and GEMOX alone. Despite the attempt of selecting patients by IHC, PCR, and Sanger sequencing for KRAS, BRAF, and PI3KCA, no significant survival differences were observed. Nevertheless, it needs to be underlined that the cohorts of these two studies were not specifically tested for enrichment in EGFR alterations [22]. In addition, a phase II clinical trial studied the efficacy of cetuximab combined with GEMOX vs. GEMOX alone in advanced BTC patients; KRAS, NRAS, and BRAF mutations and EGFR expression, were the criteria selected to stratify these patients. Despite a significant difference in progression-free survival, the study did not reach the primary endpoint (ORR) nor demonstrated a higher OS in the cetuximab arm. However, other genetic alterations involved in the EGFR pathway, i.e., ROS1, ALK, or c-MET [23], were not specifically investigated and might have a role in explaining anti-EGFR resistance.

The EGFR inhibitor erlotinib (Table 1) was studied in combination with chemotherapy regimens [24] and bevacizumab [25], but no clear survival benefits were observed when compared to current standard of care. Varlitinib, a competitive inhibitor of the tyrosine kinases EGRF and HER 2–4, is currently under investigation in monotherapy (phase II, NCT02609958) and in combination with capecitabine in advanced BTC patients (phase II/III, NCT03093870) (Table 1).

As far as the HER family is concerned, molecular profiling studies [26] have underlined the frequency of ERRB2 aberrations in p/dCCA, but evidence about the efficacy of anti-HER2 drugs in CCA has not supported their use in clinical practice so far [1]. On these bases, the feasibility of this treatment has already been demonstrated [27], and several phase II clinical trials are currently evaluating the efficacy of combination treatments with trastuzumab and tucatinib (NCT04579380) and with chemotherapy (NCT04430738).

Combination treatments with bevacizumab and gemcitabine or capecitabine have been tested in a multicenter phase II trial, given the high prevalence of VEGF overexpression in CCA [28]. Nevertheless, the patients were not selected based on their mutational profile, and this may be responsible for the poor outcome of the study.

The lack of patients' stratification may have also affected the results of different clinical trials that evaluated the multikinase inhibitor sorafenib, also targeting VEGFR2 and 3 [29]. Adding sorafenib to GEM–CIS in biliary tract cancer showed increased treatment toxicity without simultaneous clinical benefits in a phase II RCT [30] including biliary adenocarcinomas of all subtypes without taking into account histological and molecular differences. Sun et al. [31] have shown that regorafenib improved PFS of (15.6 weeks) and OS (31.8 weeks) in advanced BTC patients with disease progression after first-line therapy. Targeting neurotrophic tyrosine kinase receptor (NTKR) fusions has seemed promising, too [32]. Two phase II basket trials have investigated entrectinib [33] and larotrectinib [34]. FDA and EMA have approved larotrectinib and entrectinib as "wildcard" drugs that can be used in every kind of malignancy harboring this genetic alteration, regardless of the anatomical origin. Unfortunately, NTKR fusions are rarely detected in CCA [35].

2.4. Proteasome Inhibitors

Mutations/deletions of the PTEN gene were observed in approximately 5% of iCCAs associated with poor prognosis [6]. It was also observed that PTEN mutation/deletion is also associated with increased activity of proteasomes in iCCAs. On these bases, a phase III study (Table 1) is actually evaluating the efficacy of Bortezomib, a proteasome inhibitor, in patients with advanced iCCA who have progressed after at least two cycles of systemic chemotherapy (NCT03345303).

3. Immunotherapy

Since 2010, immunotherapy has been one of the most important strategies in the treatment of malignancies, together with surgery, chemotherapy, radiotherapy, and targeted therapy, even if its efficacy is very variable, and only a percentage of patients obtain a durable response [36]. The mechanism of immunotherapy is to enhance the anti-tumor immune response, including both adaptative cells (B and T cells) and innate cells such as macrophages, neutrophils, natural killers. Immunotherapy includes immune checkpoint inhibitors (ICIs) targeting programmed death 1 (PD-1), programmed death-ligand 1 (PD-L1), and cytotoxic T lymphocyte antigen-4 (CTLA-4), cancer vaccines, and adoptive cell transfer (ACT). Several factors can influence the effect of immunotherapy-based treatments: the environment of tumor and immune cells, vascularization, extracellular matrix, and molecular signaling pathway [37]. Several therapeutic options in patients affected by biliary tract cancers are under investigation, such as immunotherapeutic strategies with checkpoint inhibitors, peptide- and dendritic cell-based vaccines, and adoptive cell therapy, in monotherapy or in combination with targeted therapy and/or chemotherapy. Nowadays, scientific evidence on the use of immunotherapy in CCA are limited, although different trials are currently investigating the role of anti-CTLA-4 monoclonal antibodies, the targeting of PD-L1 or its receptor, PD-1, and chimeric antigen receptor T (CAR-T) cell immunotherapy. Unfortunately, checkpoint inhibitor monotherapy has shown low efficacy in CCA patients. Indeed, Pembrolizumab, a PD-L1 inhibitor, demonstrated a median progression-free survival of 1.8 months in patients affected by CCA in the phase Ib basket trial KEYNOTE 028 [38]. Checkpoint inhibitors showed encouraging results in patients with microsatellite instability or DNA mismatch repair in the KEYNOTE 158 trial [39], even if only a small percentage of patients with a positive response to this kind of treatment reported a better clinical response [40]. Pembrolizumab demonstrated good efficacy in a recent Korean study that retrospectively analyzed 51 patients with PD-L1-positive CisGem-refractory biliary tract cancer. In PD-L1-positive patients, pembrolizumab showed durable efficacy, with a 9.8% response rate with manageable adverse events. Ongoing studies and clinical trials are currently exploring combined immunotherapeutic approaches targeting both the innate and the adaptive immune system, and/or combined strategies also involving chemotherapy or radiation.

Particularly, there are many ongoing phase I–III trials exploring the role of targeting PD-L1, its receptor PD-1, anti CTL-A4 with monoclonal antibodies in monotherapy or in combination with chemotherapy, targeted therapy, local ablative therapy, and the role of CAR-T cell immunotherapy in biliary tract cancer (Tables 2 and 3). In particular, KEYNOTE-028 and KEYNOTE-158, two multicentric, non-randomized, open-label, phase IB and II trials, showed a durable antitumor activity of Pembrolizumab in 6–13% of patients with advanced BTC. In KEYNOTE-158, they observed a median progression free survival (PFS) of 2.0 months and a Median overall survival (OS) of 7.4 months; adverse events were mainly mild to moderate in severity [39]. Another immunotherapeutic agent, Nivolumab showed a response rate of 22% and a disease control rate of 59% in a Phase II multi-institutional study including 46 patients affected by advanced biliary tract cancer in second-line therapy [41].

The combination of immunotherapy and chemotherapy looks promising. Two Phase III trials are evaluating the efficacy and safety of KN035 plus Gemcitabine–Oxaliplatin compared to standard of care Gemcitabine–Oxaliplatin therapy (NCT03478488) and the association of Durvalumab and Gemcitabine plus cisplatin (NCT03875235). BilT-01, a multicenter randomized Phase II trial, described a prolonged PFS six months after the addition of nivolumab to gemcitabine and cisplatin (NCT02829918) [42]. LEAP 005 demonstrated a promising antitumor activity and manageable toxicity of Pembrolizumab in combination with Lenvatinib in 31 patients affected by BTC [43].

Regarding Adoptive Cell Therapy (ACT), a phase III, non-randomized trial is studying the role of cytokine-induced killer cells in association with radiofrequency ablation in 50 patients with CCA (NCT02482454).

Table 2. Ongoing immunotherapy trials of biliary tract cancers.

NCT	Phase	Condition or Disease	Number of Patients	Regimen	Status
ICI MONOTHERAPY					
NCT03110328	II	Advanced or refractory BTC	33	Pemrolizumab	Recruiting
NCT02054806 KEYNOTE-28	IB	Incurable advanced PD-L1 positive cancers, including BTC	477	Pembrolizumab	Completed
NCT02628067 KEYNOTE-158	IIA	Advanced, refractory solid cancer including BTC	1595	Pemrolizumab	Recruiting
NCT02829918	II	Advanced refractory BTC	54	Nivolumab	Active, not recruiting
NCT03867370	IB-II	Operable HCC o iCC	40	Toripalimab	Recruiting
DUAL ICI					
NCT03101566	II	BTC	75	Nivolumab+ Ipilimumab	Active, not recruiting
ICI IN COMBINATION WITH CHEMOTHERAPY					
NCT03473574	II	Naïve BTC	128	Durvalumab + tremelimumab + GEM or GEMCIS vs. GEMCIS chemotherapy	Active, not recruiting
NCT03046862	II	Unresectable, untreated BTC	31	Durvalumab + Tremelimumab + GEMCIS chemotherapy	Recruiting
NCT03704480	II	Advanced BTC	106	Durvalumab + tremelimumab + paclitaxel	Recruiting
NCT03875235	III	Advanced BTC	757	Durvalumab + GEMCIS vs GEMCIS + chemotherapy	Recruiting
NCT03257761	Ib	Unresecable, refractory HCC, PDAC, BTC excluding ampullary	90	Durvalumab + guadecitabine	Recruiting
NCT03111732	II	Unresecable, refractory BTC	11	Pemrolizumab + Oxaliplatine + Capecitabine	Active, not recruiting
NCT03260712	II	Unresecable, untreated BTC	50	Pemrolizumab + GEMCIS	Recruiting
NCT03796429	II	Advanced BTC	40	Gemcitabine + Toripalimab	Recruiting
NCT03101566	II	Unresecable, untreatable BTC	75	Nivolumab + Ipilimumab vs GEMCIS + Nivolumab	Active, not recruiting
NCT03785873	I/II	Unresecable, refractory BTC	40	Nivolumab + nal-irinotecan + 5-fluorouracil + leucovorin	Recruiting
NCT03478488	III	Unresecable, untreatable BTC	480	KN035 + GEMOX vs. GEMOX + chemotherapy	Recruiting
ICI IN COMBINATION WITH TARGETED THERAPY					
NCT03797326	II	Advanced, refractory solid tumours, including BTC	590	Lenvatinib + pembrolizumab	Recruiting
NCT02393248	I/II	Advanced solid tumour malignancy, including CCA		Pembrolizumab +pemigatinib	Recruiting

Table 2. *Cont.*

NCT	Phase	Condition or Disease	Number of Patients	Regimen	Status
NCT03684811	I/II	BTC, iCC and other Hepatobiliary Carcinomas with IDH1 mutation	200	Nivolumab +FT-2102	Active, not recruiting
NCT03201458	Phase II	Metastatic BTC or gallbladder cancer	76	Atezolizumab + Cobimetinib	Active, not recruiting
NCT03639935	Phase II	Advance metastatic BTC	35	Nivolumab + Rucaparib	Recruiting
NCT03991832	Phase II	Solid tumours including IDH-mutated CCA	78	Olaparib and Durvalumab	Recruiting
ICI IN COMBINATION WITH LOCAL ABLATIVE THERAPY					
NCT02821754	II	Refractory or unresecable HCC or BTC	90	Durvalumab + Tremelimumab, Durvalumab + Tremelimumab + procedure (RFA or TACE or Cryoablation)	Recruiting
NCT03898895	II	Unresecable iCCA, eligible for RT	184	Pembrolizumab + SBRT	Recruiting
NCT03482102	II	Unresecable HCC or BTC	70	Durvalumab + tremelimumab + RT	Recruiting
TME TARGETED THERAPY					
NCT03314935	I/II	Malignant tumours including BTC	149	INCB001158 + FOLFOX/gemcitabine + cisplatin/paclitaxel	Active, not recruiting
NCT03329950	I	Malignant tumours including CCA	260	CDX-1140 (CD40 antibody), either alone or in combination with CDX-301 (FLT3L), pembrolizumab, or chemotherapy	Recruiting
NCT03071757	I	Locally advanced or metastatic solid tumours including CCA	170	ABBV-368 and ABBV-368 + Budigalimab (ABBV-181)	Active, not recruiting
ACT THERAPY					
NCT03820310	II	iCC after radical resection	20	Autologous Tcm Cellular Immunotherapy Combined with Traditional Therapy	Recruiting
NCT03801083	II	Locally Advanced, Recurrent, or Metastatic BTC	59	Tumour Infiltrating Lymphocyte	Recruiting
NCT03633773	I/II	iCC	9	MUC-1 CAR-T cell immunotherapy after fludarabine and cyclophosphamide	Recruiting
NCT02482454	III	Unresected CCA, withoutextrahepatic metastasis	50	Autologous cytokine-induced killer cells (CIK) after RFA	Active, not recruiting

ACT: adoptive cellular therapy, BTC: biliary tract cancer, CAR-T cell: chimeric antigen receptor T cell, CCA: cholangiocarcinoma, FOLFOX: folinic acid (leucovorin) + 5-fluorouracil + oxaliplatin, GEM: gemcitabine, GEMCIS: gemcitabine + cisplatin, HCC: hepatocellular carcinoma, iCC: intrahepatic cholangiocarcinoma, ICI: immune-checkpoint inhibitors, MUC-1: mucin 1, PDAC: pancreatic ductal adenocarcinoma, RFA: radiofrequency ablation, RT: radiotherapy, SBRT: stereotactic body radiation therapy, TACE: trans-arterial chemo embolization, TME: tumor microenvironment.

Table 3. Ongoing immunotherapy trials for BTC with preliminary results.

NCT	Phase	Condition or Disease	N. Patients	Regimen	Results
NCT02054806 KEYNOTE-28	IB	Incurable advanced PD-L1 positive cancers, including BTC	477	Pembrolizumab	ORR: 13% Median PFS: 2 months
NCT02628067 KEYNOTE-158	IIA	Advanced, refractory solid cancer including BTC	1595	Pemrolizumab	ORR: 5.8% Median PFS: 1.8 months
NCT02829918	II	Advanced refractory BTC	54	Nivolumab	ORR: 22% Median PFS: 3.8 monthd
NCT03797326	II	Advanced, refractory solid tumours, including BTC	590	Lenvatinib + pembrolizumab	ORR: 16%

4. Clinical-Pathological and Radiomic Monotherapy Susceptibility in Patients with Cholangiocarcinoma

Within the CCA clinical-pathological spectrum, the pattern of tumor growth has been correlated with specific histological features, e.g., small-bile duct iCCAs and cholangiolocarcinoma (CLC) showed a mass-forming growth pattern, while large-bile duct iCCAs showed both a mass-forming growth pattern and a combination of a mass-forming growth pattern with a periductal infiltrative growth pattern, the latter being the typical pattern of growth of pCCA [44]. Mass-forming iCCAs showed more heterogeneous clinical-pathological characteristics than other gross types [45]. Radiologically, at dynamic contrast-enhanced imaging, all large-bile duct iCCAs showed concentric filling at the venous phase, whereas small-bile duct iCCAs/CLCs showed washout in various patterns, in a clinical-pathological study including correlates with magnetic resonance imaging [44].

The USA Food and Drug Administration approved the use of pembrolizumab for patients with advanced solid tumors lacking the expression of mismatch repair (MMR) proteins (MLH1, MSH2, MSH6, and PMS2) or having high microsatellite instability (MSI-H) [46]. MMR proteins can be inactivated through somatic or germline mutations or they can be silenced through promoter hypermethylation, e.g., of the MLH1 gene [47]. These alterations culminate to hypermutation during DNA replication (MSI) and may lead to the development of malignancies [48]. Interestingly, such molecular alterations predispose to an increase of the neoantigen load of the tumor, promoting susceptibility to immunotherapies targeting the PD-1 pathway because of the increased inflammation surrounding these tumors [40].

Given the potential for immunotherapy in patients with CCA, authors studied the expression of PD-L1/PD-1 and evaluated the presence of associated genetic alterations. For example, in 652 biliary tract cancers that comprised 77 p/dCCA, 372 iCCA, and 203 gallbladder cancer (GBC), 8.6% tumors were PD-L1-positive [GBC 12.3% (25/203), iCCA 7.3% (27/372), and p/dCCA 5.2% (4/77)]. Interestingly, there was an increase in BRAF, BRCA2, RNF43, and TP53 mutations in the PD-L1-positive group with respect to the PD-L1-negative one. Furthermore, there was an association between PD-L1 expression and certain biomarkers (TOP2A, TMB high, MSI-H). As noted by the authors, the aforementioned combinations of molecular alterations might direct the use of rational combination strategies and clinical trial development [49]. On the same line, Ju et al. analyzed 96 cases of CCA for morphology using H&E staining and for mutations of MMR genes using immunohistochemical staining. The authors found that 6% of the samples showed MMR deficiency (MMR-d). Divided by location, 10% (3 of 31) of iCCA and 5% (3 of 65) of p/dCCA were MMR-d. The best predictive factor for MMR-d was a nontypical infiltrating pattern of invasion [50].

The increasing awareness of CCA heterogeneity at the morphological and molecular levels, together with the advent of radiomic, artificial intelligence (AI), and machine learning, has revitalized the study of radiological correlates. For example, it has been shown that the magnetic resonance imaging texture signature, including three wavelets and one 3D feature, has the ability to discriminate inflamed from non-inflamed immunophenotypes based on the density of CD8+ T cells. This may be a surrogate of the response to immune checkpoint blockade [51]. The preoperative prediction of PD-1/PD-L1 expression and outcome in iCCA patients using magnetic resonance biomarkers and a machine learning approach has been attempted [52]. Utilizing qualitative and quantitative imaging traits, reasonable accuracy in predicting tumor grade and higher AJCC stage in iCCA has been shown [53].

5. Conclusions

The role of targeted therapy and immunotherapy in the treatment of CCA is currently under investigation. These options might improve survival outcomes (OS and PFS), as shown by the promising results of several clinical trials illustrated in the present review. This is even more important considering the poor therapeutic options in the management of CCA. The co-presence of driver mutations and markers of susceptibility to immunotherapy may lead to rational therapeutic combination strategies and clinical trial development. The combination of new therapeutic strategies, such as targeted therapy and immunotherapy, with conventional chemotherapy and/or locoregional treatments could be the next frontier for the treatment of advanced CCA. The evaluation of innovative strategies for the prediction of immunotherapy susceptibility, such as multi omics, preferably within longitudinal clinical trials, and the use of systems of data analysis based on the precepts of AI, may circumvent the lack of therapeutic biomarkers for immunotherapy. A better understanding of immunological-based therapeutic weapons is needed, which will lead to a form of a precision medicine strategy capable of alleviating the clinical aggressiveness and to improve the prognosis of CCA.

Author Contributions: All authors: writing—review and editing. All authors have read and agreed to the published version of the manuscript.

Funding: This research received no external funding.

Conflicts of Interest: The authors declare no conflict of interest.

References

1. Banales, J.M.; Marin, J.J.G.; Lamarca, A.; Rodrigues, P.M.; Khan, S.A.; Roberts, L.R.; Cardinale, V.; Carpino, G.; Andersen, J.B.; Braconi, C.; et al. Cholangiocarcinoma 2020: The next horizon in mechanisms and management. *Nat. Rev. Gastroenterol. Hepatol.* **2020**, *17*, 577–588. [CrossRef]
2. Khan, S.A.; Tavolari, S.; Brandi, G. Cholangiocarcinoma: Epidemiology and risk factors. *Liver Int.* **2019**, *39*, 19–31. [CrossRef]
3. Shin, H.-R.; Oh, J.-K.; Masuyer, E.; Curado, M.-P.; Bouvard, V.; Fang, Y.; Wiangnon, S.; Sripa, B.; Hong, S.-T. Comparison of incidence of intrahepatic and extrahepatic cholangiocarcinoma–focus on East and South-Eastern Asia. *Asian Pac. J. Cancer Prev.* **2010**, *11*, 1159–1166.
4. Varadhachary, G.R.; Raber, M.N. Cancer of unknown primary site. *N. Engl. J. Med.* **2014**, *371*, 757–765. [CrossRef] [PubMed]
5. Bertuccio, P.; Bosetti, C.; Levi, F.; Decarli, A.; Negri, E.; La Vecchia, C. A comparison of trends in mortality from primary liver cancer and intrahepatic cholangiocarcinoma in Europe. *Ann. Oncol.* **2013**, *24*, 1667–1674. [CrossRef] [PubMed]
6. Lamarca, A.; Barriuso, J.; McNamara, M.G.; Valle, J.W. Molecular targeted therapies: Ready for 'prime time' in biliary tract cancer. *J. Hepatol.* **2020**, *73*, 170–185. [CrossRef]
7. Valle, J.; Wasan, H.; Palmer, D.H.; Cunningham, D.; Anthoney, A.; Maraveyas, A.; Madhusudan, S.; Iveson, T.; Hughes, S.; Pereira, S.P.; et al. Cisplatin plus Gemcitabine versus Gemcitabine for Biliary Tract Cancer. *N. Engl. J. Med.* **2010**, *362*, 1273–1281. [CrossRef] [PubMed]
8. Okusaka, T.; Nakachi, K.; Fukutomi, A.; Mizuno, N.; Ohkawa, S.; Funakoshi, A.; Nagino, M.; Kondo, S.; Nagaoka, S.; Funai, J.; et al. Gemcitabine alone or in combination with cisplatin in patients with biliary tract cancer: A comparative multicentre study in Japan. *Br. J. Cancer* **2010**, *103*, 469–474. [CrossRef]
9. Nault, J.; Villanueva, A. Biomarkers for Hepatobiliary Cancers. *Hepatology* **2021**, *73*, 115–127. [CrossRef]
10. Reck, M.; Rodríguez-Abreu, D.; Robinson, A.G.; Hui, R.; Csőszi, T.; Fülöp, A.; Gottfried, M.; Peled, N.; Tafreshi, A.; Cuffe, S.; et al. Pembrolizumab versus Chemotherapy for PD-L1–Positive Non–Small-Cell Lung Cancer. *N. Engl. J. Med.* **2016**, *375*, 1823–1833. [CrossRef] [PubMed]

11. Valle, J.W.; Lamarca, A.; Goyal, L.; Barriuso, J.; Zhu, A.X. REVIEW I New horizons for precision medicine in biliary tract cancers. *Cancer Discov.* **2017**, *9*, 943–962.
12. Bekaii-Saab, T.S.; Valle, J.W.; Van Cutsem, E.; Rimassa, L.; Furuse, J.; Ioka, T.; Melisi, D.; Macarulla, T.; Bridgewater, J.; Wasan, H.; et al. FIGHT-302: First-line pemigatinib vs gemcitabine plus cisplatin for advanced cholangiocarcinoma with FGFR2 rearrangements. *Futur. Oncol.* **2020**, *16*, 2385–2399. [CrossRef]
13. Krook, M.A.; Bonneville, R.; Chen, H.-Z.; Reeser, J.W.; Wing, M.R.; Martin, D.M.; Smith, A.M.; Dao, T.; Samorodnitsky, E.; Paruchuri, A.; et al. Tumor heterogeneity and acquired drug resistance in FGFR2-fusion-positive cholangiocarcinoma through rapid research autopsy. *Mol. Case Stud.* **2019**, *5*, a004002. [CrossRef] [PubMed]
14. Bahleda, R.; Italiano, A.; Hierro, C.; Mita, A.; Cervantes, A.; Chan, N.; Awad, M.; Calvo, E.; Moreno, V.; Govindan, R.; et al. Multicenter Phase I Study of Erdafitinib (JNJ-42756493), Oral Pan-Fibroblast Growth Factor Receptor Inhibitor, in Patients with Advanced or Refractory Solid Tumors. *Clin. Cancer Res.* **2019**, *25*, 4888–4897. [CrossRef] [PubMed]
15. Hanahan, D.; Weinberg, R.A. Hallmarks of Cancer: The Next Generation. *Cell* **2011**, *144*, 646–674. [CrossRef] [PubMed]
16. Nepal, C.; O'Rourke, C.J.; Oliveira, D.N.P.; Taranta, A.; Shema, S.; Gautam, P.; Calderaro, J.; Barbour, A.; Raggi, C.; Wennerberg, K.; et al. Genomic perturbations reveal distinct regulatory networks in intrahepatic cholangiocarcinoma. *Hepatology* **2018**, *68*, 949–963. [CrossRef] [PubMed]
17. Abou-Alfa, G.K.; Macarulla, T.; Javle, M.M.; Kelley, R.K.; Lubner, S.J.; Adeva, J.; Cleary, J.M.; Catenacci, D.V.; Borad, M.J.; Bridgewater, J.; et al. Ivosidenib in IDH1-mutant, chemotherapy-refractory cholangiocarcinoma (ClarIDHy): A multicentre, randomised, double-blind, placebo-controlled, phase 3 study. *Lancet Oncol.* **2020**, *21*, 796–807. [CrossRef]
18. Uribe, M.; Marrocco, I.; Yarden, Y. EGFR in Cancer: Signaling Mechanisms, Drugs, and Acquired Resistance. *Cancers* **2021**, *13*, 2748. [CrossRef] [PubMed]
19. FDA. Approval Summary: Osimertinib for Adjuvant Treatment of Surgically Resected Non-Small Cell Lung Cancer, a Collaborative Project Orbis review I Clinical Cancer Research. 2021. Available online: https://clincancerres.aacrjournals.org/content/early/2021/07/22/1078-0432.CCR-21-1034 (accessed on 28 July 2021).
20. Xie, Y.-H.; Chen, Y.-X.; Fang, J.-Y. Comprehensive review of targeted therapy for colorectal cancer. Signal Transduct. *Target. Ther.* **2020**, *5*, 22. [CrossRef]
21. Vogel, A.; Kasper, S.; Bitzer, M.; Block, A.; Sinn, M.; Schulze-Bergkamen, H.; Moehler, M.; Pfarr, N.; Endris, V.; Goeppert, B.; et al. PICCA study: Panitumumab in combination with cisplatin/gemcitabine chemotherapy in KRAS wild-type patients with biliary cancer—a randomised biomarker-driven clinical phase II AIO study. *Eur. J. Cancer* **2018**, *92*, 11–19. [CrossRef] [PubMed]
22. Leone, F.; Marino, D.; Cereda, S.; Filippi, R.; Belli, C.; Spadi, R.; Nasti, G.; Montano, M.; Amatu, A.; Aprile, G.; et al. Panitumumab in combination with gemcitabine and oxaliplatin does not prolong survival in wild-type KRAS advanced biliary tract cancer: A randomized phase 2 trial (Vecti-BIL study). *Cancer* **2016**, *122*, 574–581.
23. Chiang, N.-J.; Hsu, C.; Chen, J.-S.; Tsou, H.-H.; Shen, Y.-Y.; Chao, Y.; Chen, M.-H.; Yeh, T.-S.; Shan, Y.-S.; Huang, S.-F.; et al. Expression levels of ROS1/ALK/c-MET and therapeutic efficacy of cetuximab plus chemotherapy in advanced biliary tract cancer. *Sci. Rep.* **2016**, *6*, 25369. [CrossRef]
24. Lee, J.; Park, S.H.; Chang, H.M.; Kim, J.S.; Choi, H.J.; Lee, M.A.; Jang, J.S.; Jeung, H.C.; Kang, J.H.; Lee, H.W.; et al. Gemcitabine and oxaliplatin with or without erlotinib in advanced biliary-tract cancer: A multicentre, open-label, randomised, phase 3 study. *Lancet Oncol.* **2012**, *13*, 181–188. [CrossRef]
25. Lubner, S.J.; Mahoney, M.R.; Kolesar, J.L.; Loconte, N.K.; Kim, G.P.; Pitot, H.C.; Philip, P.A.; Picus, J.; Yong, W.-P.; Horvath, L.; et al. Report of a multicenter phase II trial testing a combination of biweekly bevacizumab and daily erlotinib in patients with unresectable biliary cancer: A phase II Consortium study. *J. Clin. Oncol.* **2010**, *28*, 3491–3497. [CrossRef]
26. Jusakul, A.; Cutcutache, I.; Yong, C.H.; Lim, J.Q.; Ni Huang, M.; Padmanabhan, N.; Nellore, V.; Kongpetch, S.; Ng, A.W.T.; Ng, L.M.; et al. Whole-Genome and Epigenomic Landscapes of Etiologically Distinct Subtypes of Cholangiocarcinoma. *Cancer Discov.* **2017**, *7*, 1116–1135. [CrossRef]
27. Jeong, H.; Jeong, J.H.; Kim, K.-P.; Lee, S.S.; Oh, D.W.; Park, D.H.; Song, T.J.; Park, Y.; Hong, S.-M.; Ryoo, B.-Y.; et al. Feasibility of HER2-Targeted Therapy in Advanced Biliary Tract Cancer: A Prospective Pilot Study of Trastuzumab Biosimilar in Combination with Gemcitabine Plus Cisplatin. *Cancers* **2021**, *13*, 161. [CrossRef]
28. Iyer, R.V.; Pokuri, V.K.; Groman, A.; Ma, W.W.; Malhotra, U.; Iancu, D.M.; Grande, C.; Saab, T.B. A Multicenter Phase II Study of Gemcitabine, Capecitabine, and Bevacizumab for Locally Advanced or Metastatic Biliary Tract Cancer. *Am. J. Clin. Oncol.* **2018**, *41*, 649–655. [CrossRef]
29. El-Khoueiry, A.B.; Rankin, C.J.; Ben-Josef, E.; Lenz, H.-J.; Gold, P.J.; Hamilton, R.D.; Govindarajan, R.; Eng, C.; Blanke, C.D. SWOG 0514: A phase II study of sorafenib in patients with unresectable or metastatic gallbladder carcinoma and cholangiocarcinoma. Investig. *New Drugs* **2012**, *30*, 1646–1651. [CrossRef]
30. Lee, J.K.; Capanu, M.; O'Reilly, E.M.; Ma, J.; Chou, J.F.; Shia, J.; Katz, S.; Gansukh, B.; Reidylagunes, D.; Segal, N.H.; et al. A phase II study of gemcitabine and cisplatin plus sorafenib in patients with advanced biliary adenocarcinomas. *Br. J. Cancer* **2013**, *109*, 915–919. [CrossRef] [PubMed]
31. Sun, W.; Patel, A.; Normolle, D.; Patel, K.; Ohr, J.; Lee, J.J.; Bahary, N.; Chu, E.; Streeter, N.; Drummond, S. A phase 2 trial of regorafenib as a single agent in patients with chemotherapy—refractory, advanced, and metastatic biliary tract adenocarcinoma. *Cancer* **2019**, *125*, 902–909. [CrossRef]

32. Kam, A.E.; Masood, A.; Shroff, R.T. Current and emerging therapies for advanced biliary tract cancers. *Lancet Gastroenterol. Hepatol.* **2021**, *6*, 956–969. [CrossRef]

33. Doebele, R.C.; Drilon, A.; Paz-Ares, L.; Siena, S.; Shaw, A.T.; Farago, A.F.; Blakely, C.M.; Seto, T.; Cho, B.C.; Tosi, D.; et al. Entrectinib in patients with advanced or metastatic NTRK fusion-positive solid tumours: Integrated analysis of three phase 1–2 trials. *Lancet Oncol.* **2020**, *21*, 271–282. [CrossRef]

34. Drilon, A.; Laetsch, T.W.; Kummar, S.; DuBois, S.G.; Lassen, U.N.; Demetri, G.D.; Nathenson, M.; Doebele, R.C.; Farago, A.F.; Pappo, A.S.; et al. Efficacy of Larotrectinib in TRK Fusion-Positive Cancers in Adults and Children. *N. Engl. J. Med.* **2018**, *378*, 731–739. [CrossRef]

35. Boilève, A.; Verlingue, L.; Hollebecque, A.; Boige, V.; Ducreux, M.; Malka, D. Rare cancer, rare alteration: The case of NTRK fusions in biliary tract cancers. Expert Opin. *Investig. Drugs* **2021**, *30*, 401–409. [CrossRef]

36. Hellmann, M.D.; Friedman, C.F.; Wolchok, J.D. Combinatorial Cancer Immunotherapies. *Adv. Immunol.* **2016**, *130*, 251–277. [CrossRef] [PubMed]

37. Carpino, G.; Cardinale, V.; Renzi, A.; Hov, J.R.; Berloco, P.B.; Rossi, M.; Karlsen, T.H.; Alvaro, D.; Gaudio, E. Activation of biliary tree stem cells within peribiliary glands in primary sclerosing cholangitis. *J. Hepatol.* **2015**, *63*, 1220–1228. [CrossRef] [PubMed]

38. Piha-Paul, S.A.; Oh, D.; Ueno, M.; Malka, D.; Chung, H.C.; Nagrial, A.; Kelley, R.K.; Ros, W.; Italiano, A.; Nakagawa, K.; et al. Efficacy and safety of pembrolizumab for the treatment of advanced biliary cancer: Results from the KEYNOTE -158 and KEYNOTE -028 studies. *Int. J. Cancer* **2020**, *147*, 2190–2198. [CrossRef]

39. Marabelle, A.; Le, D.T.; Ascierto, P.A.; Di Giacomo, A.M.; De Jesus-Acosta, A.; Delord, J.-P.; Geva, R.; Gottfried, M.; Penel, N.; Hansen, A.R.; et al. Efficacy of Pembrolizumab in Patients With Noncolorectal High Microsatellite Instability/Mismatch Repair–Deficient Cancer: Results From the Phase II KEYNOTE-158 Study. *J. Clin. Oncol.* **2020**, *38*, 1–10. [CrossRef]

40. Le, D.T.; Uram, J.N.; Wang, H.; Bartlett, B.R.; Kemberling, H.; Eyring, A.D.; Skora, A.D.; Luber, B.S.; Azad, N.S.; Laheru, D.; et al. PD-1 Blockade in Tumors with Mismatch-Repair Deficiency. *N. Engl. J. Med.* **2015**, *372*, 2509–2520. [CrossRef] [PubMed]

41. A Phase 2 Multi-Institutional Study of Nivolumab for Patients with Advanced Refractory Biliary Tract Cancer I Gastroenterology I JAMA Oncology I JAMA Network. 2021. Available online: https://jamanetwork.com/journals/jamaoncology/fullarticle/276529 3 (accessed on 28 July 2021).

42. Sahai, V.; Griffith, K.A.; Beg, M.S.; Shaib, W.L.; Mahalingam, D.; Zhen, D.B.; Deming, D.A.; Dey, S.; Mendiratta-Lala, M.; Zalupski, M. A multicenter randomized phase II study of nivolumab in combination with gemcitabine/cisplatin or ipilimumab as first-line therapy for patients with advanced unresectable biliary tract cancer (BilT-01). *J. Clin. Oncol.* **2020**, *38*, 4582. [CrossRef]

43. Lwin, Z.; Gomez-Roca, C.; Saada-Bouzid, E.; Yanez, E.; Muñoz, F.L.; Im, S.-A.; Castanon, E.; Senellart, H.; Graham, D.; Voss, M.; et al. LBA41 LEAP-005: Phase II study of lenvatinib (len) plus pembrolizumab (pembro) in patients (pts) with previously treated advanced solid tumours. *Ann. Oncol.* **2020**, *31*, S1170. [CrossRef]

44. Komuta, M.; Govaere, O.; Vandecaveye, V.; Akiba, J.; Van Steenbergen, W.; Verslype, C.; Laleman, W.; Pirenne, J.; Aerts, R.; Yano, H.; et al. Histological diversity in cholangiocellular carcinoma reflects the different cholangiocyte phenotypes. *Hepatology* **2012**, *55*, 1876–1888. [CrossRef]

45. Chung, T.; Rhee, H.; Nahm, J.H.; Jeon, Y.; Yoo, J.E.; Kim, Y.-J.; Han, D.H.; Park, Y.N. Clinicopathological characteristics of intrahepatic cholangiocarcinoma according to gross morphologic type: Cholangiolocellular differentiation traits and inflammation- and proliferation-phenotypes. *HPB* **2020**, *22*, 864–873. [CrossRef]

46. Boyiadzis, M.M.; Kirkwood, J.M.; Marshall, J.L.; Pritchard, C.C.; Azad, N.S.; Gulley, J.L. Significance and implications of FDA approval of pembrolizumab for biomarker-defined disease. *J. Immunother. Cancer* **2018**, *6*, 35. [CrossRef] [PubMed]

47. Gong, J.; Chehrazi-Raffle, A.; Reddi, S.; Salgia, R. Development of PD-1 and PD-L1 inhibitors as a form of cancer immunotherapy: A comprehensive review of registration trials and future considerations. *J. Immunother. Cancer* **2018**, *6*, 8. [CrossRef] [PubMed]

48. Tiwari, A.; Roy, H.; Lynch, H. Lynch syndrome in the 21st century: Clinical perspectives. *Qjm Int. J. Med.* **2016**, *109*, 151–158. [CrossRef]

49. Patterns and Genomic Correlates of PD-L1 Expression in Patients with Biliary Tract Cancers—Mody. *J. Gastrointest. Oncol.* **2021**. Available online: https://jgo.amegroups.com/article/view/31932/html (accessed on 28 July 2021).

50. Ju, J.Y.; Dibbern, M.E.; Mahadevan, M.S.; Fan, J.; Kunk, P.R.; Stelow, E.B. Mismatch Repair Protein Deficiency/Microsatellite Instability Is Rare in Cholangiocarcinomas and Associated With Distinctive Morphologies. *Am. J. Clin. Pathol.* **2020**, *153*, 598–604. [CrossRef] [PubMed]

51. Zhang, J.; Wu, Z.; Zhao, J.; Liu, S.; Zhang, X.; Yuan, F.; Shi, Y.; Song, B. Intrahepatic cholangiocarcinoma: MRI texture signature as predictive biomarkers of immunophenotyping and survival. *Eur. Radiol.* **2020**, *31*, 3661–3672. [CrossRef] [PubMed]

52. Rhee, H.; Kim, M.-J.; Park, Y.N.; An, C. A proposal of imaging classification of intrahepatic mass-forming cholangiocarcinoma into ductal and parenchymal types: Clinicopathologic significance. *Eur. Radiol.* **2018**, *29*, 3111–3121. [CrossRef]

53. Yoo, J.; Kim, J.H.; Bae, J.S.; Kang, H.-J. Prediction of prognosis and resectability using MR imaging, clinical, and histopathological findings in patients with perihilar cholangiocarcinoma. *Abdom. Radiol.* **2021**, *46*, 4159–4169. [CrossRef] [PubMed]

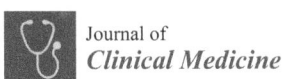

Journal of
Clinical Medicine

Review

Treatment of Hepatocellular Carcinoma with Immune Checkpoint Inhibitors and Applicability of First-Line Atezolizumab/Bevacizumab in a Real-Life Setting

Maria Corina Plaz Torres [1], Quirino Lai [2], Fabio Piscaglia [3], Eugenio Caturelli [4], Giuseppe Cabibbo [5], Elisabetta Biasini [6], Filippo Pelizzaro [7], Fabio Marra [8], Franco Trevisani [9] and Edoardo G. Giannini [1],*

[1] Gastroenterology Unit, Department of Internal Medicine, IRCCS—Ospedale Policlinico San Martino, University of Genoa, 16132 Genoa, Italy; mariacorina.plaztorres@edu.unige.it
[2] Hepatobiliary and Organ Transplantation Unit, Umberto I Polyclinic of Rome, Sapienza University of Rome, 00185 Rome, Italy; quirino.lai@uniroma1.it
[3] Internal Medicine Unit, Department of Medical and Surgical Sciences, IRCCS Azienda Ospedaliero—Universitaria di Bologna, 40138 Bologna, Italy; fabio.piscaglia@unibo.it
[4] Gastroenterology Unit, Belcolle Hospital, 01100 Viterbo, Italy; e.caturelli@tiscali.it
[5] Gastroenterology and Hepatology Unit, Department of Health Promotion, Mother and Child Care, Internal Medicine and Medical Specialties (PROMISE), University of Palermo, 90133 Palermo, Italy; giuseppe.cabibbo@policlinico.pa.it
[6] Infectious Diseases and Hepatology Unit, Azienda Ospedaliero—Universitaria di Parma, 43126 Parma, Italy; ebiasini@ao.pr.it
[7] Gastroenterology Unit, Department of Surgery, Oncology and Gastroenterology, University of Padova, 35128 Padova, Italy; filippo.pelizzaro@unipd.it
[8] Internal Medicine and Hepatology Unit, Department of Experimental and Clinical Medicine, University of Firenze, 50134 Firenze, Italy; fabio.marra@unifi.it
[9] Medical Semeiotics Unit, Department of Medical and Surgical Sciences, IRCCS Azienda Ospedaliero—Universitaria di Bologna, 40138 Bologna, Italy; franco.trevisani@unibo.it
* Correspondence: egiannini@unige.it; Tel.: +39-010-353-7950; Fax: +39-010-353-8638

Citation: Plaz Torres, M.C.; Lai, Q.; Piscaglia, F.; Caturelli, E.; Cabibbo, G.; Biasini, E.; Pelizzaro, F.; Marra, F.; Trevisani, F.; Giannini, E.G. Treatment of Hepatocellular Carcinoma with Immune Checkpoint Inhibitors and Applicability of First-Line Atezolizumab/Bevacizumab in a Real-Life Setting. *J. Clin. Med.* **2021**, *10*, 3201. https://doi.org/10.3390/jcm10153201

Academic Editors: Pierluigi Toniutto and Hidekazu Suzuki

Received: 1 June 2021
Accepted: 19 July 2021
Published: 21 July 2021

Publisher's Note: MDPI stays neutral with regard to jurisdictional claims in published maps and institutional affiliations.

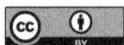
Abstract: Immune checkpoint inhibitors (ICIs) are the new frontier for the treatment of advanced hepatocellular carcinoma (HCC). Since the first trial with tremelimumab, a cytotoxic T-lymphocyte-associated protein 4 inhibitor, increasing evidence has confirmed that these drugs can significantly extend the survival of patients with advanced hepatocellular carcinoma (HCC). As a matter of fact, the overall survival and objective response rates reported in patients with advanced HCC treated with ICIs are the highest ever reported in the second-line setting and, most recently, the combination of the anti-programmed death ligand protein-1 atezolizumab with bevacizumab—an anti-vascular endothelial growth factor monoclonal antibody—demonstrated superiority to sorafenib in a Phase III randomized clinical trial. Therefore, this regimen has been approved in several countries as first-line treatment for advanced HCC and is soon expected to be widely used in clinical practice. However, despite the promising results of trials exploring ICIs alone or in combination with other agents, there are still some critical issues to deal with to optimize the prognosis of advanced HCC patients. For instance, the actual proportion of patients who are deemed eligible for ICIs in the real-life ranges from 10% to 20% in the first-line setting, and is even lower in the second-line scenario. Moreover, long-term data regarding the safety of ICIs in the population of patients with cirrhosis and impaired liver function are lacking. Lastly, no biomarkers have been identified to predict response, and thus to help clinicians to individually tailor treatment. This review aimed to summarize the state of the art immunotherapy in HCC and, by analyzing a large, multicenter cohort of Italian patients with HCC, to assess the potential applicability of the combination of atezolizumab/bevacizumab in the real-life setting.

Keywords: liver cancer; systemic treatment; immunotherapy; real-world; unresectable hepatocellular carcinoma

149

1. Introduction

Hepatocellular carcinoma (HCC) is one of the leading causes of cancer-related mortality worldwide, with approximately 800,000 deaths per year and an estimated increase to more than 1 million deaths by 2030 [1]. HCC arises predominantly in the context of liver cirrhosis, but also can be diagnosed in a not negligible proportion of patients without cirrhosis suffering from non-alcoholic steato-hepatitis who carry additional metabolic and genetic risk factors [2–5]. In the past decades, the *armamentarium* for the systemic treatment of advanced HCC was limited to the anti-vascular endothelial growth factor (VEGFR), multi-target-tyrosine kinase inhibitor (TKI) sorafenib. This drug determined a significant—though modest—survival benefit in two Phase III trials and remained the sole first-line treatment option for about 10 years, during which neither an alternative drug nor effective second-line therapies became available for patients who progressed during—or were intolerant to—sorafenib [6,7]. As a fact, lenvatinib (a TKI targeting VEGFR) became an effective alternative to sorafenib as first-line therapy for HCC in 2018, while regorafenib, cabozantinib, and ramucirumab only recently have been approved in the second-line setting [8]. With the advent of second-line treatments, the survival of patients with advanced HCC has significantly improved, with a proportion (approximately 20%) of patients reaching survival times of about 2 years with the sequential use of sorafenib-regorafenib [9]. These patients, however, belong to a small subgroup of patients who, maintaining an optimal liver function, are eligible for sequential treatment and tolerate the adverse effects of the anti-neoplastic agents [9].

In this scenario, immunotherapy has emerged as an additional promising approach potentially able to obtain even longer survival times. Research in this field is steadily increasing, also fueled by the positive results obtained in other cancer types and by the evidence of efficacy demonstrated in both first- and second-line settings [10–12]. The most recent Phase I/II trials have shown a clinically meaningful survival increase in the second-line setting for the programmed cell death protein 1 (PD-1) inhibitors nivolumab and pembrolizumab [12]. Hence, these agents have been granted accelerated conditional approval for sorafenib-experienced patients in the US, while the European Medicines Agency (EMA) maintains a more cautious attitude in approving these ICIs for the treatment of HCC. Indeed, subsequent Phase III trials testing nivolumab versus sorafenib as first-line treatment, and pembrolizumab versus placebo in second-line treatment, failed to meet their primary survival endpoints [13,14]. This notwithstanding, the results from trials testing the combination of immune checkpoint inhibitors (ICIs) with other agents, among which VEGFR-targeted therapies obtained very encouraging results, so that the combinations of pembrolizumab plus lenvatinib as well as atezolizumab (monoclonal antibody against PD-L1) plus bevacizumab (monoclonal antibody against VEGF) have both received breakthrough therapy designation from the US Food and Drug Administration (FDA). Actually, in a recent Phase III trial, the latter overperformed compared to sorafenib as first-line treatment of advanced HCC in terms of both overall (OS) and progression-free survival (PFS) [15]. Therefore, atezolizumab plus bevacizumab has been approved as the first-line treatment option for advanced HCC, thus becoming the standard of care for these patients.

Overall, the results from the trials testing ICIs alone or in combination, or combined with other agents, suggest that ICIs alone are not the best option for the treatment of HCC, while combined treatments are safe and highly effective. As such, immunotherapy-based treatments will probably soon change the landscape of advanced HCC therapy. In this review, we summarize the state of the art immunotherapy in advanced HCC, with a particular focus on the combination of atezolizumab plus bevacizumab, by assessing in a large cohort of Italian patients with HCC the potential applicability of this regimen to the real-life setting.

2. Approved Treatments for HCC before the "Era" of Immune Checkpoint Inhibitors

Until the approval of sorafenib in 2008, no systemic treatment was available for advanced HCC [6]. Sorafenib, an orally active multi-target TKI targeting different cell surface tyrosine kinases (e.g., VEGFR-1, -2, and -3 and platelet-derived growth factor (PDGFR)-β), at the dose of 400 mg twice daily, significantly improved OS in patients with HCC not amenable to surgery and locoregional procedures, who had well-preserved liver function (97% Child–Pugh A) and Eastern Cooperative Oncology Group (ECOG) performance status (PS) ≤ 2 [6]. The median OS was 10.7 months in the sorafenib group and 7.9 months in the placebo group ($p < 0.001$), whereas the median time to radiologic progression (TTP) was 5.5 months in the sorafenib arm versus 2.8 months in the placebo arm ($p < 0.001$). Of note, the median OS of patients with the Barcelona Clinic Liver Cancer (BCLC) staging system stage B HCC treated with sorafenib was 15–20 months, a finding confirmed by subsequent post-marketing studies [16,17]. In the following years, several drugs were tested against sorafenib in the first-line setting, failing to demonstrate superiority to this drug, so that sorafenib remained the sole effective systemic treatment available for HCC until 2018, when lenvatinib, an oral TKI with a biologic action similar to sorafenib, showed non-inferior OS as compared to sorafenib in the REFLECT trial, and was therefore approved as an alternative to this drug in the first-line setting [8]. Again, patients included in this trial belonged to a selected group of subjects with well-preserved liver function (Child–Pugh class A) and ECOG PS ≤ 1, while those with extensive tumor burden (≥50% of the liver), bile duct invasion, or invasion of the main portal vein were excluded. Forest plots for OS revealed that lenvatinib was more effective than sorafenib in patients with baseline AFP ≥ 200 ng/mL (Hazard ratio (HR), 0.78; 95% confidence interval (95%CI), 0.63–0.98) and less effective in patients without macrovascular invasion/extrahepatic spread and those enrolled in the Western area. Secondary endpoints (PFS, TTP, objective response rate (ORR)) were significantly and remarkably better with lenvatinib, suggesting that these surrogate endpoints poorly predict OS in HCC patients treated with these drugs.

As far as the second-line setting is concerned, regorafenib, an oral TKI targeting VEGFR-2, VEGFR-3, TIE-2, PDGFR, fibroblast growth factor receptor (FGFR)-1, and the mutant oncogenic kinases KIT, RET, and B-RAF, was the first agent able to provide a significant survival benefit in patients with tumor progression on sorafenib [18]. Compared with placebo, regorafenib improved OS with a HR of 0.63 (95%CI, 0.50–0.79; $p < 0.0001$). It has to be emphasized that this study enrolled patients who progressed on sorafenib but tolerated the drug (≥400 mg/day for ≥20 of last 28 days of treatment) and had Child–Pugh class A liver function. Median survival was 10.6 months (95%CI, 9.1–12.1) for the regorafenib group versus 7.8 months (95%CI, 6.3–8.8) for the placebo group [18]. Interestingly, the treatment sequence of the sorafenib-regorafenib group was able to determine an OS of 26 months from the start of sorafenib treatment versus 19.2 months in the sorafenib-placebo group [18]. This survival time is comparable with that of patients with intermediate stage HCC undergoing trans-arterial chemo-embolization (TACE), suggesting that in a well-selected subgroup of patients the sequential treatment with TKIs may significantly improve prognosis as compared to the standard of care [9].

Other drugs that have shown efficacy in placebo-controlled trials and have consequently been approved as second-line treatment options for HCC are cabozantinib and ramucirumab [19]. Cabozantinib is an oral TKI targeting MET in addition to VEGFR2. The CELESTIAL trial was a global Phase III trial testing cabozantinib in patients with HCC progression on sorafenib [20]. It also included patients who had received up to two prior therapies for advanced-stage HCC. The study was stopped after a second interim analysis, which revealed a median OS of 10.2 months in the cabozantinib versus 8.0 months in the placebo group (HR, 0.76; 95% CI 0.63–0.92; $p = 0.0049$). Approximately 72% of patients had received only prior sorafenib treatment and, in this subpopulation, median OS was even longer, being 11.3 months in patients in the cabozantinib group versus 7.2 months in the placebo group (HR, 0.70; 95% CI, 0.55–0.88) [20].

Ramucirumab is an anti-VEGFR2 monoclonal antibody, and its utility in subjects with advanced HCC emerged from the double-blind, Phase III REACH-2 trial comparing ramucirumab versus placebo as second-line treatment in patients progressing on sorafenib and with baseline AFP ≥ 400 ng/mL [19]. This study was designed on the basis of the results of the REACH trial that failed to demonstrate an OS advantage with ramucirumab as compared to the placebo, but in a post-hoc analysis showed a benefit of the drug—albeit small—in prolonging OS (8.5 months with ramucirumab versus 7.3 months with placebo (HR, 0.71; 95% CI, 0.53–0.95; p = 0.0199)) among patients with baseline AFP ≥ 400 ng/mL [21]. Ramucirumab is therefore the first agent with a biomarker-driven use for patients with HCC progression on sorafenib [22].

In summary, sorafenib and lenvatinib are the TKIs that have long been in use for the front-line treatment of advanced HCC, providing a median extension of survival of about 3 months compared to the placebo. The survival benefit for patients eligible for second-line treatment with regorafenib/cabozantinib or ramucirumab, although significant, still remains modest. Hence, novel treatments targeting different tumorigenic pathways have been studied and others are still under investigation with the aim of further improving the outcomes of these patients. In this context, ICIs have gained excellent results.

3. The Advent of Immune Checkpoint Inhibitors

Despite the benefit in OS with sequential TKI treatment, the prognosis of patients with advanced HCC remains poor [9,23]. The reasons for this include, besides the sub-optimal tumoricidal activity of these drugs, the progression of the underlying liver disease, the advanced median age of this cohort of patients (approximately 70 years), and the presence of substantial comorbidities, which are very frequent in these subjects and, overall, make them a particularly vulnerable cohort [24].

In this context, ICIs have increasingly been investigated in the last years, with extremely encouraging results both in the first- and second-line setting, further boosting a rising number of clinical trials using ICIs alone or combined with other anti-tumoral drugs or with locoregional treatment. The rationale for the use of ICIs in HCC relies on the fact that HCC arises in a context of chronic inflammation and an altered tumor microenvironment, with the presence of tumor-infiltrating lymphocytes expressing PD1, which is a recognized key enabling factor beyond tumor cell-intrinsic molecular aberrations [25–27]. Moreover, the presence of PD1-expressing lymphocytes in HCC samples has been correlated with this outcome [28,29]. In this regard, Sia et al. have recently proposed a novel HCC classification based upon the tumor immune status: according to this classification, about 30% of HCCs could be categorized into an 'immune class', with high levels of immune cell infiltration, expression of PD-1 and/or PD-L1, activation of interferon-γ signaling, and markers of cytolytic activity [30]. Within this class, two distinct subclasses have been identified: the 'active immune' and the 'exhausted immune' classes, characterized by markers of an adaptive T-cell response or of an exhausted immune response, respectively [30]. The latter subclass is the ideal target of immunotherapy. The in-depth description of the molecular mechanisms involved in the tumor microenvironment of HCC is beyond the aim of this article, but it is worth pointing out that interactions between cancer cell antigens and the antigen-presenting cells lead to a priming of T-cells and their eventual migration into the tumor microenvironment. Physiologically, the T-lymphocytes' recognition of neoplastic antigens is followed by a T-cell-mediated killing of cancer cells [31]. This process is finely modulated at a local and general level by several mechanisms including immune checkpoints, which play a pivotal role in such modulation, as they suppress T-cell activity to inhibit eventual over-activation of the immune system and maintain self-tolerance. Thus, immune checkpoints physiologically prevent hyperimmune responses leading to tissue damage. Malignancies exploit these molecular mechanisms (immune checkpoints) to escape from the immune system recognition. In other words, ICIs act as anti-neoplastic agents by inhibiting negative feedback pathways of the immune system that mediate immune escape.

The most largely studied immune checkpoints are PD-1 and cytotoxic T-lymphocyte-associated protein 4 (CTLA-4). The pathological activation of PD-1 by its ligands, in particular PD-L1, expressed by cancer cells, can result in the immune escape of the tumor [32,33]. CTLA-4, which is mainly expressed on T-cells, regulates T-cell activity in physiological conditions, preventing an excess in T-cell responses and a hyperactivation of the immune response. Inversely, in pathological (neoplastic) conditions, CTLA-4 activation inhibits in the activation, proliferation, and production of tumor antigen-activated T-cells in the tumor microenvironment [32,33]. In the HCC tumor microenvironment, T-regulators (T-regs) express both CTLA-4 and PD-1 [28,32].

4. Immune Checkpoint Inhibitors in HCC

Tremelimumab, a CTLA-4-blocking monoclonal antibody, was the first ICI showing benefits in the treatment of HCC. This agent was tested in 2013 by Sangro et al. in a Phase II open-label trial that enrolled 21 patients with advanced HCC who were either sorafenib-naïve (76.2%) or -experienced, and a significant proportion of them were classified as Child–Pugh class B (43%) [10]. The positive results in terms of both safety and anti-tumor activity (partial response rate (PRR) 17.6%; disease control rate (DCR) 76.4%; TTP 6.48 months (95%CI, 3.95–9.14)), were instrumental in stimulating the research in immune checkpoint blockade in both first- and second-line treatment of HCC. In the last years, the effects of ICIs in HCC have been tested alone or in combination with other ICIs or combined with agents targeting the VEGFR. Currently available immunotherapy-based regimens and those under Phase III clinical investigation are summarized in Figure 1.

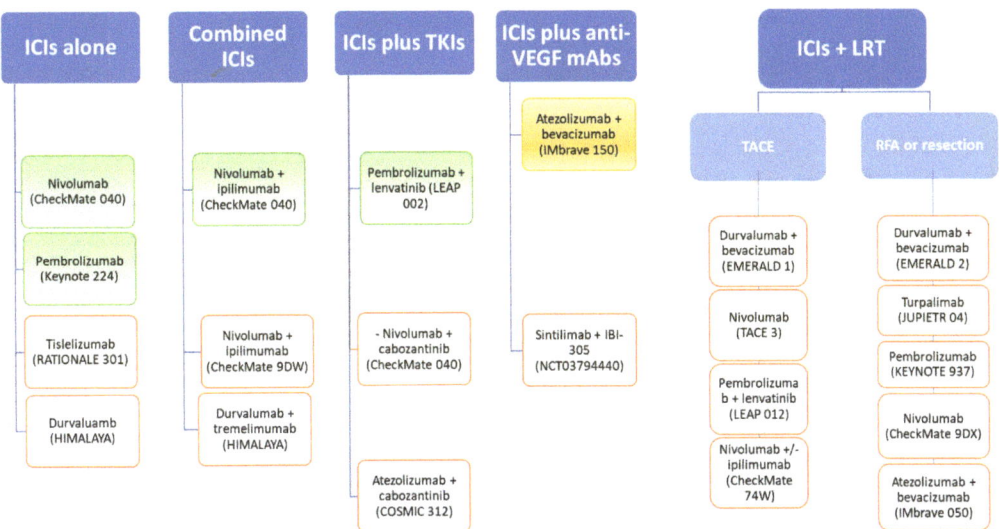

Figure 1. Possible HCC treatments with ICIs. Atezolizumab plus bevacizumab has been approved as a first-line treatment, whereas nivolumab with or without ipilimumab and pembrolizumab gained FDA approval as second-line treatments. Selected Phase III trials (orange squares) are testing ICIs alone or in combination or combined with other agents in the first and second-line setting, and in the adjuvant and neo-adjuvant setting as well.

4.1. Immune Checkpoint Inhibitors in Monotherapy

Following the encouraging results of the Phase II tremelimumab study, nivolumab, a monoclonal antibody targeting PD1, demonstrated a single-agent activity in the Phase Ib/II open-label, non-comparative, Checkmate 040 trial [11]. The initial trial included 262 sorafenib-naïve and -experienced patients assigned to a dose-escalation (48 subjects) or to a dose-expansion (214 subjects) phase. In the dose-expansion phase, the investigator-assessed overall ORR was 20%, with 3 complete responses (CR) and 39 partial responses (PR). Particularly, ORR was 22.5% for sorafenib-naive and 18.7% for sorafenib-experienced patients. Median OS was 29 months for sorafenib-naïve group and 15 months for the sorafenib-experienced group. The most impressive was the duration of response of 9.9 months amongst patients who had an objective response, which led the US FDA to grant accelerated approval to nivolumab as second-line therapy for patients with advanced-stage HCC previously treated with sorafenib [11]. In this subgroup, the ORR confirmed by blinded independent central review was 14.3% by Response Evaluation Criteria In Solid Tumors (RECIST) 1.1 and 18.2% by modified RECIST (mRECIST) criteria. Of note, the median duration of response was the longest ever seen in a second-line setting: 16.6 months [34,35]. However, the expectations raised by the results of this study were disappointed in a subsequent Phase III randomized trial (CheckMate-459) testing nivolumab versus sorafenib, as the anti-PD1 agent failed to demonstrate superiority as compared to the TKI [14]. Still, the study results confirmed clinically meaningful improvements in OS (16.4 versus 14.7 months), ORR (15% for nivolumab versus 7% for sorafenib), and CR (14 versus 5 patients). Moreover, nivolumab demonstrated a favorable safety profile, consistent with previous reports and, of particular interest, the quality of life was better in the nivolumab treatment arm [14]. The long survival of the sorafenib arm (median OS of about 15 months) was an unexpected outcome that negatively impacted the study results and that probably reflects the improved tailored management of patients with advanced HCC in the last decades, as well as physicians' familiarity with the TKI.

Another ICI that has been tested with favorable outcomes in monotherapy for advanced HCC is pembrolizumab, a monoclonal antibody targeting PD-1. Promising results came from the Phase II trial KEYNOTE 224, which showed good responses (ORR 17%, DCR 61%) and a good safety profile of pembrolizumab in patients who were intolerant to, or progressed under, sorafenib [12]. These results prompted Finn et al. to conduct the KEYNOTE-240 trial enrolling 413 patients who failed sorafenib and who were randomized 2:1 to pembrolizumab or placebo [13]. The survival in the pembrolizumab arm was among the highest ever reached in the second-line setting, being approximately 14 months (95%CI, 11.6–16.0) for pembrolizumab versus 10 months (95%CI, 8.3–13.5) for placebo (HR, 0.781; 95%CI, 0.611–0.998; $p = 0.0238$). Nevertheless, even this study failed to reach statistical significance due to the long survival of the control arm, reflecting once more the advances in the clinical management of advanced HCC. The safety profile of the drug was good, confirming the positive results of the Phase II study and the previous experience with nivolumab.

Despite the apparently "negative" results of these studies, likely due to issues related to their design requesting an overwhelming superiority of the tested ICIs over sorafenib, several positive aspects capturing the attention of researchers and clinicians were the overall objective response to nivolumab and pembrolizumab in 15–20% of cases, the durable antitumor responses, and the long-term OS in responding patients. Based on these peculiar results, the FDA granted conditional approval for these ICIs in the second-line setting.

Currently, results from the ongoing Phase III non-inferiority trial testing tislelizumab, a monoclonal antibody targeting PD-1, versus sorafenib (RATIONALE-301 trial) and those of the Phase III HIMALAYA study, testing durvalumab—an anti-PD-L1 monoclonal antibody—alone or in combination with tremelimumab versus sorafenib, are eagerly awaited [36].

As far as the safety profile of ICIs is concerned, the results of the pilot study by Sangro et al. on tremelimumab and those of the CheckMate and Keynote trials showed reassuring safety profiles for these agents, coherent with previous reports testing the use of these drugs in other cancer types [10–12,37]. As compared with the standard of care (i.e., sorafenib and lenvatinib), ICIs are generally better tolerated and have comparable or even lower rates of toxicity. The pathophysiology of adverse events (AEs) occurring during immunotherapy is related to their mechanism of action as the inhibition of physiological immune checkpoints may trigger immune-related AEs (irAEs) targeting the skin, gut, thyroid, adrenal glands, lung, and the liver itself, which may be a particularly worrisome complication in a population with an already impaired liver function [38,39]. Most frequent any grade AEs in patients treated with ICIs for other cancer types are skin AEs (rash and pruritus), colitis, hyper- or hypothyroidism, hepatitis, and pneumonitis. Skin AEs occur in about 13–35% of cases, being grade > 3 only in a minority of cases (<3%) [38,40]. Grade 1 and 2 skin AEs are usually easily managed with emollients, oral anti-histamines, and topical steroids, whereas grade ≥ 3 reactions require oral corticosteroids administration and the discontinuation of the immunotherapy until the skin AE has reverted to grade 1 [38]. Thyroid dysfunction has been reported in a variable proportion of cases (5–20%), but these events are rarely severe and rarely require treatment discontinuation or hormonal replacement treatment or corticosteroids administration [38]. The frequency of colitis ranges from 2% to 22% [38,40], being more frequent and severe in patients treated with anti-CTLA4 agents [38,40]. Again, the incidence of high-grade colitis is very low, being around 1–2% [40]. Patients with non-severe diarrhea should be treated with anti-diarrheal, fluid replacement, and electrolytes; conversely, patients with grade ≥3 diarrhea or persistent grade 2 diarrhea should discontinue ICIs and receive intravenous (i.v.) corticosteroids. In case of lack of response to corticosteroids, infliximab should be prescribed [38]. Pneumonitis occurs in 2–4% of patients, with grade ≥ 3 events representing only 1% to 2% of cases [38,40], and the frequency of fatal pneumonitis and that of treatment discontinuation (due to this AE) are extremely low (0.2% and 0.2–4%, respectively) [38]. In the case of documented or high suspicion of immune-related pneumonitis, immunosuppressive treatment should be started immediately. In grade 1 to 2 pneumonitis, treatment consists of oral steroids (prednisone 1 mg/kg daily), whilst patients with grade 3 to 4 pneumonitis should be hospitalized and treatment should consist of high-dose i.v. corticosteroids. In these severe cases, immunotherapy should be permanently discontinued. With regards to the occurrence of treatment-related hepatitis, which occurs in a proportion of 5% to 10% of patients (among which 1–2% are grade 3) [38,40], in the presence of grade ≤ 2 transaminases elevation, checkpoint inhibitor therapy should be withheld and transaminases and bilirubin should be measured twice weekly. Persistent grade 2 elevation lasting longer than 2 weeks, after having ruled out other causes, should be treated with corticosteroids at a dose of 1 mg/kg/day (methyl)prednisolone or equivalent. Upon improvement, re-challenge with ICIs may be attempted after corticosteroid tapering. In the absence of improvement despite the initiation of corticosteroids, the dose should be increased to 2 mg/kg/day of (methyl)prednisolone or equivalent and checkpoint inhibitor therapy should permanently be discontinued [38]. In the instance of grade 3 or 4 transaminase or total bilirubin elevation, checkpoint inhibitor therapy should be permanently discontinued, and corticosteroids started at 1–2 mg/kg/day (methyl)prednisolone or equivalent. If the absence of response to corticosteroids within 2–3 days, mycophenolate mofetil should be added at 1000 mg twice daily. If no improvement is seen, liver biopsy should be considered. However, ICI-related hepatitis usually resolves within 4–6 weeks with appropriate treatment; therefore, if no improvement is detected in this time frame, other contributory causes should be reconsidered and the initial diagnostic work-up should be repeated.

Overall, the available evidence suggests that, although common, irAEs can be easily managed in most cases by delaying the subsequent scheduled administrations, and with the administration of corticosteroids in severe cases [39]. In HCC studies, approximately 90–98% of patients experienced any AE during treatment, with up to 50% of them being grade 3 or higher [10–14]. However, similar rates of AEs have been recorded in randomized controlled trials in the respective placebo arms as well [13]. With regards to treatment-related AEs, grade ≥ 3 AEs have been reported in approximately 20% of cases for nivolumab and pembrolizumab monotherapy [13,14]; among them, the most frequent AE in the Keynote-240 and CheckMate-040 studies was aminotransferase increase (about 4–5% and 6–10%, respectively) [11,13]. This event is of particular concern in patients with cirrhosis due to the potential deterioration of liver function and to the peculiar risk of corticosteroid-related AEs in these subjects. However, current data show that ICIs are safe in well-selected cohorts of patients with cirrhosis and preserved liver function (Child–Pugh class A), with no safety alerts as compared with patients without cirrhosis treated with ICIs for other cancer types [9,41]. The available evidence thus suggests that cirrhotic patients with HCC should not be at increased risk of liver irAEs, but close monitoring of liver function tests should be performed in cirrhotic patients treated with ICIs. Treatment-related serious AEs such as pneumonitis and colitis occurred in a minority of patients (<1%), as reported in the literature for immunotherapy in other cancer types [11,12]. Definite data on the safety and tolerability of ICIs in Child–Pugh class B patients, which represent a significant proportion of advanced HCC patients, are lacking. However, those from the CheckMate-040 trial are reassuring, since only 4 out of 49 patients with Child–Pugh class B reported treatment-related hepatic events, and only 2 of them needed treatment discontinuation [38]. Moreover, similar results regarding the safety of nivolumab and pembrolizumab in patients with Child–Pugh class B have been observed by Scheiner et al. in a real-life cohort of HCC patients [41]. Taken together, the available evidence suggests the safety profile of ICIs in the HCC population is good in selected cases with well-preserved liver function and that ICIs may be safely administered in Child–Pugh class B patients as well.

4.2. Dual Immune Chechpoint Blockade

Based on the hypothesis that anti-PD-1 and anti-CTLA4 agents may have a synergistic effect by inhibiting two different steps of the immune checkpoint system, combinations of anti-PD1 and anti-CTLA4 are underway. A Phase III trial with dual treatment with nivolumab plus ipilimumab, a CTLA-4 monoclonal antibody, in the first-line setting (CheckMate 9DW, NCT04039607) is underway. This trial was supported by the positive results observed in the cohort 4 (nivolumab plus ipilimumab) of the Checkmate-040 trial in the second-line setting [42]. In this study, patients were randomized 1:1:1 to either nivolumab 1 mg/kg plus ipilimumab 3 mg/kg, administered every 3 weeks (4 doses), followed by nivolumab 240 mg every 2 weeks (arm A); nivolumab 3 mg/kg plus ipilimumab 1 mg/kg, administered every 3 weeks (4 doses), followed by nivolumab 240 mg every 2 weeks (arm B); or nivolumab 3 mg/kg every 2 weeks plus ipilimumab 1 mg/kg every 6 weeks (arm C). Treatment combination had manageable safety, promising ORR, and durable responses. The arm A regimen showed the greatest benefits in terms of ORR (32% versus 27% and 29% in arms B and C, respectively) and OS (22.8 months (95%CI, 9.4—not reached) in arm A versus 12.5 months (95%CI, 7.6–16.4) in arm B and 12.7 months in arm C (95%CI, 7.4–33.0) [43]. Any grade treatment-related AE occurred in 94% of cases in arm A, 71% in arm B, and 79% of cases in arm C. Among them, 53% of patients in arm A, 29% of patients in arm B, and 31% of patients in arm C had grade 3 or 4 treatment-related AEs. Arm A also had higher rates of irAEs and irAEs leading to treatment discontinuation (18%), as compared with arms B and C (6% and 4%, respectively). Consequently, in arm A, 16% of patients stopped treatment: 6% of them due to treatment-related hepatitis, 6% due to pneumonitis, and 4% due to diarrhea/colitis [43]. However, most cases of patients presenting AEs continued treatment and the AEs resolved with standard management, while only 1 treatment-related death due to pneumonitis was reported (0.6%) [43]. Importantly, among patients who were re-challenged with nivolumab or ipilimumab after experiencing an irAE in any category, no patients experienced an event recurrence after the re-challenge [43]. Considering the outstanding OS and ORR obtained in arm A, these results suggest that nivolumab plus ipilimumab may provide improved efficacy in terms of ORR, and, potentially, of survival with an acceptable safety profile. Based on this evidence, this dual treatment received accelerated approval in the US as second-line treatment for HCC.

In the first-line setting, a Phase III trial (HIMALAYA) is testing the PD-L1 inhibitor durvalumab alone and in combination with tremelimumab, compared with sorafenib. This study was designed on the basis of the findings from a Phase I/II, randomized, open-label study that included patients progressing under, intolerant to, or refusing sorafenib [44]. Patients were randomized 1:2 to different tremelimumab plus durvalumab combinations, and safety was the primary endpoint. Patients assigned to the high-dose tremelimumab arm (i.e., tremelimumab 300 mg plus durvalumab 1500 mg 1 dose followed by durvalumab every 4 weeks) had the highest confirmed ORR (duration of response not reached) and longest OS (18.7 months (10.8—not reached)) [44]. Grade 3 or 4 treatment-related AEs rates were comparable to those occurring in the nivolumab plus ipilimumab trials, being 35% in the high-dose (300 mg) tremelimumab arm and 25% in the low-dose (75 mg) tremelimumab arm. Discontinuation of the study drug due to AEs was 10.8% and 6% in the high- and low-dose arm, respectively, but no deaths were attributed to treatment.

In summary, dual checkpoint blockade may improve OS in HCC patients, but consistent evidence is still scarce. As might have been expected, the trials testing ICIs in dual treatment reported higher rates of AEs in comparison with ICIs used in monotherapy, but in most cases, the safety profile was consistent in presentation and management with that of monotherapy. Taking into consideration the poor prognosis of patients with advanced HCC, the benefit/risk ratio may still favor the dual treatment strategy. Current trials with dual checkpoint blockade are reported in Table 1.

Table 1. Ongoing clinical trials with immune checkpoint inhibitors, alone or in combination with other agents, in HCC.

Trial Name	Phase	Line of Treatment	Design	Patients Enrolled	Endpoints	ClinicalTrial.gov	Company	Status
GO30140	I	First-line	Atezolizumab + Bevacizumab (arm A) Atezolizumab + Bevacizumab (arm F1) Atezolizumab (arm F2)	430	Safety, efficacy, pharmacokinetics	NCT02715531	Hoffmann-La Roche	Active, not recruiting
-	I	No restriction	Ramucirumab + MEDI4736 [HCC] (arm C)	114	DLTs	NCT02572687	Eli Lilly & Co/Astra Zeneca	Active, not recruiting
NUANCE	I	Second-line	Nivolumab + bevacizumab	1	Safety and tolerability	NCT03382886	University of Utah	Terminated
-	I	Neo-adjuvant	Nivolumab + cabozantinib	15	Safety and tolerability	NCT 03299946	Sidney Kimmel Compehensive Cancer Center at John Hopkins	Active, not recruiting
-	Ib	First-line	Regorafenib + pembrolizumab	57	Safety and tolerability	NCT03347292	Bayer	Recruiting
-	Ib	First-line	Pembrolizumab + lenvatinib	104	Safety and tolerability	NCT 03006926	Eisai Co., Ltd.	Active, not recruiting
-	Ib	First-line	Nivolumab + lenvatinib	30	Safety and tolerability	NCT03418922	Eisai Co., Ltd.	Active, not recruiting
-	Ib	Second-line	Sintilimab + IBI305	47	AEs/ORR	NCT04401813	Innovent Biologics (Suzhou) Co., Ltd.	Recruiting
-	I/IIa	First-line	Nivolumab + Pexastimogene devacirepvec		Safety and tolerability	NCT03071094	Transgene	Active, not recruiting
CheckMate 040	I/II	Second-line	Cohort 4: Nivolumab + ipilimumab Cohort 6: Nivolumab + cabozantinib	148	Safety and tolerability	NCT01658878	Bristol-Myers Squibb/Ono Pharmaceutical Co., Ltd.	Active, not recruiting
-	I/II	Second-line	SHR-1210 + apatinib	60	OS	NCT02942329	The Affiliated Hospital of the Chinese Academy of Military Medical Sciences	Unknown
-	Ib/II	First-line	Pembrolizumab + talimogene laherarepvec	244	ORR/DLTs	NCT02509507	Amgen	Recruiting
-	II	First-line and Second-line	Durvalumab + tremelimmumab [regimen 1] (arm A) Durvalumab (arm B) Tremelimumab (arm C) Durvalumab + tremelimumab [regimen 2] (arm D) Durvalumab + bevacizumab (arm E)	545	Safety and tolerability	NCT02519348	MedImmune, LLC	Active, not recruiting

Table 1. *Cont.*

RESCUE	II	Second-line	SHR-1210 + apatinib	190	ORR	NCT03463876	Jiangsu HengRui Medicine Co., Ltd.	Active, not recruiting
-	II	First-line/Second-line	SHR1210 + apatinib (arm A) SHR1210 + FOLFOX4 or GEMOX regimen (arm B)	152	Safety and tolerability	NCT03092895	Jiangsu HengRui Medicine Co., Ltd.	Unknown
IMMUNIB	II	First-line	Nivolumab + lenvatinib	50	ORR/safety and tolerability	NCT03841201	Institut fur Klinische Krebsforschung IKF GmbH	Recruiting
-	II	First-line/Second-line	Nivolumab + Ipilimumab vs. nivolumab		Safety and tolerability	NCT03222076	MD Anderson Cancer Center	Active, not recruiting
-	II/III	First-line	Sintilimab + IBI305	566	OS/PFS	NCT03794440	Innovent Biologics (Suzhou) Co., Ltd.	Recruiting
IMbrave150	III	First-line	Atezolizumab + bevacizumab (arm A) Sorafenib (arm B)	480	OS/PFS	NCT03434379	Hoffmann-La Roche	Active, not recruiting
COSMIC-312	III	First-line	Cabozantinib + atezolizumab (arm A) Sorafenib (arm B) Cabozantinib (arm C)	740	PFS/OS	NCT03755791	Exelixis	Recruiting
LEAP-002	III	First-line	Pembrolizumab + Lenvatinib vs. placebo + lenvatinib	750	PFS/OS	NCT03713593	Merck Sharp & Dohme Corp.	Active, not recruiting
-	III	First-line	SHR-1210 + FOLFOX4 vs. sorafenib or FOLFOX4	448	OS	NCT03605706	Jiangsu HengRui Medicine Co., Ltd.	Recruiting
HIMALAYA	III	First-line	Durvalumab (arm A) Durvalumab + tremelimumab [regimen 1] (arm B) Durvalumab + tremelimumab [regimen 2] (arm C) Sorafenib (arm D)	1310	OS	NCT03298451	AstraZeneca	Active, not recruiting
-	III	First-line	CS1003 + lenvatinib vs. placebo + lenvatinib	525	PFS/OS	NCT04194775	CStone Pharmaceuticals	Recruiting

HCC, hepatocellular carcinoma; DLTs, dose-limiting toxicities; AEs, adverse events; OS, overall survival; PFS progression-free survival; ORR, overall response rate.

4.3. Immune Checkpoint Inhibitors Combined with Tyrosine Kinase Inhibitors

In addition to its well-known stimulating effect on angiogenesis, VEGF can promote immune evasion by directly and indirectly inhibiting infiltration and function of cytotoxic T-lymphocytes and increasing PD-1 expression on intra-tumoral CD8+ T-cells. In other words, the VEGF pathway is involved in the recruitment of immunosuppressive T-reg cells into the tumor. Thus, VEGF inhibition through TKIs or VEGFR-directed monoclonal antibodies might increase local antitumor immunity and favorably modify the immuno-suppressive tumor microenvironment, thus enhancing the effects of ICIs [45]. On this basis, several Phase I/II trials testing combinations of anti-PD1/PD-L1 with anti-VEGFRs were undertaken and have already shown promising results in this research field, paving the way for Phase III trials that are currently in progress (Table 1) [46].

Among these studies, one trial tested the combination of nivolumab plus cabozantinib, with or without ipilimumab, reporting preliminary clinically meaningful responses [47]. As of today, the results of this study, which included 71 patients randomized to either nivolumab plus cabozantinib (*n* = 36) or nivolumab plus ipilimumab and cabozantinib (*n* = 35), are only partially available, and show that investigator-assessed ORR was comparable with that of nivolumab alone for the dual treatment arm (17%, 6 patients with PR) but reached 26% (9 patients with PR) in the triple treatment arm. The diseased control rate was good and similar in the two groups, being 81% for the dual treatment arm and 83% for the triple treatment arm. It is noteworthy that the median OS was not reached in either arm [47]. With regards to safety, grade 3 or 4 treatment-related AEs were observed in 42% of cases in the dual treatment arm and in 71% of cases in the triple treatment arm, leading to treatment discontinuation in 3% and 20% of patients, respectively. However, no new safety signals were observed in either arm. Based on these promising findings, complete and updated results of this trial are eagerly awaited.

Another combination that is currently under investigation in patients with advanced HCC is that of pembrolizumab plus lenvatinib, which, in a Phase Ib study, showed good results with a median OS of 22 months and a 46% confirmed ORR [48]. Hence, this combination has been granted a breakthrough therapy designation by the FDA for advanced HCC patients who are not amenable to locoregional treatment, and it is currently being tested in a Phase III, international, multicenter clinical study (LEAP-002).

4.4. Immune Checkpoint Inhibitors Combined with Anti-VEGFR Agents

Recently, Finn et al. tested the combination of atezolizumab, a monoclonal antibody targeting PD-L1, plus bevacizumab, an anti-VEGF monoclonal antibody, as a front-line treatment of advanced HCC. The trial (IMbrave-150) showed a clear superiority of the dual therapy over sorafenib [15]. The intention-to-treat population included 336 patients in the atezolizumab plus bevacizumab group and 165 patients in the sorafenib group. At the time of the primary interim analysis, the HR for death with atezolizumab plus bevacizumab as compared with sorafenib was 0.58 (95%CI, 0.42–0.79; $p < 0.001$). The reported 12-month OS was 67.2% (95%CI, 61.3–73.1) with atezolizumab plus bevacizumab versus 54.6% (95%CI, 45.2–64.0) with sorafenib. Median PFS was 6.8 months (95%CI, 5.7 to 8.3) and 4.3 months (95%CI, 4.0–5.6) in the respective groups (HR for disease progression or death: 0.59; 95%CI, 0.47–0.76; $p < 0.001$) [15]. Hypertension, proteinuria, and fatigue were the top three treatment-related AEs in the combination arm. Upper gastrointestinal bleeding, a known AE of bevacizumab and a main concern in patients with cirrhosis, occurred in 7% of patients in this group, which is well within the range of previous studies evaluating the use of bevacizumab in HCC [49,50]. Esophageal varices hemorrhage occurred in 2.4% of cases, but only 1.8% were grade ≥3 and less than 1% of cases needed treatment discontinuation. Of note, in this study, causality was reported only in <1% of patients [15]. In this respect, it is important to emphasize that patients intended to receive the combination of atezolizumab plus bevacizumab had undergone endoscopic variceal screening, as per the study protocol. Given the increased bleeding risk associated with bevacizumab, patients with gastro-esophageal varices at risk of bleeding received adequate prophylactic treatment, as must be done in standard care of cirrhotic patients with esophageal varices [51,52]. Increases in aminotransferases and pruritus were other common AEs attributable to atezolizumab but, again, only a few patients (0.6% of cases) needed to stop treatment and developed immune-mediated liver damage. The proportion of patients who discontinued any treatment component because of AEs was 15.5% in the atezolizumab plus bevacizumab group (7% discontinued both components) and 10.3% in the sorafenib group [15]. Overall, AEs leading to dose modification or interruption occurred in 49.5% of patients who received atezolizumab plus bevacizumab and in 60.9% of those who received sorafenib. Therefore, this study provided the first and strong—evidence of the benefit provided by combining an ICI and a VEGFR inhibitor for patients with advanced HCC, and its superiority over sorafenib has undoubtedly already changed the standard of care for these patients, where it has substituted sorafenib as first-line treatment in most cases. Nevertheless, as only patients with Child–Pugh class A were included in this study, which is standard practice in HCC trials, so no consistent data are available regarding efficacy and safety of this combination in patients with a greater impairment in liver function. To date, only one study has reported the outcomes for four Child–Pugh class B patients treated with atezolizumab plus bevacizumab in a Japanese cohort of patients [53]. Among these patients, all patients could be treated without the development of severe AEs until tumor progression and efficacy was comparable to that of Child–Pugh class A patients. These results are undoubtedly important, but further research in larger cohorts of patients is needed before a recommendation can be made for the use of this immunotherapy in patients with Child–Pugh class B liver function. However, we could argue that well selected patients with Child–Pugh class B7 liver function may be treated safely with atezolizumab plus bevacizumab but close monitoring of biochemistry and close clinical monitoring should be performed and patients should be informed that the benefit of this treatment in the Child–Pugh class B population still has to be determined.

The role of sorafenib and that of lenvatinib and, more in general, the treatment algorithms for the systemic treatment of HCC, will soon need to be reviewed in order to be optimized. Whether TKIs are going to be part of the second-line treatment alternatives, alone or in combination with other agents, is still unknown and extensive research is ongoing to try to adequately frame treatment sequences.

4.5. Immune Checkpoint Inhibitors Combined with Locoregional Treatments for HCC

To date, no systemic treatment tested in combination with locoregional treatments for HCC has demonstrated benefit in terms of OS. Conversely, ICIs might revolutionize the therapeutic panorama of early and intermediate stage HCC, thus achieving a role not only in the setting of palliative treatment, but also in the curative one. The rationale for their use in combination with radiofrequency ablation (RFA) and TACE relies on the fact that ablative and intra-arterial techniques indirectly induce a peripheral immune response that can enhance the effect of ICIs [54,55] (Figure 2). Namely, the RFA- and TACE-induced necrosis of tumor cells favors the release of tumor antigens and the activation of immune-mediated death of tumor cells, which, in turn, stimulate a peripheral systemic immune response that can potentially be amplified by immune checkpoint blockade [56–61]. Arayu et al. showed that alpha-fetoprotein-specific CD4+ T-cell responses to three immune-dominant epitopes in HCC patients were significantly expanded during and after embolization ($p < 0.002$). Specifically, the development of alpha-fetoprotein-specific CD4+ T-cells after treatment was significantly associated with the induction of >50% necrosis of tumor and an improved clinical outcome ($p < 0.007$) [57]. Similarly, Mizokushiet al, evaluating T-cell responses in patients with HCC undergoing RFA, observed immune responses to antigens for which no T-cell response was detected before RFA [60]. Interestingly, the number of tumor-specific T-cells after RFA correlated with the prevention of HCC recurrence in patients treated with curative intent [60]. Moreover, RFA ablation not only provides activating signals for T-cell responses against HCC, but also augments the pool of circulating natural killer (NK) lymphocytes and enhances preferential expression of NK cells' activating receptors and NK cells' cytotoxicity, and all these effects are seen as soon as one week after treatment [61].

Although very limited data exist in patients with very early or early HCC (BCLC 0 or BCLC A stage) and intermediate HCC (BCLC B stage) treated with ICIs in the adjuvant and neo-adjuvant setting, preliminary data are promising. With regards to the neo-adjuvant setting, a recent pilot randomized, Phase II trial showed that dual treatment with nivolumab plus ipilimumab prior to surgery leads to a complete pathological response rate in 33.3% of cases [62]. An increase in T-cell infiltration and upregulation of cytotoxic and effector memory cell markers in tissue after treatment was also seen, as compared with before treatment [62]. Two other small studies investigated tumor-specific immune responses after combined TACE and RFA treatment, or after each individual treatment, confirming that ablative therapies induce tumor-specific T-cell responses in individual patients upon ablative therapies [59,63].

Combined ICIs plus TACE or RFA are not the only treatments under investigation, as some reports regarding the combination of trans-arterial Y^{90}-radioembolization (TARE) and immune checkpoint blockade have been presented at recent oncological meetings with promising results. In particular, Tai et al. reported the results of a Phase II, open-label, single-center, non-randomized trial regarding the effects of a combined therapy with TARE and nivolumab for advanced HCC in an Asian cohort. Their results showed that this combination had a synergistic effect, with an ORR of 30.5% and with good safety and tolerability profiles [64].

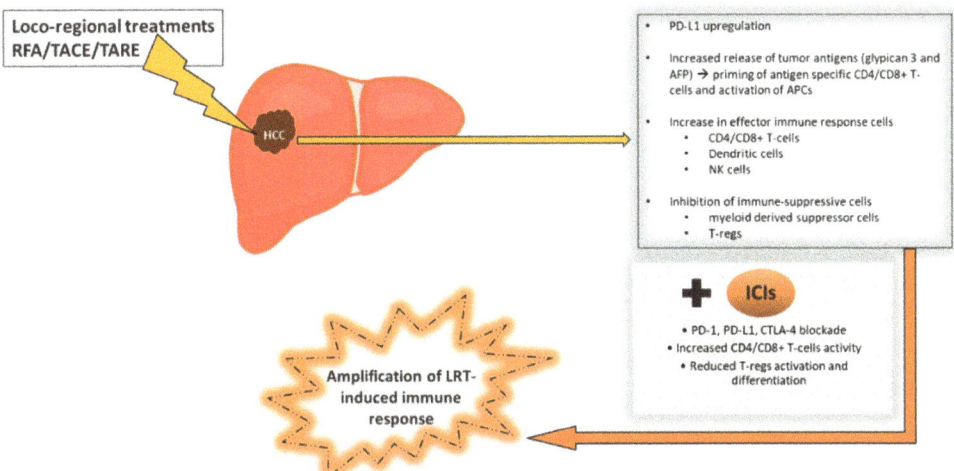

Figure 2. Locoregional treatments applied to hepatocellular carcinoma (HCC) induce immunological effects in the tumor microenvironment, which can be amplified by immune checkpoint inhibitors. After radiofrequency ablation (RFA) or trans-arterial chemo-embolization (TACE) or radio-embolization (TARE), necrosis of tumor cells induces increased tumor-antigen release, thus facilitating the recruitment and activation of cytotoxic T-cells and dendritic cells. These effects can be exploited by administering immune checkpoint inhibitors (ICIs) to transform an immunosuppressive microenvironment in an immune-supportive one, in which systemic therapies might be more effective.

Based on these findings, several trials are ongoing to test the efficacy of combined ICIs and locoregional treatments in HCC. This strategy might significantly decrease recurrence rates after treatment with ablative techniques, thus ameliorating long-term prognosis of patients with very early/early HCC. Similarly, ICIs may potentially enhance responses after trans-arterial treatments; this implicates that patients with intermediate stage HCC may be effectively down-staged and might therefore become qualified for curative treatments. Hence, if ongoing studies in this field obtain good results in terms of safety and efficacy, ICIs would not only play a role in the setting of advanced HCC, but would also become a fundamental component of the management of the earlier stages of this tumor.

5. Amenability to Atezolizumab Plus Bevacizumab in Real-Life Setting

Given the expected upcoming change in the standard of care for the treatment of patients with advanced HCC, with a preferential use of the combination of atezolizumab plus bevacizumab as first-line treatment, we aimed to explore the actual estimates of the potential applicability in clinical practice of this dual treatment in the Western HCC population. In order to do so, we applied the inclusion and exclusion criteria of the atezolizumab plus bevacizumab IMBrave-150 study to the HCC population recorded in the Italian Liver Cancer (ITA.LI.CA) database. We used this database as it is representative of the real-life setting of HCC patients in Italy: the ITA.LI.CA database, indeed, includes more than 10,000 patients with newly diagnosed or recurrent HCC, with various underlying liver disease etiologies at all stages, who are managed in a large number of Italian centers with different levels of expertise (secondary and tertiary referral centers). Thus, it provides a reliable insight into the characteristics of HCC patients in Western regions and allows for predicting figures of the potential utilization of newly available HCC drugs in real-life clinical practice [39].

In order to carry this out, within the ITA.LI.CA database, we excluded patients diagnosed before 2008—that is the year of availability of sorafenib in clinical practice in Italy—and we applied the inclusion and exclusion criteria, listed in Table 2, set forth in the Phase III IMbrave-150 trial in patients with advanced HCC. In the studied period

(2008–2019), 7529 cases of HCC were reported overall and, among them, a total of 5203 cases had a newly diagnosed HCC, whereas 2326 presented the first recurrence after surgery and/or locoregional treatment; we then calculated the eligibility rate to atezolizumab plus bevacizumab in the overall cohort and, separately, in the two subgroups of naïve patients with HCC or with an HCC recurrence after surgery or locoregional treatment (Figure 3).

Table 2. Criteria of eligibility for the management of unresectable HCC with atezolizumab plus bevacizumab as a first-line therapy.

IMBrave-150 Inclusion Criteria
Age $\geq$ 18 years
Locally advanced or metastatic and/or unresectable HCC
No prior systemic therapy for HCC
Disease that is not amenable to curative surgical and/or locoregional therapies, or progressive disease after surgical and/or locoregional therapies
At least one measurable (per RECIST 1.1) untreated lesion
Patients who received prior local therapy (e.g., radiofrequency ablation, percutaneous ethanol or acetic acid injection, cryoablation, high-intensity focused ultrasound, transarterial chemoembolization, transarterial embolization, etc.) are eligible provided the target lesion(s) have not been previously treated with local therapy or the target lesion(s) within the field of local therapy have subsequently progressed in accordance with RECIST version 1.1
ECOG PS 0-1
Child–Pugh class A
ANC $\geq$ 1.5 $\times$ 10^9/L (1500/mcL) without granulocyte colony-stimulating factor support
Lymphocyte count $\geq$ 0.5 $\times$ 109/L (500/µL)
Platelet count $\geq$ 75 $\times$ 109/L (75,000/µL) without transfusion
Hemoglobin $\geq$ 90 g/L (9 g/dL)
AST, ALT, and alkaline phosphatase (ALP) $\leq$ 5 $\times$ upper limit of normal (ULN)
Serum bilirubin $\leq$ 3 $\times$ ULN
Serum creatinine $\leq$ 1.5 $\times$ ULN or creatinine clearance $\geq$ 50 mL/min (Cockcroft–Gault formula)
Serum albumin $\geq$ 28 g/L
For patients not receiving therapeutic anticoagulation: INR or aPTT $\leq$ -2 $\times$ ULN
Urine dipstick for proteinuria < 2+
Negative HIV test at screening
In case of active HBV, HBV DNA < 500 IU/mL and anti-HBV treatment for a minimum of 14 days prior to study entry
No history of leptomeningeal disease
No active or history of autoimmune disease or immune deficiency
No history of idiopathic pulmonary fibrosis, organizing pneumonia, drug-induced pneumonitis, or idiopathic pneumonitis, or evidence of active pneumonitis
No active tuberculosis
No significant cardiovascular disease ($\geq$NYHA Class II)
No major surgical procedure, other than for diagnosis, within 4 weeks
No history of malignancy other than HCC within 5 years prior to screening
No severe infection within 4 weeks prior to initiation of study treatment
No treatment with therapeutic oral or IV antibiotics within 2 weeks prior to initiation of study treatment
No prior allogeneic stem cell or solid organ transplantation
No known fibrolamellar HCC, sarcomatoid HCC, or mixed cholangiocarcinoma and HCC
No untreated or incompletely treated varices with bleeding or high risk for bleeding
No moderate or severe ascites
No history of hepatic encephalopathy
No co-infection of HBV and HCV
No symptomatic, untreated, or actively progressing central nervous system (CNS) metastases
No uncontrolled pleural effusion, pericardial effusion, or ascites requiring recurrent drainage procedures
No uncontrolled or symptomatic hypercalcemia
No treatment with systemic immunosuppressive medication
No inadequately controlled arterial hypertension
No significant vascular disease
No history of intra-abdominal inflammatory process

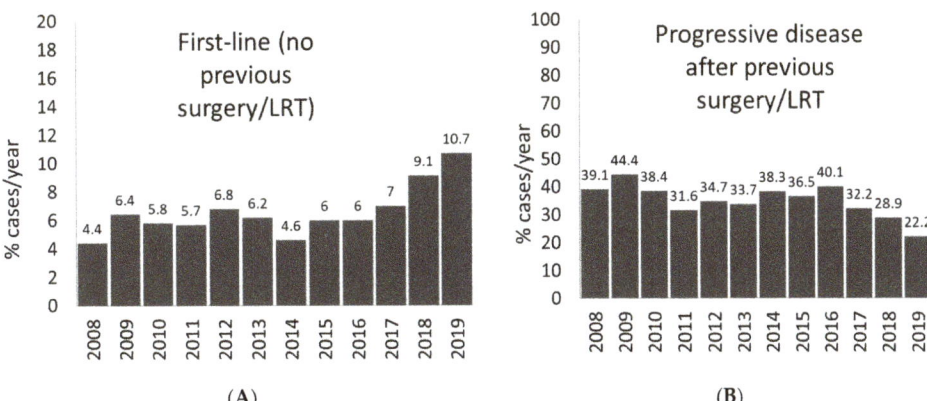

Figure 3. (**A**,**B**) Proportion of patients with new onset HCC or with HCC recurrence after surgery or locoregional treatment, which is amenable to first-line treatment with atezolizumab plus bevacizumab, per year, in the ITA.LI.CA database.

As far as the subgroup of naive patients with HCC is concerned, the overall proportion of patients deemed eligible for atezolizumab plus bevacizumab was 7.1%, ranging from 5.3% to 5.4% (2008–2014) up to 10.7% (2019), with a median eligibility rate for the novel therapy in this group of patients of 7.5%, and with an increasing trend observed in the most recent years (Figure 3A). With regard to patients with HCC recurrence after surgery or locoregional treatment, after excluding those not eligible for the treatment with ate-zolizumab plus bevacizumab as per the study inclusion and exclusion criteria, the overall eligibility rate to this ICI-based therapy was 36.3%, with a median eligibility rate across the whole period of 36.5% (range, 28.9% to 44.4%), with a decreasing trend observed in the most recent years (Figure 3B).

Taking into account all the patients included in the ITA.LI.CA database in the period 2008–2019, irrespective of previous locoregional treatment, approximately 16% of cases were considered eligible for the newly approved dual treatment. This figure is in accordance with estimates from other reports on ICI-based treatments [39].

Among patients with newly diagnosed HCC, 1.4% of patients were excluded solely due to the presence of untreated, or incompletely treated, esophageal varices at high risk of bleeding, while this figure among patients with recurrence following locoregional treatment or surgery was 4.0%. However, the presence of esophageal varices at high risk of bleeding should not be considered a strict exclusion criterion, as primary prevention of variceal bleeding can and must be performed with either non-selective beta-blockers or endoscopic banding ligation as part of the standard of care of patients with cirrhosis [51,52]. Ligation, which might be preferred due to the possibility of an objective assessment of treatment success, may delay by several weeks the beginning of anti-tumor treatment due to the need to fully evaluate the eradication of varices in a proportion of patients ranging from 1.4% to 4.0%. These considerations need to be taken into account in the therapeutic decision process, as overall approximately 13% of patients with HCC harbor large esophageal varices, a finding keeping with the overall prevalence of at-risk varices in this study population (i.e., 15.0%) before the application of the inclusion/exclusion criteria of the atezolizumab plus bevacizumab study [65]. Moreover, besides representing an issue to be solved before the beginning of treatment, the presence of varices has an inherent meaning that needs to be underscored in these patients, as it pinpoints a subpopulation of patients that—despite having similar inclusion criteria—presents a more advanced liver disease, characterized by clinically significant portal hypertension. This finding is not negligible when patients' prognosis is assessed, as the presence of esophageal varices is an independent prognostic determinant, also considering the stage of liver disease and HCC stage [51,65–67]. Therefore, the prognosis of patients with advanced HCC and esophageal varices will be poorer than that of patients without varices, regardless of the efficacy of the anti-tumoral drug (Figure 4) [65]; as such, screening and treatment (either with band ligation or beta-blockers, selected on a case by case basis) is strongly recommended and must be performed in all patients with HCC, independently from the tumor stage and prior to the initiation of any anti-tumoral treatment.

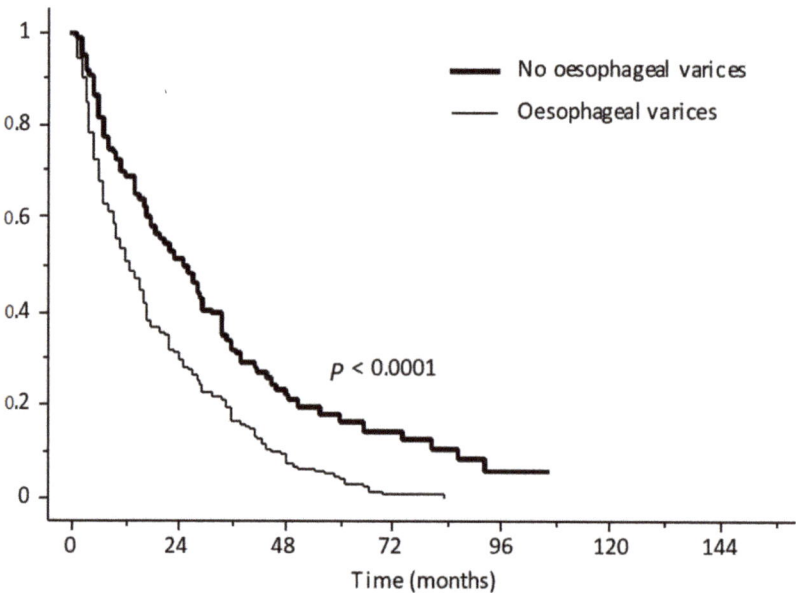

Figure 4. Overall survival of patients with advanced hepatocellular carcinoma, subdivided according to the presence of esophageal varices. Reprinted with permission from ref. [65]. Copyright 2006 American Gastroenterological Association.

6. Conclusions

Immunotherapy certainly represents a new, exciting frontier in the treatment of advanced, unresectable HCC, and might play a role as an adjuvant or neo-adjuvant treatment of patients with early-stage HCC as well, giving them the chance to decrease the risk of tumor recurrence. New ICI-based treatment strategies with dual, or even triple, combinations of immune-targeting agents, or combinations of immunotherapy and TKIs or other anti-neoplastic agents, will probably be available in the foreseeable future. Thus, it is currently difficult to predict the future algorithm for the systemic treatment of advanced HCC and to state whether sorafenib and lenvatinib, as single agents, will still be listed among the first-line treatment options for this cancer. However, despite the understandable enthusiasm for immunotherapy, some unmet needs remain and require further, extensive research to be resolved. First, as many as 30–40% of patients with HCC do not respond to ICIs, and biomarkers predicting treatment response are lacking. This is a particular challenging issue as data about histological or serological biomarkers related to the effectiveness of ICIs in HCC have not been clearly identified, and, even if a histological marker was identified, biopsy sampling of HCC is not standard clinical practice for this tumor, which is mostly diagnosed on the basis of its radiological hallmarks; therefore, in the future, the role of liver biopsy in HCC might need to be revisited [68]. Secondly, we have shown that in real-life, also taking into consideration previous treatments, only approximately one-tenth to one-third of patients with HCC are eligible for the recently approved combination of atezolizumab plus bevacizumab. Moreover, the safety and utility of immunotherapy in patients with a greater impairment in liver function, such as Child–Pugh class B patients, still has to be demonstrated, as most trials have explored the safety of these drugs in patients with well-preserved liver function (Child–Pugh class A) and, even though some reports have described an acceptable safety profile of some ICIs in Child–Pugh class B patients, consistent data regarding this topic are lacking, so that no strong recommendation can be made in this regard for the time being. Finally, ICIs are highly expensive drugs and this may represent a serious threat to the worldwide treatment implementation in clinical practice, since a large share of patients with HCC are diagnosed in developing countries, where available economic resources cannot support their use [69].

Taken together, the available evidence clearly shows that ICIs are going to play a pivotal role in the treatment of HCC and will improve the prognosis of patients with advanced HCC and, presumably, of those at earlier stages of the disease as well. We can assume that in the foreseeable future the current treatment algorithms will need revisions based on the most recent evidence. However, considering that in real-life settings a high proportion of patients will probably not be eligible for ICI-based regimens, much effort is still needed in order to optimize treatment strategies for patients with advanced, unresectable HCC.

Funding: This research received no external funding.

Institutional Review Board Statement: Not applicable.

Informed Consent Statement: Not applicable.

Data Availability Statement: Data available on request due to restrictions. The data presented in this study are available on request from the corresponding author. The data are not publicly available due to the rules of the ITA.LI.CA consortium.

Acknowledgments: We acknowledged Italian Liver Cancer (ITA.LI.CA) Group and the Italian Association for the Study of the Liver—Hepatocellular Carcinoma Special Interest Group (AISF HCC-SIG). **Others members of the ITA.LI.CA group: Maurizio Biselli, Laura Bucci, Paolo Caraceni, Annagiulia Gramenzi, Lorenzo Lani, Davide Rampoldi, Nicola Reggidori, Valentina Santi, Benedetta Stefanini:** *Semeiotics Unit, Department of Medical and Surgical Sciences, IRCCS Azienda Ospedaliero-Universitaria di Bologna, University of Bologna, Bologna, Italy.* **Donatella Magalotti, Marco Zoli:** *Medicina Interna, Malattie neurovascolari e epatometaboliche, IRCCS Azienda Ospedaliero-Universitaria di Bologna, University of Bologna, Bologna, Italy.* **Alessandro Granito, Luca Muratori, Francesco Tovoli:** *Internal Medicine, Department of Medical and Surgical Sciences, IRCCS Azienda Ospedaliero-Universitaria di Bologna, University of Bologna, Bologna, Italy.* **Francesco Azzaroli, Elton Dajti, Federico Ravaioli:** *Gastroenterology Unit, Department of Surgical and Medical Sciences, IRCCS Azienda Ospedaliero-Universitaria di Bologna, University of Bologna, Bologna, Italy.* **Alberta Cappelli, Rita Golfieri, Cristina Mosconi, Matteo Renzulli:** *Radiology Unit, Department of Specialist, Diagnostic and Experimental Medicine, IRCCS Azienda Ospedaliero-Universitaria di Bologna, University of Bologna, Bologna, Italy.* **Fabio Farinati, Barbara Penzo:** *Gastroenterology Unit, Department of Surgery, Oncology and Gastroenterology, University of Padova, Padova, Italy.* **Rodolfo Sacco, Ester Marina Cela, Antonio Facciorusso:** *Gastroenterology and Digestive Endoscopy Unit, Foggia University Hospital, Foggia, Italy.* **Giulia Pieri, Edoardo Casagrande, Mattia Vanello.** *Gastroenterology Unit, Department of Internal Medicine, IRCCS Ospedale Policlinico San Martino, University of Genova, Genova, Italy.* **Antonio Gasbarrini, Gianludovico Rapaccini, Francesca Romana Ponziani, Nicoletta de Matthaeis:** *Gastroenterology Unit, IRCCS Fondazione Policlinico Universitario A. Gemelli, Roma, Italy.* **Gianluca Svegliati Baroni, Gloria Allegrini:** *Liver Injury and Transplant Unit, Polytechnic University of Marche, Ancona, Italy.* **Valentina Lauria, Giorgia Ghittoni, Giorgio Pelecca:** *Gastroenterology Unit, Belcolle Hospital, Viterbo, Italy.* **Fabrizio Chegai, Fabio Coratella, Mariano Ortenzi:** *Vascular and Interventional Radiology Unit, Belcolle Hospital, Viterbo, Italy.* **Serena Dell'Isola:** *Infectious Disease Unit, Belcolle Hospital, Viterbo, Italy.* **Gabriele Missale, Elisabetta Biasini, Andrea Olivani:** *Infectious Diseases and Hepatology Unit, Department of Medicine and Surgery, University of Parma and Azienda Ospedaliero-Universitaria of Parma, Parma, Italy.* **Alberto Masotto, Alessandro Inno, Fabiana Marchetti:** *Gastroenterology Unit, IRCCS Sacro Cuore Don Calabria Hospital, Negrar, Italy.* **Maria Di Marco:** *Medicine Unit, Bolognini Hospital, Seriate, Italy.* **Andrea Mega:** *Gastroenterology Unit, Bolzano Regional Hospital, Bolzano, Italy.* **Ciro Celsa, Mauro Grova, Caterina Stornello, Anita Busacca, Calogero Cammà, Giacomo Emanuele Maria Rizzo:** *Gastroenterology and Hepatology Unit, Department of Health Promotion, Mother and Child Care, Internal Medicine and Medical Specialties, PROMISE, University of Palermo, Palermo, Italy.* **Maria Stella Franzè, Giovanni Raimondo,**

Carlo Saitta: *Clinical and Molecular Hepatology Unit, Department of Clinical and Experimental Medicine, University of Messina, Messina, Italy.* **Gianpaolo Vidili, Assunta Sauchella**: *Department of Medical, Surgical and Experimental Sciences, Azienda Ospedaliero-Universitaria of Sassari, Sassari, Italy.* **Francesco Giuseppe Foschi, Lucia Napoli, Vittoria Bevilacqua, Dante Berardinelli, Alberto Borghi, Andrea Casadei Gardini, Fabio Conti, Alessandro Cucchetti, Anna Chiara Dall'Aglio, Giorgio Ercolani**: *Department of Internal Medicine, Ospedale per gli Infermi di Faenza, Faenza, Italy.* **Claudia Campani, Chiara Di Bonaventura, Stefano Gitto, Valentina Adotti**: *Internal Medicine and Hepatology Unit, Department of Experimental and Clinical Medicine, University of Firenze, Firenze, Italy.* **Gerardo Nardone, Pietro Coccoli, Antonio Malerba**: *Hepato-Gastroenterology Unit, Department of Clinical Medicine and Surgery, University of Napoli "Federico II", Napoli, Italy.* **Filomena Morisco, Maria Guarino, Mario Capasso**: *Gastroenterology Unit, Department of Clinical Medicine and Surgery, University of Napoli "Federico II", Napoli, Italy.* **Mauriza Rossana Brunetto, Filippo Oliveri, Veronica Romagnoli**: *Hepatology and Liver Physiopathology Laboratory, Department of Clinical and Experimental Medicine, University Hospital of Pisa, Pisa, Italy.* **Members of the Associazione Italiana per lo Studio del Fegato Special Interest Group on Hepatocellular Carcinoma (AISF SIG-HCC):** Aglitti A., Baccarani U.,Bhoori S., Borzio M., Brancaccio G., Burra P., Carrai P., Conti F., Cozzolongo R, Cucchetti A., D'Ambrosio R., Dell'Unto C., De Matthaeis N., Di Costanzo G.G., Di Sandro S., Famularo S, Fucilli F., Galati G., Gambato M., Giuliante F., Ghinolfi D., Grieco A., Gruttadauria S., Iavarone M., Kostandini A., Lenci I., Levi Sandri G.V., Losito F., Lupo L.G., Marasco G, Manzia T.M., Mazzocato S., Masarone M., Melandro F., Mescoli C., Miele L., Muley M., Nicolini D., Pagano D, Persico M., Pompili M., Pravisani R., Rendina M., Renzulli M., Romano F, Rossi M., Rreka E., Russo F.P., Sangiovanni A., Sessa A., Simonetti N., Sposito C., Tortora R., Viganò L., Viganò M., Villa E., Vincenzi V., Violi P., Vitale A.

Conflicts of Interest: The authors declare no conflict of interest.

References

1. Villanueva, A. Hepatocellular Carcinoma. *N. Engl. J. Med.* **2019**, *380*, 1450–1462. [CrossRef]
2. Mittal, S.; El-Serag, H.B.; Sada, Y.H.; Kanwal, F.; Duan, Z.; Temple, S.; May, S.; Kramer, J.R.; Richardson, P.A.; Davila, J.A. Hepatocellular Carcinoma in the Absence of Cirrhosis in United States Veterans Is Associated with Nonalcoholic Fatty Liver Disease. *Clin. Gastroenterol. Hepatol.* **2016**, *14*, 124–131.e1. [CrossRef]
3. Kanwal, F.; Kramer, J.R.; Mapakshi, S.; Natarajan, Y.; Chayanupatkul, M.; Richardson, P.A.; Li, L.; Desiderio, R.; Thrift, A.P.; Asch, S.M.; et al. Risk of Hepatocellular Cancer in Patients with Non-Alcoholic Fatty Liver Disease. *Gastroenterology* **2018**, *155*, 1828–1837.e2. [CrossRef] [PubMed]
4. Torres, M.C.P.; Bodini, G.; Furnari, M.; Marabotto, E.; Zentilin, P.; Strazzabosco, M.; Giannini, E.G. Surveillance for Hepatocellular Carcinoma in Patients with Non-Alcoholic Fatty Liver Disease: Universal or Selective? *Cancers* **2020**, *12*, 1422. [CrossRef]
5. Torres, M.C.P.; Aghemo, A.; Lleo, A.; Bodini, G.; Furnari, M.; Marabotto, E.; Miele, L.; Giannini, E.G. Mediterranean Diet and NAFLD: What We Know and Questions That Still Need to Be Answered. *Nutrients* **2019**, *11*, 2971. [CrossRef]
6. Llovet, J.M.; Ricci, S.; Mazzaferro, V.; Hilgard, P.; Gane, E.; Blanc, J.F.; De Oliveira, A.C.; Santoro, A.; Raoul, J.L.; Forner, A.; et al. Sorafenib in Advanced Hepatocellular Carcinoma. *N. Engl. J. Med.* **2008**, *359*, 378–390. [CrossRef]
7. Cheng, A.-L.; Kang, Y.-K.; Chen, Z.; Tsao, C.-J.; Qin, S.; Kim, J.S.; Luo, R.; Feng, J.; Ye, S.; Yang, T.-S.; et al. Efficacy and safety of sorafenib in patients in the Asia-Pacific region with advanced hepatocellular carcinoma: A phase III randomised, double-blind, placebo-controlled trial. *Lancet Oncol.* **2009**, *10*, 25–34. [CrossRef]
8. Cheng, A.-L.; Finn, R.S.; Qin, S.; Han, K.-H.; Ikeda, K.; Piscaglia, F.; Baron, A.D.; Park, J.-W.; Han, G.; Jassem, J.; et al. Phase III trial of lenvatinib (LEN) vs sorafenib (SOR) in first-line treatment of patients (pts) with unresectable hepatocellular carcinoma (uHCC). *J. Clin. Oncol.* **2017**, *35*, 4001. [CrossRef]
9. Kirstein, M.M.; Scheiner, B.; Marwede, T.; Wolf, C.; Voigtländer, T.; Semmler, G.; Wacker, F.; Manns, M.P.; Hinrichs, J.B.; Pinter, M.; et al. Sequential systemic treatment in patients with hepatocellular carcinoma. *Aliment. Pharmacol. Ther.* **2020**, *52*, 205–212. [CrossRef] [PubMed]
10. Sangro, B.; Gomez-Martin, C.; de la Mata, M.; Iñarrairaegui, M.; Garralda, E.; Barrera, P.; Riezu-Boj, J.-I.; Larrea, E.; Alfaro, C.; Sarobe, P.; et al. A clinical trial of CTLA-4 blockade with tremelimumab in patients with hepatocellular carcinoma and chronic hepatitis C. *J. Hepatol.* **2013**, *59*, 81–88. [CrossRef]
11. El-Khoueiry, A.B.; Sangro, B.; Yau, T.C.C.; Crocenzi, T.S.; Kudo, M.; Hsu, C.; Kim, T.-Y.; Choo, S.-P.; Trojan, J.; Welling, T.H.; et al. Nivolumab in patients with advanced hepatocellular carcinoma (CheckMate 040): An open-label, non-comparative, phase 1/2 dose escalation and expansion trial. *Lancet* **2017**, *389*, 2492–2502. [CrossRef]
12. Zhu, A.X.; Finn, R.S.; Edeline, J.; Cattan, S.; Ogasawara, S.; Palmer, D.; Verslype, C.; Zagonel, V.; Fartoux, L.; Vogel, A.; et al. Pembrolizumab in patients with advanced hepatocellular carcinoma previously treated with sorafenib (KEYNOTE-224): A non-randomised, open-label phase 2 trial. *Lancet Oncol.* **2018**, *19*, 940–952. [CrossRef]

13. Finn, R.S.; Ryoo, B.-Y.; Merle, P.; Kudo, M.; Bouattour, M.; Lim, H.Y.; Breder, V.; Edeline, J.; Chao, Y.; Ogasawara, S.; et al. Pembrolizumab As Second-Line Therapy in Patients with Advanced Hepatocellular Carcinoma in KEYNOTE-240: A Randomized, Double-Blind, Phase III Trial. *J. Clin. Oncol.* **2020**, *38*, 193–202. [CrossRef] [PubMed]

14. Yau, T.; Park, J.W.; Finn, R.S.; Cheng, A.L.; Mathurin, P.; Edeline, J.; Kudo, M.; Han, K.H.; Harding, J.J.; Merle, P.; et al. CheckMate 459: A randomized, multi-center phase III study of nivolumab (NIVO) vs sorafenib (SOR) as first-line (1L) treatment in patients (pts) with advanced hepatocellular carcinoma (aHCC). *Ann. Oncol.* **2019**, *30*, v874–v875. [CrossRef]

15. Finn, R.S.; Qin, S.; Ikeda, M.; Galle, P.R.; Ducreux, M.; Kim, T.-Y.; Kudo, M.; Breder, V.; Merle, P.; Kaseb, A.O. Atezolizumab plus Bevacizumab in Unresectable Hepatocellular Carcinoma. *N. Engl. J. Med.* **2020**, *382*, 1894–1905. [CrossRef]

16. Iavarone, M.; Cabibbo, G.; Piscaglia, F.; Zavaglia, C.; Grieco, A.; Villa, E.; Camma', C.; Colombo, M.; on behalf of the SOFIA (SOraFenib Italian Assessment) study group. Field-practice study of sorafenib therapy for hepatocellular carcinoma: A prospective multicenter study in Italy. *Hepatology* **2011**, *54*, 2055–2063. [CrossRef] [PubMed]

17. Ganten, T.M.; Stauber, R.E.; Schott, E.; Malfertheiner, P.; Buder, R.; Galle, P.R.; Göhler, T.; Walther, M.; Koschny, R.; Gerken, G. Sorafenib in Patients with Hepatocellular Carcinoma—Results of the Observational INSIGHT Study. *Clin. Cancer Res.* **2017**, *23*, 5720–5728. [CrossRef]

18. Bruix, J.; Qin, S.; Merle, P.; Granito, A.; Huang, Y.-H.; Bodoky, G.; Pracht, M.; Yokosuka, O.; Rosmorduc, O.; Breder, V.; et al. Regorafenib for patients with hepatocellular carcinoma who progressed on sorafenib treatment (RESORCE): A randomised, double-blind, placebo-controlled, phase 3 trial. *Lancet* **2017**, *389*, 56–66. [CrossRef]

19. Zhu, A.X.; Kang, Y.-K.; Yen, C.-J.; Finn, R.S.; Galle, P.R.; Llovet, J.M.; Assenat, E.; Brandi, G.; Lim, H.Y.; Pracht, M.; et al. REACH-2: A randomized, double-blind, placebo-controlled phase 3 study of ramucirumab versus placebo as second-line treatment in patients with advanced hepatocellular carcinoma (HCC) and elevated baseline alpha-fetoprotein (AFP) following first-line sorafenib. *J. Clin. Oncol.* **2018**, *36*, 4003. [CrossRef]

20. Abou-Alfa, G.K.; Meyer, T.; Cheng, A.-L.; El-Khoueiry, A.B.; Rimassa, L.; Ryoo, B.-Y.; Cicin, I.; Merle, P.; Chen, Y.; Park, J.-W.; et al. Cabozantinib in Patients with Advanced and Progressing Hepatocellular Carcinoma. *N. Engl. J. Med.* **2018**, *379*, 54–63. [CrossRef]

21. Zhu, A.X.; Park, J.O.; Ryoo, B.-Y.; Yen, C.-J.; Poon, R.; Pastorelli, D.; Blanc, J.-F.; Chung, H.; Baron, A.D.; Pfiffer, T.E.F.; et al. Ramucirumab versus placebo as second-line treatment in patients with advanced hepatocellular carcinoma following first-line therapy with sorafenib (REACH): A randomised, double-blind, multicentre, phase 3 trial. *Lancet Oncol.* **2015**, *16*, 859–870. [CrossRef]

22. Giannini, E.G.; Trevisani, F. Ramucirumab as a second-line treatment for hepatocellular carcinoma: Reaching out further to patients with elevated alpha-fetoprotein. *Hepatobiliary Surg. Nutr.* **2019**, *8*, 515–518. [CrossRef]

23. Lai, E.; Astara, G.; Ziranu, P.; Pretta, A.; Migliari, M.; Dubois, M.; Donisi, C.; Mariani, S.; Liscia, N.; Impera, V.; et al. Introducing immunotherapy for advanced hepatocellular carcinoma patients: Too early or too fast? *Crit. Rev. Oncol.* **2021**, *157*, 103167. [CrossRef]

24. Garuti, F.; Neri, A.; Avanzato, F.; Gramenzi, A.; Rampoldi, D.; Rucci, P.; Farinati, F.; Giannini, E.G.; Piscaglia, F.; Rapaccini, G.L.; et al. The changing scenario of hepatocellular carcinoma in Italy: An update. *Liver Int.* **2021**, *41*, 585–597. [CrossRef]

25. Hoshida, Y.; Villanueva, A.; Kobayashi, M.; Peix, J.; Chiang, D.Y.; Camargo, A.; Gupta, S.; Moore, J.; Wrobel, M.J.; Lerner, J.; et al. Gene Expression in Fixed Tissues and Outcome in Hepatocellular Carcinoma. *N. Engl. J. Med.* **2008**, *359*, 1995–2004. [CrossRef]

26. Pikarsky, E.; Porat, R.M.; Stein, I.; Abramovitch, R.; Amit, S.; Kasem, S.; Gutkovich-Pyest, E.; Urieli-Shoval, S.; Galun, E.; Ben-Neriah, Y. NF-κB functions as a tumour promoter in inflammation-associated cancer. *Nature* **2004**, *431*, 461–466. [CrossRef]

27. Llovet, J.M.; Montal, R.; Sia, D.; Finn, R.S. Molecular therapies and precision medicine for hepatocellular carcinoma. *Nat. Rev. Clin. Oncol.* **2018**, *15*, 599–616. [CrossRef] [PubMed]

28. Prieto, J.; Melero, I.; Sangro, B. Immunological landscape and immunotherapy of hepatocellular carcinoma. *Nat. Rev. Gastroenterol. Hepatol.* **2015**, *12*, 681–700. [CrossRef] [PubMed]

29. Shi, F.; Shi, M.; Zeng, Z.; Qi, R.-Z.; Liu, Z.-W.; Zhang, J.-Y.; Yang, Y.-P.; Tien, P.; Wang, F.-S. PD-1 and PD-L1 upregulation promotes CD8+ T-cell apoptosis and postoperative recurrence in hepatocellular carcinoma patients. *Int. J. Cancer* **2010**, *128*, 887–896. [CrossRef] [PubMed]

30. Sia, D.; Jiao, Y.; Martinez-Quetglas, I.; Kuchuk, O.; Villacorta-Martin, C.; de Moura, M.C.; Putra, J.; Camprecíós, G.; Bassaganyas, L.; Akers, N.; et al. Identification of an Immune-specific Class of Hepatocellular Carcinoma, Based on Molecular Features. *Gastroenterology* **2017**, *153*, 812–826. [CrossRef] [PubMed]

31. Chen, D.S.; Mellman, I. Oncology Meets Immunology: The Cancer-Immunity Cycle. *Immunity* **2013**, *39*, 1–10. [CrossRef]

32. Ringelhan, M.; Pfister, D.; O'Connor, T.; Pikarsky, E.; Heikenwalder, M. The immunology of hepatocellular carcinoma. *Nat. Immunol.* **2018**, *19*, 222–232. [CrossRef]

33. Postow, M.A.; Callahan, M.K.; Wolchok, J.D. Immune Checkpoint Blockade in Cancer Therapy. *J. Clin. Oncol.* **2015**, *33*, 1974–1982. [CrossRef] [PubMed]

34. El-Khoueiry, A.B.; Melero, I.; Yau, T.C.; Crocenzi, T.S.; Kudo, M.; Hsu, C.; Choo, S.; Trojan, J.; Welling, T.; Meyer, T.; et al. Impact of antitumor activity on survival outcomes, and nonconventional benefit, with nivolumab (NIVO) in patients with advanced hepatocellular carcinoma (aHCC): Subanalyses of CheckMate-040. *J. Clin. Oncol.* **2018**, *36*, 475. [CrossRef]

35. Crocenzi, T.S.; El-Khoueiry, A.B.; Yau, T.C.; Melero, I.; Sangro, B.; Kudo, M.; Hsu, C.; Trojan, J.; Kim, T.-Y.; Choo, S.-P.; et al. Nivolumab (nivo) in sorafenib (sor)-naive and -experienced pts with advanced hepatocellular carcinoma (HCC): CheckMate 040 study. *J. Clin. Oncol.* **2017**, *35*, 4013. [CrossRef]

36. Abou-Alfa, G.K.; Chan, S.; Furuse, J.; Galle, P.R.; Kelley, R.K.; Qin, S.; Armstrong, J.; Darilay, A.; Vlahovic, G.; Negro, A.; et al. A randomized, multicenter phase 3 study of durvalumab (D) and tremelimumab (T) as first-line treatment in patients with unresectable hepatocellular carcinoma (HCC): HIMALAYA study. *J. Clin. Oncol.* **2018**, *36*, TPS4144. [CrossRef]

37. Kudo, M.; Matilla, A.; Santoro, A.; Melero, I.; Gracian, A.C.; Acosta-Rivera, M.; Choo, S.P.; El-Khoueiry, A.B.; Kuromatsu, R.; El-Rayes, B.F.; et al. Checkmate-040: Nivolumab (NIVO) in patients (pts) with advanced hepatocellular carcinoma (aHCC) and Child-Pugh B (CPB) status. *J. Clin. Oncol.* **2019**, *37*, 327. [CrossRef]

38. Haanen, J.; Carbonnel, F.; Robert, C.; Kerr, K.; Peters, S.; Larkin, J.; Jordan, K. Management of toxicities from immunotherapy: ESMO Clinical Practice Guidelines for diagnosis, treatment and follow-up. *Ann. Oncol.* **2017**, *28*, iv119–iv142. [CrossRef] [PubMed]

39. Giannini, E.G.; Aglitti, A.; Borzio, M.; Gambato, M.; Guarino, M.; Iavarone, M.; Lai, Q.; Sandri, G.B.L.; Melandro, F.; Morisco, F.; et al. Overview of Immune Checkpoint Inhibitors Therapy for Hepatocellular Carcinoma, and The ITA.LI.CA Cohort Derived Estimate of Amenability Rate to Immune Checkpoint Inhibitors in Clinical Practice. *Cancers* **2019**, *11*, 1689. [CrossRef]

40. De Velasco, G.; Je, Y.; Bossé, D.; Awad, M.M.; Ott, P.A.; Moreira, R.B.; Schutz, F.; Bellmunt, J.; Sonpavde, G.P.; Hodi, F.S.; et al. Comprehensive Meta-analysis of Key Immune-Related Adverse Events from CTLA-4 and PD-1/PD-L1 Inhibitors in Cancer Patients. *Cancer Immunol. Res.* **2017**, *5*, 312–318. [CrossRef]

41. Scheiner, B.; Kirstein, M.M.; Hucke, F.; Finkelmeier, F.; Schulze, K.; Von Felden, J.; Koch, S.; Schwabl, P.; Hinrichs, J.B.; Waneck, F.; et al. Programmed cell death protein-1 (PD-1)-targeted immunotherapy in advanced hepatocellular carcinoma: Efficacy and safety data from an international multicentre real-world cohort. *Aliment. Pharmacol. Ther.* **2019**, *49*, 1323–1333. [CrossRef]

42. Yau, T.; Kang, Y.-K.; Kim, T.-Y.; El-Khoueiry, A.B.; Santoro, A.; Sangro, B.; Melero, I.; Kudo, M.; Hou, M.-M.; Matilla, A.; et al. Nivolumab (NIVO) + ipilimumab (IPI) combination therapy in patients (pts) with advanced hepatocellular carcinoma (aHCC): Results from CheckMate. *J. Clin. Oncol.* **2019**, *37* (Suppl. S15), 4012. [CrossRef]

43. Yau, T.; Kang, Y.-K.; Kim, T.-Y.; El-Khoueiry, A.B.; Santoro, A.; Sangro, B.; Melero, I.; Kudo, M.; Hou, M.-M.; Matilla, A.; et al. Efficacy and Safety of Nivolumab Plus Ipilimumab in Patients with Advanced Hepatocellular Carcinoma Previously Treated with Sorafenib. *JAMA Oncol.* **2020**, *6*, e204564. [CrossRef] [PubMed]

44. Kelley, R.K.; Sangro, B.; Harris, W.P.; Ikeda, M.; Okusaka, T.; Kang, Y.-K.; Qin, S.; Tai, W.M.D.; Lim, H.Y.; Yau, T.; et al. Efficacy, tolerability, and biologic activity of a novel regimen of tremelimumab (T) in combination with durvalumab (D) for patients (pts) with advanced hepatocellular carcinoma (aHCC). *J. Clin. Oncol.* **2020**, *38*, 4508. [CrossRef]

45. Tai, D.; Choo, S.P.; Chew, V. Rationale of Immunotherapy in Hepatocellular Carcinoma and Its Potential Biomarkers. *Cancers* **2019**, *11*, 1926. [CrossRef]

46. Liu, L.; Qin, S.; Zhang, Y. The Evolving Landscape of Checkpoint Inhibitor Combination Therapy in the Treatment of Advanced Hepatocellular Carcinoma. *Target. Oncol.* **2021**, *16*, 153–163. [CrossRef]

47. Yau, T.; Zagonel, V.; Santoro, A.; Acosta-Rivera, M.; Choo, S.P.; Matilla, A.; He, A.R.; Gracián, A.C.; El-Khoueiry, A.B.; Sangro, B.; et al. Nivolumab (NIVO) + ipilimumab (IPI) + cabozantinib (CABO) combination therapy in patients (pts) with advanced hepatocellular carcinoma (aHCC): Results from CheckMate 040. *J. Clin. Oncol.* **2020**, *38*, 478. [CrossRef]

48. Finn, R.S.; Ikeda, M.; Zhu, A.X.; Sung, M.W.; Baron, A.D.; Kudo, M.; Okusaka, T.; Kobayashi, M.; Kumada, H.; Kaneko, S.; et al. Phase Ib Study of Lenvatinib Plus Pembrolizumab in Patients with Unresectable Hepatocellular Carcinoma. *J. Clin. Oncol.* **2020**, *38*, 2960–2970. [CrossRef] [PubMed]

49. Pinter, M.; Ulbrich, G.; Sieghart, W.; Kölblinger, C.; Reiberger, T.; Li, S.; Ferlitsch, A.; Müller, C.; Lammer, J.; Peck-Radosavljevic, M. Hepatocellular Carcinoma: A Phase II Randomized Controlled Double-Blind Trial of Transarterial Chemoembolization in Combination with Biweekly Intravenous Administration of Bevacizumab or a Placebo. *Radiology* **2015**, *277*, 903–912. [CrossRef] [PubMed]

50. Siegel, A.B.; Cohen, E.I.; Ocean, A.; Lehrer, D.; Goldenberg, A.; Knox, J.J.; Chen, H.; Clark-Garvey, S.; Weinberg, A.; Mandeli, J.; et al. Phase II Trial Evaluating the Clinical and Biologic Effects of Bevacizumab in Unresectable Hepatocellular Carcinoma. *J. Clin. Oncol.* **2008**, *26*, 2992–2998. [CrossRef]

51. Angeli, P.; Bernardi, M.; Villanueva, C.; Francoz, C.; Mookerjee, R.; Trebicka, J.; Krag, A.; Laleman, W.; Gines, P. EASL Clinical Practice Guidelines for the management of patients with decompensated cirrhosis. *J. Hepatol.* **2018**, *69*, 406–460. [CrossRef]

52. Giannini, E.G.; Trevisani, F. Improving survival of cirrhosis patients with hepatocellular carcinoma through application of standard of care. *Hepatology* **2014**, *60*, 1446–1447. [CrossRef]

53. Iwamoto, H.; Shimose, S.; Noda, Y.; Shirono, T.; Niizeki, T.; Nakano, M.; Okamura, S.; Kamachi, N.; Suzuki, H.; Sakai, M.; et al. Initial Experience of Atezolizumab Plus Bevacizumab for Unresectable Hepatocellular Carcinoma in Real-World Clinical Practice. *Cancers* **2021**, *13*, 2786. [CrossRef] [PubMed]

54. Greten, T.F.; Duffy, A.G.; Korangy, F. Hepatocellular Carcinoma from an Immunologic Perspective. *Clin. Cancer Res.* **2013**, *19*, 6678–6685. [CrossRef] [PubMed]

55. Singh, P.; Toom, S.; Avula, A.; Kumar, V.; E Rahma, O. The Immune Modulation Effect of Locoregional Therapies and Its Potential Synergy with Immunotherapy in Hepatocellular Carcinoma. *J. Hepatocell. Carcinoma* **2020**, *7*, 11–17. [CrossRef] [PubMed]

56. Duffy, A.G.; Ulahannan, S.; Makorova-Rusher, O.; Rahma, O.; Wedemeyer, H.; Pratt, D.; Davis, J.L.; Hughes, M.S.; Heller, T.; ElGindi, M.; et al. Tremelimumab in combination with ablation in patients with advanced hepatocellular carcinoma. *J. Hepatol.* **2017**, *66*, 545–551. [CrossRef] [PubMed]

57. Ayaru, L.; Pereira, S.; Alisa, A.; Pathan, A.A.; Williams, R.; Davidson, B.; Burroughs, A.K.; Meyer, T.; Behboudi, S. Unmasking of α-Fetoprotein-Specific CD4+ T Cell Responses in Hepatocellular Carcinoma Patients Undergoing Embolization. *J. Immunol.* **2007**, *178*, 1914–1922. [CrossRef]

58. Hänsler, J.; Hä, J.; Nsler, T.; Wissniowski, D.S.U.T. Activation and dramatically increased cytolytic activity of tumor specific T lymphocytes after radio-frequency ablation in patients with hepatocellular carcinoma and colorectal liver metastases. *World J. Gastroenterol.* **2006**, *12*, 3716–3721. [CrossRef] [PubMed]

59. Hiroishi, K.; Eguchi, J.; Baba, T.; Shimazaki, T.; Ishii, S.; Hiraide, A.; Sakaki, M.; Doi, H.; Uozumi, S.; Omori, R.; et al. Strong CD8+ T-cell responses against tumor-associated antigens prolong the recurrence-free interval after tumor treatment in patients with hepatocellular carcinoma. *J. Gastroenterol.* **2009**, *45*, 451–458. [CrossRef]

60. Mizukoshi, E.; Nakamoto, Y.; Arai, K.; Yamashita, T.; Sakai, A.; Sakai, Y.; Kagaya, T.; Yamashita, T.; Honda, M.; Kaneko, S. Comparative analysis of various tumor-associated antigen-specific t-cell responses in patients with hepatocellular carcinoma. *Hepatology* **2011**, *53*, 1206–1216. [CrossRef]

61. Zerbini, A.; Pilli, M.; Laccabue, D.; Pelosi, G.; Molinari, A.; Negri, E.; Cerioni, S.; Fagnoni, F.; Soliani, P.; Ferrari, C.; et al. Radiofrequency Thermal Ablation for Hepatocellular Carcinoma Stimulates Autologous NK-Cell Response. *Gastroenterology* **2010**, *138*, 1931–1942.e2. [CrossRef]

62. Kaseb, A.O.; Vence, L.; Blando, J.; Yadav, S.S.; Ikoma, N.; Pestana, R.C.; Vauthey, J.N.; Allison, J.P.; Sharma, P. Immunologic Correlates of Pathologic Complete Response to Preoperative Immunotherapy in Hepatocellular Carcinoma. *Cancer Immunol. Res.* **2019**, *7*, 1390–1395. [CrossRef] [PubMed]

63. Nakatsura, T.; Nobuoka, D.; Motomura, Y.; Shirakawa, H.; Yoshikawa, T.; Kuronuma, T.; Takahashi, M.; Nakachi, K.; Ishii, H.; Furuse, J.; et al. Radiofrequency ablation for hepatocellular carcinoma induces glypican-3 peptide-specific cytotoxic T lymphocytes. *Int. J. Oncol.* **2011**, *40*, 63–70. [CrossRef] [PubMed]

64. Tai, W.M.D.; Loke, K.S.H.; Gogna, A.; Tan, S.H.; Ng, D.C.E.; Hennedige, T.P.; Irani, F.; Lee, J.J.X.; Too, C.W.; Ng, M.C.; et al. A phase II open-label, single-center, nonrandomized trial of Y90-radioembolization in combination with nivolumab in Asian patients with advanced hepatocellular carcinoma: CA 209-678. *J Clin. Oncol.* **2020**, *38*, 4590. [CrossRef]

65. Giannini, E.G.; Risso, D.; Testa, R.; Trevisani, F.; Di Nolfo, M.A.; Del Poggio, P.; Benvegnù, L.; Rapaccini, G.L.; Farinati, F.; Zoli, M.; et al. Prevalence and Prognostic Significance of the Presence of Esophageal Varices in Patients with Hepatocellular Carcinoma. *Clin. Gastroenterol. Hepatol.* **2006**, *4*, 1378–1384. [CrossRef] [PubMed]

66. European Association for the Study of the Liver. EASL Clinical Practice Guidelines: Management of hepatocellular carcinoma. *J. Hepatol.* **2018**, *69*, 182–236. [CrossRef]

67. D'Amico, G.; Pasta, L.; Morabito, A.; Caltagirone, M.; Malizia, G.; Tinè, F.; Giannuoli, G.; Traina, M.; Vizzini, G.; Politi, F.; et al. Competing risks and prognostic stages of cirrhosis: A 25-year inception cohort study of 494 patients. *Aliment. Pharmacol. Ther.* **2014**, *39*, 1180–1193. [CrossRef]

68. Russo, F.P.; Imondi, A.; Lynch, E.N.; Farinati, F. When and how should we perform a biopsy for HCC in patients with liver cirrhosis in 2018? A review. *Dig. Liver Dis.* **2018**, *50*, 640–646. [CrossRef]

69. Dimitroulis, D.; Damaskos, C.; Valsami, S.; Davakis, S.; Garmpis, N.; Spartalis, E.; Athanasiou, A.; Moris, D.; Sakellariou, S.; Kykalos, S.; et al. From diagnosis to treatment of hepatocellular carcinoma: An epidemic problem for both developed and developing world. *World J. Gastroenterol.* **2017**, *23*, 5282–5294. [CrossRef]

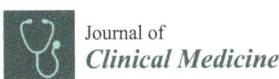

Journal of
Clinical Medicine

Review

Liver Transplantation in Patients with Hepatocellular Carcinoma beyond the Milan Criteria: A Comprehensive Review

Pierluigi Toniutto *, Elisa Fumolo, Ezio Fornasiere and Davide Bitetto

Hepatology and Liver Transplantation Unit, Azienda Sanitaria Universitaria Integrata, 33100 Udine, Italy; elisa.fumolo@asufc.sanita.fvg.it (E.F.); ezio.fornasiere@asufc.sanita.fvg.it (E.F.); davide.bitetto@asufc.sanita.fvg.it (D.B.)
* Correspondence: pierluigi.toniutto@uniud.it; Tel.: +39-0432-552636; Fax: +39-0432-559487

Abstract: The Milan criteria (MC) were developed more than 20 years ago and are still considered the benchmark for liver transplantation (LT) in patients with hepatocellular carcinoma (HCC). However, the strict application of MC might exclude some patients who may receive a clinical benefit of LT. Several expanded criteria have been proposed. Some of these consider pretransplant morphological and biological variables of the tumor, others consider post-LT variables such as the histology of the tumor, and others combine pre- and post-LT variables. More recently, the HCC response to locoregional treatments before transplantation emerged as a surrogate marker of the biological aggressiveness of the tumor to be used as a better selection criterion for LT in patients beyond the MC at presentation. This essential review aims to present the current data on the pretransplant selection criteria for LT in patients with HCC exceeding the MC at presentation based on morphological and histological characteristics of the tumor and to critically discuss those that have been validated in clinical practice. Moreover, the role of HCC biological markers and the tumor response to downstaging procedures as new tools for selecting patients with a tumor burden outside of the MC for LT is evaluated.

Keywords: hepatocellular carcinoma; liver transplantation; Milan criteria; alpha-fetoprotein

Citation: Toniutto, P.; Fumolo, E.; Fornasiere, E.; Bitetto, D. Liver Transplantation in Patients with Hepatocellular Carcinoma beyond the Milan Criteria: A Comprehensive Review. *J. Clin. Med.* **2021**, *10*, 3932. https://doi.org/10.3390/jcm10173932

Academic Editor: Tatsuo Kanda

Received: 24 July 2021
Accepted: 29 August 2021
Published: 31 August 2021

Publisher's Note: MDPI stays neutral with regard to jurisdictional claims in published maps and institutional affiliations.

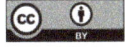
1. Introduction

Hepatocellular carcinoma (HCC) is the fifth most common cancer and the third most common cause of cancer-related mortality [1]. The incidence of HCC has progressively increased during recent decades due to the increased number of patients with liver cirrhosis caused by chronic hepatitis C (HCV), hepatitis B (HBV), and alcohol abuse, as well as patients with metabolic syndrome-induced liver disease [2]. Fewer than half of HCC cases are diagnosed at an early stage, which allows them to receive curative treatments such as surgical resection, locoregional ablative therapy, and liver transplantation (LT) [3]. LT is considered the best treatment option for HCC because removal of the native liver simultaneously eliminates the tumor and the underlying liver disease [4].

In the second half of the 1960s, LT programs were developed in humans with the aim of offering radical treatment of unresectable liver tumors [5]. However, the initial enthusiasm for these experiences quickly dwindled, as it appeared evident that post-transplant survival was unsatisfactory due to the unsustainable tumor recurrence rates in the transplanted liver, which predicted poor survival [6]. These unsatisfactory results stemmed from a lack of precise selection criteria for patients to undergo transplantation, which were based on the tumor type and on the intrahepatic burden of the neoplastic disease [7]. Thus, the dramatic change that allowed improvement of the post-transplant survival in patients with HCC was the introduction of more accurate selection criteria. In 1996, Mazzaferro et al. published for the first time the Milan criteria (MC), which are still largely used as

J. Clin. Med. **2021**, *10*, 3932. https://doi.org/10.3390/jcm10173932

https://www.mdpi.com/journal/jcm

the reference benchmark to select patients with HCC for LT in many countries. The MC were based on HCC morphological characteristics evaluable before LT (up to three HCC nodules the largest < 3 cm in diameter or a single HCC nodule up to 5 cm in diameter), without macrovascular invasion or extrahepatic spread of the tumor [8]. Patients fulfilling MC experienced a 4-year survival rate of 75%. Several studies confirmed these results and demonstrated that the overall post-transplant survival of HCC patients transplanted within MC was not unlike that of patients transplanted for decompensated liver cirrhosis without HCC [9]. However, even in patients transplanted within MC, HCC recurrence was described in 10–16% of cases and was the main cause of death [10,11]. These data showed that despite the careful selection of HCC patients for transplantation, based on tumor morphological criteria, the risk of HCC recurrence remained consistent. This may be explained by the dissemination of circulating cancer cells and micrometastases before or during transplant operation [12]. Thus, the key issue in the success of LT for HCC is to select candidates that present as the least likely to experience tumor recurrence after transplantation and who maintain a comparable post-LT survival expectancy to that of non-HCC recipients [13].

Although the MC are still largely applied to candidate LT patients with HCC, a growing number of studies have shown that acceptable post-LT may be obtained in patients exceeding the MC at baseline [14–17]. This evidence is of paramount importance, suggesting that the strict application of the MC in all LT candidates could take away the possibility of transplantation in some patients who instead would have an important clinical benefit of LT [18]. The reasons why the MC did not allow accurate prediction of the outcome after LT in all patients stem from the fact that they were based exclusively on tumor morphological characteristics, such as the size and number of nodules. To overcome this limitation, several selection criteria that sought to expand the MC were proposed [19]. Some of these criteria were constructed using morphological and biological variables of the tumor obtainable pretransplant (Tables 1 and 2), others on variables obtainable only after transplantation (for example, the full histology of the tumor), and others by combining variables obtainable in both the pre- and post-transplantation periods. More recently, it has been proposed that the response of HCC to locoregional treatment (LRT) before transplantation may represent a surrogate marker of biological aggressiveness of the tumor to be used to improve patient selection for transplantation and overcome the limitations of criteria based exclusively on tumor morphology. This concept shifts the current paradigm to select for LT-only patients fulfilling the MC at baseline and offers the possibility of considering all patients with an HCC outside the MC at baseline that may be downstaged with locoregional treatments to within the MC as potentially suitable for LT (Figure 1).

Table 1. The preoperative selection criteria for liver transplantation (LT) in patients with hepatocellular carcinoma (HCC) based on morphological characteristics of the tumor. Only the externally validated selection criteria are reported in the table.

Authors	Criterion Name	Country	No. of Patients	HCC Morphology	Post-LT Survival	Post-LT RFS
Mazzaferro et al. [8]	Milan	Italy	48	Up to 3 nodules <3 cm in diameter or up to 5 cm in diameter in the case of a single nodule	75% at 4 years	83% at 4 years
Fan et al. [20]	Shanghai Fudan	China	1078	Single nodule ≤ 9 cm in diameter, no more than 3 nodules with the largest ≤5 cm, a total tumor diameter ≤ 9 cm, without MVI or EHS	80% at 3 years	88% at 3 years
Yao et al. [14]	UCSF	US	168	Single nodule ≤ 6 cm in diameter or 2–3 nodules ≤ 4.5 cm, with a total tumor diameter ≤ 8 cm	-	80.7% at 5 years

RFS: recurrence-free survival; MVI: macrovascular invasion; EHS: extrahepatic spread; UCSF: University of California, San Francisco.

Table 2. The preoperative selection criteria for liver transplantation (LT) in patients with hepatocellular carcinoma (HCC) based on the addition of the biological serum markers and/or histological differentiation grade to the morphological characteristics of the tumor. Only the externally validated selection criteria are reported in the table.

Authors	Criterion Name	Country	No. of Patients	HCC Characteristics	Post-LT Survival	Post-LT RFS
Du Bay et al. [21]	Toronto	Canada	294	HCC confined to the liver, AFP serum levels < 400 ng/mL, no poor histologic differentiation	70% at 5years	66% at 5 years
Zheng et al. [22]	Hangzhou	China	195	HCC ≤ 8 cm in diameter or >8 cm if associated with AFP serum levels <400 ng/mL and histological grade I–II	70.7% at 5 years	62.4% at 5 years
Toso et al. [23]	Toso	Canada Swiss UK	233	Total tumor volume ≤ 115 cm³ and AFP serum levels ≤ 400 ng/mL	74.6% at 4 years	68% at 4 years
Duvoux et al. [24]	French	France	972	Nodule diameters ≤ 3 cm, between 3–6 cm, or ≥6 cm and AFP serum levels ≤ 100, between 100–1000, or >1000 ng/mL	69.9% at 5 years	66.6% at 5 years
Mazzaferro et al. [25]	Metroticket 2.0	Italy China	1359	The sum of the size (in cm) of the larger HCC and the number of nodules not exceeding 7, without MVI	74.9% at 5 years	77.9% at 5 years
* Kaido et al. [26]	Kyoto	Japan	198	Up to 10 HCCs with a diameter ≤ 5 cm and DCP serum levels ≤400 mAU/mL	82% at 5 years	-
* Lee et al. [27]	MoRAL	Korea	566	Simultaneous evaluation of DCP and AFP serum levels	86% at 5 years	66.3% at 5 years

RFS: recurrence-free survival; AFP: alpha-fetoprotein; MVI: macrovascular invasion; DCP: des-gamma-carboxyprothrombin. * The criteria were evaluated in living donor liver transplantation.

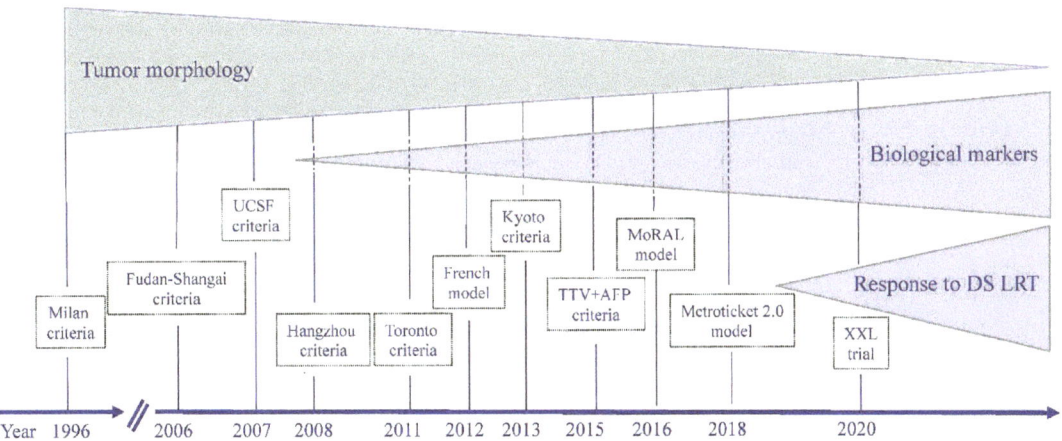

Figure 1. Evolving concepts in the selection of patients with HCC for liver transplantation. After the discovery of the Milan criteria in 1996, the subsequently expanded criteria for liver transplantation in patients with HCC were mainly based on the morphological characteristics of the tumor. Starting in 2008, with the Hangzhou criteria, the addition of biological markers to tumor morphologic criteria allowed expansion of the original Milan criteria, maintaining a good clinical outcome of liver transplanted patients with HCC. More recently, the new way to select patients to be transplanted for HCC who are beyond the Milan criteria at presentation has been to qualify those who can be traced back to the Milan criteria after successful downstaging after locoregional and/or systemic treatments. UCSF: University California, San Francisco; TTV: total tumor volume; AFP: alpha-fetoprotein; DS: downstaging; LRT: locoregional treatment.

It should be considered that the expansion of the transplant criteria for HCC will progressively increase the number of potential candidates on the waiting list. This imposes three main questions when contemplating expansion of the MC for LT in patients with HCC: (a) What upper limit of the tumor burden beyond the MC could be accepted for LT? (b) What could be the minimal acceptable overall survival after LT? (c) How could markers of tumor biology, in addition to the tumor burden, be incorporated to better select patients for LT?

This essential review aims to present the current data on the pretransplant selection criteria for LT in patients with HCC exceeding the MC at presentation based on morphological and histological characteristics of the tumor and to critically discuss those that have been validated in clinical practice. Moreover, the role of HCC biological markers and the tumor response to downstaging procedures as new tools for selecting patients for LT with a baseline tumor burden outside of the MC will be evaluated.

2. Selection Criteria for LT Based on HCC Morphological Characteristics

A common theme in the morphological criteria adopted to select patients with HCC was to exclude those patients presenting HCC with macrovascular invasion and/or extrahepatic spread. The main reason why morphological pre-LT criteria improved the accuracy in the selection of patients with HCC for LT derives from the demonstration that both the number and the size of HCC nodules can be considered surrogate markers of histologic microvascular invasion (MVI) and/or poor tumor differentiation [28,29], which are the main determinants of HCC recurrence and death after LT [30]. In addition to MC, two pretransplant expansive morphological criteria were adopted and validated in cohorts of patients of various geographical origins. The Shanghai Fudan criteria were originally developed in patients with chronic HBV infection. Patients transplanted with a single HCC nodule ≤ 9 cm in diameter or with up to three lesions (the largest ≤ 5 cm) but with a maximum tumor diameter of ≤9 cm experienced 1- and 3-year post-LT survival and HCC recurrence-free survival comparable with those transplanted within the MC [20]. These criteria were subsequently validated in more than 1000 patients enrolled in liver transplant centers in Shanghai [31]. In the United States, a further criterion aimed at expanding the original MC was developed at the University of California, San Francisco (UCSF) [14]. The UCSF criteria were developed after the observation that patients transplanted with a single nodule of HCC ≤ 6.5 cm or with up to 2–3 lesions ≤ 4.5 cm each, maintaining the total tumor diameter ≤ 8 cm, experienced a 5-year post-LT recurrence-free survival of 80.7%, which was not significantly different than that obtained in patients transplanted within the MC.

Both new criteria increased, albeit slightly, the size and/or the number of HCC nodules to select patients for LT compared to what was originally established by the MC. The certainty of always being able to carry out an accurate and reproducible measurement of the size and number of nodules to capture millimeter differences with respect to the MC probably represents the greatest limitation of the new criteria based exclusively on the morphological characteristics of HCC. There is great heterogeneity and different accuracies of liver imaging techniques applied to detect liver nodules and to properly characterize them, such as contrast-enhanced computed tomography (CT) or magnetic resonance imaging (MRI) [19]. Several reports have indicated that as many as 20–25% of patients undergoing LT for HCC have been inaccurately staged when only imaging techniques were used [32,33]. To overcome this important drawback, the American College of Radiology created the Liver Imaging Reporting and Data System (LI-RADS), aimed at standardizing the process of acquisition, interpretation, reporting, and data collection for liver imaging [34]. LI-RADS stratified the characteristics of liver lesions into five categories starting from LR-1 (definitely benign) to LR-5 (definitely HCC). This system is adopted in many countries to allow a standardized differential diagnosis of liver nodules in patients at high risk of HCC. Despite this improvement in the radiological categorization of liver nodules, a recent meta-analysis showed that LI-RADS was only 67% sensitive and 92% specific in diagnosing HCC [35].

3. Selection Criteria for LT Based on HCC Histological Characteristics

In patients transplanted beyond MC, a greater incidence of MVI, which is associated with higher post-LT tumor recurrence and death, has been demonstrated [36]. When the explanted livers of patients within and outside the MC were compared, MVI was present in 11% of the former group and in 42% of the latter group [37]. A potential tool to detect the presence of MVI of HCC before LT is to perform liver biopsy of the nodules. Liver biopsy of confirmed HCC in the explanted liver was performed before LT in a series of 155 patients [33]. MVI was significantly more frequent in patients with larger nodules or with multinodular HCC; furthermore, 68% of patients who experienced HCC recurrence after LT were positive for MVI. In addition to the detection of MVI, another potential tool employing liver biopsy of HCC is to evaluate tumor histological grading. It has been demonstrated that well-differentiated HCCs may be successfully transplanted, assuring a recipient 5-year post-LT survival of 75% despite approximately 30% of these patients being beyond MC at the explant [38]. Although the clinical usefulness of pre-LT histologic assessment of tumor grading and MVI may be important, routine biopsy of HCC is not often feasible, mainly due to the presence of multiple nodules or the risk of promoting seeding of cancer cells [39].

The current challenging question is whether the presence of MVI may be predicted by means of noninvasive methods. To answer this question, several authors propose the use of imaging techniques such 18F-FDG PET/CT or gadoxetic acid enhanced dynamic MRI as noninvasive methods to predict the presence of MVI [40,41]. The rationale for using 18F-FDG PET/CT in detecting MVI derives from the observation that the HCC growth rate and the activity of glycolytic enzymes are related [42]. This explains why poorly differentiated HCC shows low glucose-6 phosphatase activity and high 18F-FDG uptake [43]. It has been proposed that good cutoff values for the SUVmax of HCC (SUVmax T) and SUVmax of the normal liver (SUVmax L) in predicting the presence of MVI may be 3.80 and 1.49, respectively [44]. The SUVmax T/SUVmean L ratio $\geq$ 1.2 was demonstrated to be significantly associated with the presence of MVI [45]. Compared with 18F-FDG PET/CT alone, the addition of gadoxetic acid enhanced dynamic MRI is a promising technology that may further improve the sensitivity and specificity of MVI detection. This was confirmed by applying the combination of MRI and PET/CT, as the sensitivity and specificity in predicting the presence of MVI were 78.6% and 80%, respectively [40]. These observations have been confirmed in clinical studies conducted in Asia in living donor liver transplantation. In Japan, 182 living donor liver transplanted patients with HCC were studied by means of 18F-FDG PET/CT and the serum levels of alpha-fetoprotein (AFP) before LT. In recipients transplanted beyond MC who presented negative 18F-FDG PET/CT and AFP serum levels < 115 ng/mL, the 5-year HCC recurrence rate was comparable to those transplanted within MC [46]. Very similar results were obtained in a Korean study also conducted in patients transplanted outside the Milan and UCSF criteria using living donors. The authors demonstrated that these two groups of patients, if they presented a negative 18F-FDG PET/CT, experienced 5-year post-LT HCC-free survival rates of 73.3% and 72.8%, respectively [47]. Although these results are encouraging, it is necessary to confirm them in populations of different ethnic groups, where the causes of LT are often different from those present in Asia, as well as in patients transplanted using deceased donors. At the present time, the combined use of 18F-FDG PET/CT and gadoxetic acid enhanced MRI could be applied in addition to the morphological and biological characteristics of HCC to stratify the risk of MVI.

4. Selection Criteria Based on Serum Biological Marker Measurements

The measurement of serum markers referring to biological tumor characteristics and/or to host immune system reactivity has been considered a fascinating approach to overcome the limits of morphological criteria. Three main categories of measurable biological markers are currently available: (a) serum markers related to the biological characteristics of HCC, such as AFP and des-gamma-carboxyprothrombin (DCP); (b) markers reflecting systemic host inflammation (neutrophil-to-lymphocyte ratio and platelet-to-lymphocyte ratio); and (c) molecular biomarkers that may be measured both in liver tissue and in serum (genetic mutations, enzymes, and microRNAs). In relation to the clinical purpose of this review, only serum markers will be discussed, as there is still no solid evidence justifying the use of inflammation and molecular biomarkers in clinical practice.

5. Selection Criteria Based on the Addition of AFP and/or DCP Serum Level Measurements to HCC Morphology

AFP is considered a marker of HCC differentiation and vascular invasion; thus, the measurement of its serum levels pre-LT has been proposed as a potential tool to identify HCC patients with a higher risk of tumor recurrence and poor post-LT survival who should be excluded from transplantation [48]. The limitations of this approach became immediately evident, since it was very difficult to apply AFP measurement in a standardized and reproducible timeframe. For example, in deceased donor liver transplantation, the date of the transplant is never predictable. Thus, the optimal time interval between transplantation and AFP measurement that would make it a predictive marker of recurrence was unclear [19]. Instead of adopting cutoff values of AFP, an interesting approach is to consider multiple AFP measurements to calculate a trend in the increase or decrease in its serum levels. Patients experiencing an increase in serum AFP > 15 ng/mL/month had a higher frequency of waitlist dropout or significantly worse post-LT survival than those with a lower ($\leq$15 ng/mL/month) increase in AFP (54% vs. 94%) [49]. These results suggest that the variations in AFP serum levels, rather than the last AFP level available before LT, may be more accurate in predicting post-LT outcome. [50]. This concept is incorporated to increase the accuracy of the assessment of tumor downstaging before LT. For example, a rapid increase in AFP serum levels after a presumed successful downstaging, assessed by radiologic imaging, should be considered a predictor of poor post-transplant outcome.

A very attractive way to select in patients beyond MC at baseline those with a higher risk of HCC recurrence is to add AFP serum levels to the morphologic characteristics of HCC [51]. The Toronto criteria [21] were developed assuming that all patients with HCC may have acceptable post-LT survival independent of the number and/or size of the nodules if HCC was confined to the liver, well differentiated at histology, and without macrovascular invasion. These criteria identified AFP serum levels > 400 IU/mL at the time of transplant as an independent predictor of worse 5-year disease-free survival. The Toronto criteria were subsequently validated, confirming that AFP serum levels before LT were strongly associated with post-LT survival and HCC recurrence [52].

Similar results, combining the morphology and histology of HCC with AFP serum levels, have been obtained in China, where the Hangzhou criteria were developed [22]. These criteria selected HCC patients for LT in the absence of portal vein tumor invasion and with either HCC $\leq$ 8 cm in diameter or with HCC $\geq$ 8 cm in diameter but with concurrent AFP serum levels < 400 ng/mL and histological grade I or II. Patients fulfilling the Hangzhou criteria experienced 1- and 3-year survival rates very similar to those reported in patients transplanted within the MC. The combination of AFP serum levels and morphologic characteristics of the tumor also inspired European authors to expand the MC for selecting patients with HCC for LT. Toso et al. [53] evaluated a large cohort of 6000 European LT patients and demonstrated that the subgroup of recipients who presented a total tumor volume (TTV) of $\leq$115 cm^3 and AFP serum levels $\leq$ 400 ng/mL experienced a lower risk of HCC recurrence and better survival after LT. It should be highlighted that these expanded criteria were more effective than both the Milan and UCSF criteria in selecting patients with a low risk of HCC recurrence for LT. The TTV-AFP criteria were subsequently validated in cohorts of patients in countries outside Europe and in Canada [23]. A further model that combined AFP serum levels and morphologic characteristics of HCC, known as the AFP model, was proposed by the Liver Transplantation French Group [24]. The AFP model merges AFP serum levels and the size and the number of nodules, attributing different scores for each variable. Tumor sizes of 0, 1, or 4 points were assigned if the largest tumor diameter was $\leq$3 cm, 3–6 cm, or >6 cm, respectively. Moreover, 0 or 2 points were assigned if the number of nodules was $\leq$3 or $\geq$4. Regarding the AFP serum levels, 0, 2, or 3 points were assigned if AFP serum levels were $\leq$100, 100–1000, or >1000 ng/mL, respectively. The maximum score sum of the AFP model is 9. Patients may be divided into low risk of HCC recurrence if the final score is up to 2 points and high risk of HCC recurrence if the final score is ≥3. A very innovative observation of the study was that in patients presenting AFP serum levels > 1000 ng/mL, 3 points are attributed, irrespective of the number or size of nodules; thus, they may be immediately considered at high risk of HCC recurrence. The AFP model was validated in different countries and in living donor liver transplantation, confirming its clinical utility in stratifying the recurrence risk of HCC after LT in a better way than MC [54–57]. The Metroticket 2.0 model [25], developed in Italy, was based on the measurement of the sum of the number and size of nodules and the $\log_{10}$ AFP level. Recipients with AFP levels < 200 ng/mL and with the sum of the number and size of tumors (in centimeters) not exceeding 7 presented a post-LT survival probability of 70%, which was comparable to that observed in patients transplanted within MC. To maintain this excellent clinical outcome in the presence of AFP levels of 200–400 ng/mL, the sum of the number and size of tumors should be reduced to ≤5, and if AFP levels are 400–1000 ng/mL, the sum of the number and size of tumors should be further reduced to ≤4. This model outperformed the original MC, UCSF, and AFP French models in identifying patients with excellent 5-year post-LT survival.

The results obtained by combining the morphological characteristics of the tumor and the AFP values made it possible to develop selection criteria for LT that definitively exceeded those of Milan. These models introduced many innovations to more accurately select patients with HCC for LT. First, these selection criteria made it possible to offer LT to many patients with HCC who would have been excluded by application of the MC, assuring excellent post-transplant survival. Second, the calculation of both the size and number of nodules and the AFP serum levels appears simple and available in every context, making these models applicable in different geographical contexts and with all types of patients. Third, these models may be used "dynamically", in addition to the assessment of the HCC response to neoadjuvant treatments, to more accurately select patients who will undergo tumor downstaging before LT.

The interest in measuring DCP serum levels was derived from the observation that some HCCs expressed normal levels of AFP but increased levels of DCP. These subtypes of HCCs present a poor grade of differentiation and frequent MVI [58,59]. The combination of morphological characteristics of HCC (up to 10 nodules ≤ 5 cm in diameter) and DCP serum levels (≤400 mAU/mL) are the key elements included in the Kyoto criteria [26,60,61]. Patients beyond MC who fulfilled the Kyoto criteria at the time of LT had similar post-LT prognoses in terms of survival and HCC recurrence compared to those within MC [60]. In the context of living donor liver transplantation, the Kyushu criteria [62] that are considered suitable for LT patients with any number of HCC < 5 cm in diameter and DCP serum levels < 300 mAU/mL were developed. These criteria appeared more accurate for predicting HCC recurrence than both the Kyoto and UCSF criteria but only when living donation was considered [63,64].

Another interesting way to construct a prediction model of post-LT clinical outcome in patients with HCC beyond MC is to combine DCP and AFP serum levels. Starting from this assumption, the MoRAL model was developed in living donor liver transplant patients exceeding the MC [27]. Both AFP and DCP serum levels were significantly associated with the time elapsed from transplantation to HCC recurrence. In the group of recipients exceeding the MC, a MoRAL score ≤ 314.8 was predictive to select patients with significantly longer (66.3%) 5-year recurrence-free and overall (82.1%) survival. In contrast, the group of recipients fulfilling the MC but with a MoRAL score > 314.8 showed a higher risk of HCC recurrence and lower post-LT survival than patients beyond MC with a low MoRAL score. A retrospective study evaluating the combination of DCP and AFP serum levels in predicting clinical outcome in liver transplant patients outside the MC was also conducted in the United States [65]. In this study, AFP and DCP serum levels ≥ 250 ng/mL and ≥7.5 ng/mL, respectively, were predictive of more frequent HCC recurrence. When AFP and DCP were combined with MC, the hazard ratio of HCC recurrence risk increased from 2.6 for patients beyond MC to 8.6 when AFP serum levels were ≥250 ng/mL and to

7.2 when DCP serum levels were ≥ 7.5 ng/mL. The encouraging results deriving from the use of DCP as post-transplant survival as well as post-transplant HCC recurrence predictor should be analyzed with caution. It should be emphasized that more than 90% of the published papers related to DCP have been produced in Asian countries and refer to living donor liver transplanted patients for liver diseases mainly related to HBV infection [66]. Thus, solid data on the role of DCP in conditioning the clinical outcome of patients with HCC transplanted with deceased donors and with liver diseases due to nonviral etiologies are still lacking. Considering these limitations, among all biological markers that have been studied, AFP remains the only one that has proven useful in predicting the clinical outcome in patients transplanted for HCC. The prognostic models of post-transplant survival that incorporate pre-LT AFP serum levels and HCC morphological characteristics remain the most widely used to accurately select patients beyond MC for LT. In addition, the evaluation of AFP serum level variations induced by locoregional therapies and HCC downstaging modalities is becoming the most promising strategy to select patients to be transplanted with HCC beyond the MC with even greater accuracy.

6. Selection Criteria Based on the Response of HCC to Bridging and Downstaging Treatments

A very innovative approach to select patients for LT presenting at baseline beyond the MC is to evaluate the characteristics of tumor response after LRT and consider it a surrogate marker of biological HCC aggressiveness and of the risk of recurrence [19]. When LRT is used to control tumor growth with the aim of reducing the risk of waiting list dropout, it may be considered a "bridge" treatment to LT. The efficacy of LRT in reducing waiting list dropout has been demonstrated if the waiting time for LT is at least 6 months [67]. Patients whose tumor progression occurs despite LRT within 6 months have a worse post-LT outcome than those who achieved treatment response or the stability of HCC following LRT [49,68,69]. These observations suggest that the response to LRT might be influenced not only by the treatment modality but also, more importantly, by the biological behavior of the tumor.

The term "downstaging" is used by attributing the possibility of LRT decreasing the baseline tumor burden until it meets the criteria for LT (ideally within MC) and to assure acceptable post-LT outcomes [36]. This concept was derived from some studies suggesting that post-LT outcomes in patients successfully downstaged to the MC were comparable with those observed in transplanting patients with MC at presentation [70,71]. The potential explanation of these findings is that a close correlation exists between successful downstaging and better explant histologic characteristics of the tumor [70–72].

As indicated by the Barcelona Clinic Liver Cancer (BCLC) staging system [73], among the LRT modalities that may be employed to perform downstaging of HCC, transarterial chemoembolization (TACE) is the most commonly utilized. Transarterial radioembolization (TARE) and ablative techniques may be often proposed [74].

It should be emphasized that there are important potential safety concerns of TACE and TARE in generating hepatic decompensation. In accordance with the guidelines for TACE [3], it has been strongly suggested that only patients with preserved liver function (Child–Pugh score A/B and bilirubin ≤ 3 mg/dL) should be considered for downstaging procedures [75]. Although TACE is the recommended first-line treatment for downstaging objectives in most studies [75–77], TARE may be considered an alternative treatment to TACE, particularly in larger HCCs, where the results are encouraging. However, this treatment modality requires further studies to confirm its real utility as a downstaging procedure [78]. The major limitation of downstaging protocols is that they can be applied only in a subgroup of patients who present simultaneously compensated cirrhosis complicated with HCC but cannot be applied in patients with decompensated cirrhosis with HCC.

A very challenging issue will soon be the potential role of neoadjuvant treatments combining systemic drugs such tyrosine kinase and checkpoint inhibitors in downstaging protocols [79]. In a recent clinical trial, the combination of atezolizumab plus bevacizumab in the treatment of unresectable HCC was able to induce a complete and partial response to therapy in 18% and 71% of treated patients, respectively [80]. These results open the critical question of whether systemic treatments may be adopted in combination and/or sequentially with traditional LRT to increase the chances of obtaining successful HCC downstaging.

A further critical element that must be considered in the application of downstaging procedures is the objective measurement of the treatment response. The modified Response Evaluation Criteria in Solid Tumors (mRECIST) were developed for the assessment of treatment response by measuring tumor shrinkage. These criteria divided the rate of response to treatment into four categories: (1) complete response (CR—disappearance of arterial enhancement in tumor(s), (2) partial response (PR—a minimum 30% reduction in the sum of diameters of viable tumors compared with baseline), (3) stable disease (SD—not meeting PR or progressive disease), and (4) progressive disease (PD—an increase of at least 20% in the sum of diameters of viable tumors compared with baseline or the appearance of new lesions) [81]. The usefulness of the mRECIST criteria in the evaluation of response to LRT after downstaging protocols in patients with HCC has been confirmed both in those within and beyond the MC. In a small series of 33 patients presenting HCC outside the MC who underwent LT after downstaging performed by TACE, the 5-year survival was significantly higher in those who achieved CR (94.4%) than in those who had PR (45.4%) and SD (50%). These significant differences were explained by a progressive increase in HCC recurrence rates from patients with CR (15.5%) to those with SD (50%) to those with PR (53.3%) [82]. Similar results were obtained in the study performed by Kim et al., which evaluated HCC recipients within and beyond MC after the TACE procedure [83]. The 5-year HCC recurrence rate was 5.3% in patients who achieved CR or PR after TACE compared with 17.6% in those who achieved SD or PD. It should be noted that although the mRECIST criteria are sufficiently detailed, they may not be systematically adopted among different transplant centers, such that the results obtained by LRT may not be comparable [19].

In addition to the quality of the response to LRT, the duration of response is increasingly used as a surrogate marker to identify HCC with more aggressive behavior. Starting from this assumption, many liver transplant centers adopted the strategy to "ablate and wait" to assess the type and duration of response to LRT [9]. It has been suggested that the success of downstaging should be assessed, demonstrating the absence of tumor progression during an observation period of at least 3 months after the procedure. A successful downstaging procedure allows the selection of candidates with more favorable tumor biology and better post-LT survival [84]. This strategy avoided early post-LT recurrences, as demonstrated in patients with HCC beyond MC transplanted after short waiting times [85]. Thus, the guidelines of both the American and European associations for the study of the liver are concordant in recommending the adoption of LRT in patients with HCC beyond MC and the consideration of those who achieved successful downstaging for at least 3–6 months as suitable candidates for LT [3–86].

The question at this time is what the baseline and the final burdens of HCC obtained after successful downstaging that may be considered sufficient to perform LT should be. In the United States, the UCSF downstaging protocol [70] has recently been employed as a national policy both for the graduation of urgency to transplantation and to try to answer this question. In this protocol, the baseline selection criteria for patients with HCC who may benefit from LRT downstaging procedures before LT were as follows: a single HCC ≤ 8 cm in diameter; up to three lesions < 5 cm in diameter; or up to five nodules, all of them <3 cm in diameter, but in any case with a total tumor diameter < 8 cm. Retrospectively analyzing the UNOS database, the 3819 liver transplanted patients with HCC were divided as always within the MC or achieved UNOS downstaging criteria (UNOS-DS). The 3-year post-LT survival was 83.2% in patients always within MC and 79.1% in those fulfilling UNOS-DS. Moreover, the 3-year HCC recurrence rate was 6.9% in recipients who were always within MC and 12.8% for those within UNOS-DS. A very interesting issue that emerged from this study was that AFP serum levels ≥ 100 ng/mL were the only independent predictor of post-LT HCC recurrence in downstaged groups [87].

To date, only one randomized clinical trial (the XXL trial) has evaluated the clinical outcome of patients presenting at baseline with HCC beyond MC who were successfully downstaged by means of LRT and subsequently transplanted compared with those who received only LRT [88]. This study was conducted in Italy and enrolled 74 patients with HCC beyond the MC, without macrovascular invasion or extrahepatic spread, with a 5-year expected post-LT survival of at least 50% (estimated by Metroticket calculator [37]) and preserved liver function (Child–Pugh classes A5–B7). All patients initially underwent tumor downstaging with LRT or systemic therapies, according to a multidisciplinary decision. After an observation period of 3 months, during which treatment with sorafenib was allowed, patients presenting CR or PR, assessed by means of the mRECIST criteria, were randomly assigned (1:1) to LT or to continue LRT or systemic treatments (control group). Of note, in patients with baseline AFP values ≥ 400 ng/mL, a radiological tumor response was confirmed only in case of a parallel percentage decrease in AFP concentrations. In contrast, in patients with AFP serum levels < 400 ng/mL at recruitment, an increase in AFP concentrations above that cutoff value at the end of the downstaging phase or during the observation period was considered tumor progression, independent of radiological assessment. The primary endpoints of the study were the evaluation of 5-year tumor-event-free survival and overall survival. The first result of the study was that 29/74 (39.1%) of the patients dropped out before randomization; thus, only 45 (60.9%) patients were finally included in the study (23 underwent LT, and 22 maintained LRT or systemic treatments). Despite the high rate of dropout, after a median follow-up of 71 months, a significantly higher 5-year tumor-event-free survival was observed in the LT group (76.8%) than in the control group (18.3%). Regarding the 5-year overall survival, the figures were quite similar, indicating a better overall survival in the LT group (77.5%) than in the control group (31.2%). Tumor progression was the main cause of death in both groups, while in the LT group, HCC recurrence was detected in 22% of cases. The results of this study provide additional evidence to previous results demonstrating comparable post-LT outcomes in patients with HCC beyond the MC who underwent successful downstaging within the MC and in those who underwent LT fulfilling the MC at presentation. A further very important message from this study is that different schedules of LRT and systemic treatments may be employed in patients with HCC beyond the MC to achieve successful and durable downstaging to permit them to be suitable for LT.

7. Conclusions

LT must be considered the best treatment option for patients with unresectable HCC [89]. Since the number of donors is insufficient to satisfy all requests for transplantation for HCC, it is essential to perform careful selection of transplant candidates. For approximately 25 years, MC have been the benchmark for offering patients with HCC the opportunity for transplantation, but as recently demonstrated, they excluded a subset of patients who could have benefited from LT. For this reason, several other more extended selection criteria to offer LT to an increasing number of patients with HCC have been evaluated. In the beginning, many of the expanded criteria evaluable in the pre-LT period were based on the morphological characteristics of the tumor as the original strategy adopted for constructing the MC. Subsequently, the addition of biological markers, predominantly AFP serum levels, to the morphological characteristics of the tumor emerged as the more solid and reproducible criteria for patient selection beyond the MC for LT, assuring excellent post-LT outcomes. Downstaging HCC to MC by means of LRT and/or systemic therapies is becoming a valid and increasingly utilized method of patient selection for LT. Adopting this approach, the surrogates of tumor biology can be assessed, such as the response rate to LRT and its maintenance for a sufficient time during the waiting list before transplant. The measurement of AFP serum levels or AFP slope during or after downstaging protocols can be considered a further important option to identify those patients at higher risk of

HCC recurrence that should be excluded from LT. It appears clear that the risk of failure of successful downstaging is related to both the tumor burden and to AFP serum levels at baseline.

It is important to highlight that the selection of HCC patients for LT by means of the expanded criteria may be difficult to adopt in areas of the world with severe organ shortages. In these areas, the selection criteria based on the utility principle that assures the maximum post-transplant survival, such as the MC, will remain preponderant, rather than expanded criteria that could reduce access to LT for patients with better post-LT prognosis [67–90]. This justified that not all liver transplant centers around the world adopt the same criteria to select patients with HCC for LT [3–74]. Each country developed, based on its scientific experiences, some selection criteria for transplanting patients with HCC beyond MC. A common thread that links the various selection criteria adopted in different countries is to consider the morphological characteristics of the tumor (number and size of nodules) and the values of some biological markers, mainly AFP, as main determinants of the selection process. In the United States and in Europe, the concept to not necessarily set a baseline HCC limit size to consider patients potentially transplantable, except for the presence of macrovascular invasion or extrahepatic spread, appears to be more accepted. Thus, the downstaging process will probably become the main selection tool for LT, enabling clinicians to postpone the transplantation decision from tumor presentation to the assessment of final response to LRT [91]. The effectiveness of downstaging procedures should be considered as having brought the tumor back within the MC for a period of at least 3–6 months before enlisting [84].

In summary, to try to answer the key questions reported in the introduction, the following proposals can be suggested: (a) it seems proven that in the absence of macrovascular invasion and extrahepatic spread, no upper limit of tumor burden beyond MC should be established "a priori" to determine transplant eligibility for HCC; (b) to justify a policy to transplant patients with HCC beyond MC at presentation, the minimal expected 5-year post-LT survival probability, estimated by Metroticket calculator, should be at least 50% [37]; (c) the response to neoadjuvant LRT and/or systemic treatments in addition to the dynamic evaluation of AFP serum levels are expected to replace conventional morphological criteria for selecting patients with HCC for LT in the near future.

Author Contributions: Conceptualization, P.T.; methodology, E.F. (Elisa Fumolo); data curation, E.F. (Ezio Fornasiere), D.B.; writing—original draft preparation, P.T., E.F. (Elisa Fumolo), E.F. (Ezio For-nasiere), and D.B.; writing—review and editing, P.T. All authors have read and agreed to the published version of the manuscript.

Funding: This research received no external funding.

Institutional Review Board Statement: Ethical review and approval were waived for this study due to the fact that it refers to a review of the scientific literature in the field.

Informed Consent Statement: Not applicable.

Conflicts of Interest: The authors declare no conflict of interest.

References

1. White, D.L.; Thrift, A.P.; Kanwal, F.; Davila, J.; El-Serag, H.B. Incidence of Hepatocellular Carcinoma in All 50 United States, from 2000 through 2012. *Gastroenterology* **2017**, *152*, 812–820.e5. [CrossRef] [PubMed]
2. Kulik, L.; El-Serag, H.B. Epidemiology and Management of Hepatocellular Carcinoma. *Gastroenterology* **2019**, *156*, 477–491. [CrossRef] [PubMed]
3. European Association for the Study of the Liver. EASL Clinical Practice Guidelines: Management of hepatocellular carcinoma. *J. Hepatol.* **2018**, *69*, 182–236. [CrossRef]
4. Vibert, E.; Schwartz, M.; Olthoff, K.M. Advances in resection and transplantation for hepatocellular carcinoma. *J. Hepatol.* **2020**, *72*, 262–276. [CrossRef]
5. Starzl, T.E.; Marchioro, T.L.; Vonkaulla, K.N.; Hermann, G.; Brittain RSWaddell, W.R. Homotransplantation of the Liver in Humans. *Surg. Gynecol. Obs.* **1963**, *117*, 659–676.

6. Starzl, T.E.; Groth, C.G.; Brettschneider, L.; Penn, I.; Fulginiti, V.A.; Moon, J.B.; Blanchard, H.; Martin, A.J., Jr.; Porter, K.A. Orthotopic homotransplantation of the human liver. *Ann. Surg.* **1968**, *168*, 392–415. [CrossRef]

7. Iwatsuki, S.; Gordon, R.D.; Shaw, B.W., Jr.; Starzl, T.E. Role of liver transplantation in cancer therapy. *Ann. Surg.* **1985**, *202*, 401–407. [CrossRef]

8. Mazzaferro, V.; Regalia, E.; Doci, R.; Andreola, S.; Pulvirenti, A.; Bozzetti, F.; Montalto, F.; Ammatuna, M.; Morabito, A.; Gennari, L. Liver transplantation for the treatment of small hepatocellular carcinomas in patients with cirrhosis. *N. Engl. J. Med.* **1996**, *334*, 693–699. [CrossRef]

9. Lingiah, V.A.; Niazi, M.; Olivo, R.; Paterno, F.; Guarrera, J.V.; Pyrsopoulos, N.T. Liver Transplantation Beyond Milan Criteria. *J. Clin. Transl. Hepatol.* **2020**, *8*, 69–75. [CrossRef] [PubMed]

10. Plessier, A.; Codes, L.; Consigny, Y.; Sommacale, D.; Dondero, F.; Cortes, A.; Degos, F.; Brillet, P.Y.; Vilgrain, V.; Paradis, V.; et al. Underestimation of the influence of satellite nodules as a risk factor for post-transplantation recurrence in patients with small hepatocellular carcinoma. *Liver Transplant.* **2004**, *10*, S86–S90. [CrossRef] [PubMed]

11. Escartin, A.; Sapisochin, G.; Bilbao, I.; Vilallonga, R.; Bueno, J.; Castells, L.; Dopazo, C.; Castro, E.; Caralt, M.; Balsells, J. Recurrence of hepatocellular carcinoma after liver transplantation. *Transplant. Proc.* **2007**, *39*, 2308–2310. [CrossRef] [PubMed]

12. Roayaie, S.; Schwartz, J.D.; Sung, M.W.; Emre, S.H.; Miller, C.M.; Gondolesi, G.E.; Krieger, N.R.; Schwartz, M.E. Recurrence of hepatocellular carcinoma after liver transplant: Patterns and prognosis. *Liver Transplant.* **2004**, *10*, 534–540. [CrossRef]

13. Bruix, J.; Fuster, J.; Llovet, J.M. Liver transplantation for hepatocellular carcinoma: Foucault pendulum versus evidence-based decision. *Liver Transplant.* **2003**, *9*, 700–702. [CrossRef] [PubMed]

14. Yao, F.Y.; Xiao, L.; Bass, N.M.; Kerlan, R.; Ascher, N.L.; Roberts, J.P. Liver transplantation for hepatocellular carcinoma: Validation of the UCSF-expanded criteria based on preoperative imaging. *Am. J. Transplant.* **2007**, *7*, 2587–2596. [CrossRef]

15. Herrero, J.I.; Sangro, B.; Pardo, F.; Quiroga, J.; Inarrairaegui, M.; Rotellar, F.; Montiel, C.; Alegre, F.; Prieto, J. Liver transplantation in patients with hepatocellular carcinoma across Milan criteria. *Liver Transplant.* **2008**, *14*, 272–278. [CrossRef]

16. Silva, M.; Moya, A.; Berenguer, M.; Sanjuan, F.; Lopez-Andujar, R.; Pareja, E.; Torres-Quevedo, R.; Aguilera, V.; Montalva, E.; De Juan, M.; et al. Expanded criteria for liver transplantation in patients with cirrhosis and hepatocellular carcinoma. *Liver Transplant.* **2008**, *14*, 1449–1460. [CrossRef]

17. Guiteau, J.J.; Cotton, R.T.; Washburn, W.K.; Harper, A.; O'Mahony, C.A.; Sebastian, A.; Cheng, S.; Klintmalm, G.; Ghobrial, M.; Halff, G.; et al. An early regional experience with expansion of Milan Criteria for liver transplant recipients. *Am. J. Transplant.* **2010**, *10*, 2092–2098. [CrossRef]

18. Costentin, C.E.; Bababekov, Y.J.; Zhu, A.X.; Yeh, H. Is It Time to Reconsider the Milan Criteria for Selecting Patients With Hepatocellular Carcinoma for Deceased-Donor Liver Transplantation? *Hepatology* **2019**, *69*, 1324–1336. [CrossRef]

19. Toniutto, P.; Fornasiere, E.; Fumolo, E.; Bitetto, D. Risk factors for hepatocellular carcinoma recurrence after liver transplantation. *Hepatoma Res.* **2020**, *6*, 50–71. [CrossRef]

20. Fan, J.; Zhou, J.; Xu, Y.; Qiu, S.J.; Wu, Z.Q.; Yu, Y.; Huang, X.W.; Tang, Z.Y.; Wang, Y.Q. Indication of liver transplantation for hepatocellular carcinoma: Shanghai Fudan Criteria. *Zhonghua Yi Xue Za Zhi* **2006**, *86*, 1227–1231.

21. DuBay, D.; Sandroussi, C.; Sandhu, L.; Cleary, S.; Guba, M.; Cattral, M.S.; McGilvray, I.; Ghanekar, A.; Selzner, M.; Greig, P.D.; et al. Liver transplantation for advanced hepatocellular carcinoma using poor tumor differentiation on biopsy as an exclusion criterion. *Ann. Surg.* **2011**, *253*, 166–172. [CrossRef]

22. Zheng, S.S.; Xu, X.; Wu, J.; Chen, J.; Wang, W.L.; Zhang, M.; Liang, T.B.; Wu, L.M. Liver transplantation for hepatocellular carcinoma: Hangzhou experiences. *Transplantation* **2008**, *85*, 1726–1732. [CrossRef]

23. Toso, C.; Meeberg, G.; Hernandez-Alejandro, R.; Dufour, J.F.; Marotta, P.; Majno, P.; Kneteman, N.M. Total tumor volume and alpha-fetoprotein for selection of transplant candidates with hepatocellular carcinoma: A prospective validation. *Hepatology* **2015**, *62*, 158–165. [CrossRef]

24. Duvoux, C.; Roudot-Thoraval, F.; Decaens, T.; Pessione, F.; Badran, H.; Piardi, T.; Francoz, C.; Compagnon, P.; Vanlemmens, C.; Dumortier, J.; et al. Liver transplantation for hepatocellular carcinoma: A model including alpha-fetoprotein improves the performance of Milan criteria. *Gastroenterology* **2012**, *143*, 986–994 e3. [CrossRef]

25. Mazzaferro, V.; Sposito, C.; Zhou, J.; Pinna, A.D.; De Carlis, L.; Fan, J.; Cescon, M.; Di Sandro, S.; Yi-Feng, H.; Lauterio, A.; et al. Metroticket 2.0 Model for Analysis of Competing Risks of Death After Liver Transplantation for Hepatocellular Carcinoma. *Gastroenterology* **2018**, *154*, 128–139. [CrossRef]

26. Kaido, T.; Ogawa, K.; Mori, A.; Fujimoto, Y.; Ito, T.; Tomiyama, K.; Takada, Y.; Uemoto, S. Usefulness of the Kyoto criteria as expanded selection criteria for liver transplantation for hepatocellular carcinoma. *Surgery* **2013**, *154*, 1053–1060. [CrossRef]

27. Lee, J.H.; Cho, Y.; Kim, H.Y.; Cho, E.J.; Lee, D.H.; Yu, S.J.; Lee, J.W.; Yi, N.J.; Lee, K.W.; Kim, S.H.; et al. Serum Tumor Markers Provide Refined Prognostication in Selecting Liver Transplantation Candidate for Hepatocellular Carcinoma Patients Beyond the Milan Criteria. *Ann. Surg.* **2016**, *263*, 842–850. [CrossRef]

28. Shah, S.A.; Tan, J.C.; McGilvray, I.D.; Cattral, M.S.; Levy, G.A.; Greig, P.D.; Grant, D.R. Does microvascular invasion affect outcomes after liver transplantation for HCC? A histopathological analysis of 155 consecutive explants. *J. Gastrointest. Surg.* **2007**, *11*, 464–471. [CrossRef]

29. Zhang, X.; Li, J.; Shen, F.; Lau, W.Y. Significance of presence of microvascular invasion in specimens obtained after surgical treatment of hepatocellular carcinoma. *J. Gastroenterol. Hepatol.* **2018**, *33*, 347–354. [CrossRef] [PubMed]

30. Jonas, S.; Bechstein, W.O.; Steinmuller, T.; Herrmann, M.; Radke, C.; Berg, T.; Settmacher, U.; Neuhaus, P. Vascular invasion and histopathologic grading determine outcome after liver transplantation for hepatocellular carcinoma in cirrhosis. *Hepatology* **2001**, *33*, 1080–1086. [CrossRef]

31. Fan, J.; Yang, G.S.; Fu, Z.R.; Peng, Z.H.; Xia, Q.; Peng, C.H.; Qian, J.M.; Zhou, J.; Xu, Y.; Qiu, S.J.; et al. Liver transplantation outcomes in 1,078 hepatocellular carcinoma patients: A multi-center experience in Shanghai, China. *J. Cancer Res. Clin. Oncol.* **2009**, *135*, 1403–1412. [CrossRef]

32. Sotiropoulos, G.C.; Malago, M.; Molmenti, E.; Paul, A.; Nadalin, S.; Brokalaki, E.; Kuhl, H.; Dirsch, O.; Lang, H.; Broelsch, C.E. Liver transplantation for hepatocellular carcinoma in cirrhosis: Is clinical tumor classification before transplantation realistic? *Transplantation* **2005**, *79*, 483–487. [CrossRef]

33. Shah, S.A.; Tan, J.C.; McGilvray, I.D.; Cattral, M.S.; Cleary, S.P.; Levy, G.A.; Greig, P.D.; Grant, D.R. Accuracy of staging as a predictor for recurrence after liver transplantation for hepatocellular carcinoma. *Transplantation* **2006**, *81*, 1633–1639. [CrossRef]

34. Kierans, A.S.; Song, C.; Gavlin, A.; Roudenko, A.; Lu, L.; Askin, G.; Hecht, E.M. Diagnostic Performance of LI-RADS Version 2018, LI-RADS Version 2017, and OPTN Criteria for Hepatocellular Carcinoma. *AJR Am. J. Roentgenol.* **2020**, *215*, 1085–1092. [CrossRef]

35. Lee, S.; Kim, S.S.; Roh, Y.H.; Choi, J.Y.; Park, M.S.; Kim, M.J. Diagnostic Performance of CT/MRI Liver Imaging Reporting and Data System v2017 for Hepatocellular Carcinoma: A Systematic Review and Meta-Analysis. *Liver Int.* **2020**, *40*, 1488–1497. [CrossRef]

36. Rudnick, S.R.; Russo, M.W. Liver transplantation beyond or downstaging within the Milan criteria for hepatocellular carcinoma. *Expert Rev. Gastroenterol. Hepatol.* **2018**, *12*, 265–275. [CrossRef]

37. Mazzaferro, V.; Llovet, J.M.; Miceli, R.; Bhoori, S.; Schiavo, M.; Mariani, L.; Camerini, T.; Roayaie, S.; Schwartz, M.E.; Grazi, G.L.; et al. Predicting survival after liver transplantation in patients with hepatocellular carcinoma beyond the Milan criteria: A retrospective, exploratory analysis. *Lancet Oncol.* **2009**, *10*, 35–43. [CrossRef]

38. Cillo, U.; Vitale, A.; Bassanello, M.; Boccagni, P.; Brolese, A.; Zanus, G.; Burra, P.; Fagiuoli, S.; Farinati, F.; Rugge, M.; et al. Liver transplantation for the treatment of moderately or well-differentiated hepatocellular carcinoma. *Ann. Surg.* **2004**, *239*, 150–159. [CrossRef]

39. Cuccurullo, V.; Di Stasio, G.D.; Mazzarella, G.; Cascini, G.L. Microvascular Invasion in HCC: The Molecular Imaging Perspective. *Contrast Media Mol. Imaging* **2018**, *2018*, 9487938. [CrossRef]

40. Yaprak, O.; Acar, S.; Ertugrul, G.; Dayangac, M. Role of pre-transplant 18F-FDG PET/CT in predicting hepatocellular carcinoma recurrence after liver transplantation. *World J. Gastrointest. Oncol.* **2018**, *10*, 336–343. [CrossRef] [PubMed]

41. Choi, S.H.; Byun, J.H.; Kwon, H.J.; Ha, H.I.; Lee, S.J.; Kim, S.Y.; Won, H.J.; Kim, P.N. The usefulness of gadoxetic acid-enhanced dynamic magnetic resonance imaging in hepatocellular carcinoma: Toward improved staging. *Ann. Surg. Oncol.* **2015**, *22*, 819–825. [CrossRef]

42. Sweeney, M.J.; Ashmore, J.; Morris, H.P.; Weber, G. Comparative Biochemistry Hepatomas. Iv. Isotope Studies of Glucose and Fructose Metabolism in Liver Tumors of Different Growth Rates. *Cancer Res.* **1963**, *23*, 995–1002. [PubMed]

43. Torizuka, T.; Tamaki, N.; Inokuma, T.; Magata, Y.; Sasayama, S.; Yonekura, Y.; Tanaka, A.; Yamaoka, Y.; Yamamoto, K.; Konishi, J. In vivo assessment of glucose metabolism in hepatocellular carcinoma with FDG-PET. *J. Nucl. Med.* **1995**, *36*, 1811–1817. [PubMed]

44. Lin, C.Y.; Liao, C.W.; Chu, L.Y.; Yen, K.Y.; Jeng, L.B.; Hsu, C.N.; Lin, C.L.; Kao, C.H. Predictive Value of 18F-FDG PET/CT for Vascular Invasion in Patients With Hepatocellular Carcinoma Before Liver Transplantation. *Clin. Nucl. Med.* **2017**, *42*, e183–e187. [CrossRef]

45. Ahn, S.Y.; Lee, J.M.; Joo, I.; Lee, E.S.; Lee, S.J.; Cheon, G.J.; Han, J.K.; Choi, B.I. Prediction of microvascular invasion of hepatocellular carcinoma using gadoxetic acid-enhanced MR and (18)F-FDG PET/CT. *Abdom. Imaging* **2015**, *40*, 843–851. [CrossRef] [PubMed]

46. Takada, Y.; Kaido, T.; Shirabe, K.; Nagano, H.; Egawa, H.; Sugawara, Y.; Taketomi, A.; Takahara, T.; Wakabayashi, G.; Nakanishi, C.; et al. Significance of preoperative fluorodeoxyglucose-positron emission tomography in prediction of tumor recurrence after liver transplantation for hepatocellular carcinoma patients: A Japanese multicenter study. *J. Hepatobiliary Pancreat. Sci.* **2017**, *24*, 49–57. [CrossRef]

47. Lee, S.D.; Kim, S.H.; Kim, S.K.; Kim, Y.K.; Park, S.J. Clinical Impact of 18F-Fluorodeoxyglucose Positron Emission Tomography/Computed Tomography in Living Donor Liver Transplantation for Advanced Hepatocellular Carcinoma. *Transplantation* **2015**, *99*, 2142–2149. [CrossRef]

48. Hakeem, A.R.; Young, R.S.; Marangoni, G.; Lodge, J.P.; Prasad, K.R. Systematic review: The prognostic role of alpha-fetoprotein following liver transplantation for hepatocellular carcinoma. *Aliment. Pharmacol. Ther.* **2012**, *35*, 987–999. [CrossRef]

49. Lai, Q.; Avolio, A.W.; Graziadei, I.; Otto, G.; Rossi, M.; Tisone, G.; Goffette, P.; Vogel, W.; Pitton, M.B.; Lerut, J.; et al. Alpha-fetoprotein and modified response evaluation criteria in solid tumors progression after locoregional therapy as predictors of hepatocellular cancer recurrence and death after transplantation. *Liver Transplant.* **2013**, *19*, 1108–1118. [CrossRef]

50. Dumitra, T.C.; Dumitra, S.; Metrakos, P.P.; Barkun, J.S.; Chaudhury, P.; Deschenes, M.; Paraskevas, S.; Hassanain, M.; Tchervenkov, J.I. Pretransplantation alpha-fetoprotein slope and milan criteria: Strong predictors of hepatocellular carcinoma recurrence after transplantation. *Transplantation* **2013**, *95*, 228–233. [CrossRef]

51. Burra, P.; Giannini, E.G.; Caraceni, P.; Ginanni Corradini, S.; Rendina, M.; Volpes, R.; Toniutto, P. Specific issues concerning the management of patients on the waiting list and after liver transplantation. *Liver Int.* **2018**, *38*, 1338–1362. [CrossRef] [PubMed]

52. Sapisochin, G.; Goldaracena, N.; Laurence, J.M.; Dib, M.; Barbas, A.; Ghanekar, A.; Cleary, S.P.; Lilly, L.; Cattral, M.S.; Marquez, M.; et al. The extended Toronto criteria for liver transplantation in patients with hepatocellular carcinoma: A prospective validation study. *Hepatology* **2016**, *64*, 2077–2088. [CrossRef]
53. Toso, C.; Asthana, S.; Bigam, D.L.; Shapiro, A.M.; Kneteman, N.M. Reassessing selection criteria prior to liver transplantation for hepatocellular carcinoma utilizing the Scientific Registry of Transplant Recipients database. *Hepatology* **2009**, *49*, 832–838. [CrossRef]
54. Notarpaolo, A.; Layese, R.; Magistri, P.; Gambato, M.; Colledan, M.; Magini, G.; Miglioresi, L.; Vitale, A.; Vennarecci, G.; Ambrosio, C.D.; et al. Validation of the AFP model as a predictor of HCC recurrence in patients with viral hepatitis-related cirrhosis who had received a liver transplant for HCC. *J. Hepatol.* **2017**, *66*, 552–559. [CrossRef] [PubMed]
55. Varona, M.A.; Soriano, A.; Aguirre-Jaime, A.; Garrido, S.; Oton, E.; Diaz, D.; Portero, J.; Bravo, P.; Barrera, M.A.; Perera, A. Risk factors of hepatocellular carcinoma recurrence after liver transplantation: Accuracy of the alpha-fetoprotein model in a single-center experience. *Transplant. Proc.* **2015**, *47*, 84–89. [CrossRef]
56. Pinero, F.; Tisi Bana, M.; de Ataide, E.C.; Hoyos Duque, S.; Marciano, S.; Varon, A.; Anders, M.; Zerega, A.; Menendez, J.; Zapata, R.; et al. Liver transplantation for hepatocellular carcinoma: Evaluation of the alpha-fetoprotein model in a multicenter cohort from Latin America. *Liver Int.* **2016**, *36*, 1657–1667. [CrossRef]
57. Rhu, J.; Kim, J.M.; Choi, G.S.; Kwon, C.H.D.; Joh, J.W. Validation of the alpha-fetoprotein Model for Hepatocellular Carcinoma Recurrence After Transplantation in an Asian Population. *Transplantation* **2018**, *102*, 1316–1322. [CrossRef] [PubMed]
58. Okuda, H.; Nakanishi, T.; Takatsu, K.; Saito, A.; Hayashi, N.; Yamamoto, M.; Takasaki, K.; Nakano, M. Comparison of clinicopathological features of patients with hepatocellular carcinoma seropositive for alpha-fetoprotein alone and those seropositive for des-gamma-carboxy prothrombin alone. *J. Gastroenterol. Hepatol.* **2001**, *16*, 1290–1296. [CrossRef]
59. Hong, Y.M.; Cho, M.; Yoon, K.T.; Chu, C.W.; Yang, K.H.; Park, Y.M.; Rhu, J.H. Risk factors of early recurrence after curative hepatectomy in hepatocellular carcinoma. *Tumour Biol.* **2017**, *39*, 1010428317720863. [CrossRef]
60. Takada, Y.; Ito, T.; Ueda, M.; Sakamoto, S.; Haga, H.; Maetani, Y.; Ogawa, K.; Ogura, Y.; Oike, F.; Egawa, H.; et al. Living donor liver transplantation for patients with HCC exceeding the Milan criteria: A proposal of expanded criteria. *Dig. Dis.* **2007**, *25*, 299–302. [CrossRef] [PubMed]
61. Fujiki, M.; Takada, Y.; Ogura, Y.; Oike, F.; Kaido, T.; Teramukai, S.; Uemoto, S. Significance of des-gamma-carboxy prothrombin in selection criteria for living donor liver transplantation for hepatocellular carcinoma. *Am. J. Transplant.* **2009**, *9*, 2362–2371. [CrossRef]
62. Soejima, Y.; Taketomi, A.; Yoshizumi, T.; Uchiyama, H.; Aishima, S.; Terashi, T.; Shimada, M.; Maehara, Y. Extended indication for living donor liver transplantation in patients with hepatocellular carcinoma. *Transplantation* **2007**, *83*, 893–899. [CrossRef]
63. Shirabe, K.; Itoh, S.; Yoshizumi, T.; Soejima, Y.; Taketomi, A.; Aishima, S.; Maehara, Y. The predictors of microvascular invasion in candidates for liver transplantation with hepatocellular carcinoma-with special reference to the serum levels of des-gamma-carboxy prothrombin. *J. Surg. Oncol.* **2007**, *95*, 235–240. [CrossRef]
64. Shirabe, K.; Taketomi, A.; Morita, K.; Soejima, Y.; Uchiyama, H.; Kayashima, H.; Ninomiya, M.; Toshima, T.; Maehara, Y. Comparative evaluation of expanded criteria for patients with hepatocellular carcinoma beyond the Milan criteria undergoing living-related donor liver transplantation. *Clin. Transplant.* **2011**, *25*, E491–E498. [CrossRef]
65. Chaiteerakij, R.; Zhang, X.; Addissie, B.D.; Mohamed, E.A.; Harmsen, W.S.; Theobald, P.J.; Peters, B.E.; Balsanek, J.G.; Ward, M.M.; Giama, N.H.; et al. Combinations of biomarkers and Milan criteria for predicting hepatocellular carcinoma recurrence after liver transplantation. *Liver Transplant.* **2015**, *21*, 599–606. [CrossRef]
66. Lai, Q.; Iesari, S.; Levi Sandri, G.B.; Lerut, J. Des-gamma-carboxy prothrombin in hepatocellular cancer patients waiting for liver transplant: A systematic review and meta-analysis. *Int. J. Biol. Markers* **2017**, *32*, e370–e374. [CrossRef]
67. Clavien, P.A.; Lesurtel, M.; Bossuyt, P.M.; Gores, G.J.; Langer, B.; Perrier, A.; The OLT for HCC Consensus Group. Recommendations for liver transplantation for hepatocellular carcinoma: An international consensus conference report. *Lancet Oncol.* **2012**, *13*, e11–e22. [CrossRef]
68. Otto, G.; Herber, S.; Heise, M.; Lohse, A.W.; Monch, C.; Bittinger, F.; Hoppe-Lotichius, M.; Schuchmann, M.; Victor, A.; Pitton, M. Response to transarterial chemoembolization as a biological selection criterion for liver transplantation in hepatocellular carcinoma. *Liver Transplant.* **2006**, *12*, 1260–1267. [CrossRef]
69. Millonig, G.; Graziadei, I.W.; Freund, M.C.; Jaschke, W.; Stadlmann, S.; Ladurner, R.; Margreiter, R.; Vogel, W. Response to preoperative chemoembolization correlates with outcome after liver transplantation in patients with hepatocellular carcinoma. *Liver Transplant.* **2007**, *13*, 272–279. [CrossRef] [PubMed]
70. Yao, F.Y.; Mehta, N.; Flemming, J.; Dodge, J.; Hameed, B.; Fix, O.; Hirose, R.; Fidelman, N.; Kerlan, R.K., Jr.; Roberts, J.P. Downstaging of hepatocellular cancer before liver transplant: Long-term outcome compared to tumors within Milan criteria. *Hepatology* **2015**, *61*, 1968–1977. [CrossRef] [PubMed]
71. Ravaioli, M.; Grazi, G.L.; Piscaglia, F.; Trevisani, F.; Cescon, M.; Ercolani, G.; Vivarelli, M.; Golfieri, R.; D'Errico Grigioni, A.; Panzini, I.; et al. Liver transplantation for hepatocellular carcinoma: Results of down-staging in patients initially outside the Milan selection criteria. *Am. J. Transplant.* **2008**, *8*, 2547–2557. [CrossRef]
72. Mehta, N.; Guy, J.; Frenette, C.T.; Dodge, J.L.; Osorio, R.W.; Minteer, W.B.; Roberts, J.P.; Yao, F.Y. Excellent Outcomes of Liver Transplantation Following Down-Staging of Hepatocellular Carcinoma to Within Milan Criteria: A Multicenter Study. *Clin. Gastroenterol. Hepatol.* **2018**, *16*, 955–964. [CrossRef]

73. Bruix, J.; Reig, M.; Sherman, M. Evidence-Based Diagnosis, Staging, and Treatment of Patients With Hepatocellular Carcinoma. *Gastroenterology* **2016**, *150*, 835–853. [CrossRef]

74. Marrero, J.A.; Kulik, L.M.; Sirlin, C.B.; Zhu, A.X.; Finn, R.S.; Abecassis, M.M.; Roberts, L.R.; Heimbach, J.K. Diagnosis, Staging, and Management of Hepatocellular Carcinoma: 2018 Practice Guidance by the American Association for the Study of Liver Diseases. *Hepatology* **2018**, *68*, 723–750. [CrossRef]

75. Yao, F.Y.; Fidelman, N. Reassessing the boundaries of liver transplantation for hepatocellular carcinoma: Where do we stand with tumor down-staging? *Hepatology* **2016**, *63*, 1014–1025. [CrossRef] [PubMed]

76. Parikh, N.D.; Waljee, A.K.; Singal, A.G. Downstaging hepatocellular carcinoma: A systematic review and pooled analysis. *Liver Transplant.* **2015**, *21*, 1142–1152. [CrossRef]

77. Mehta, N.; Bhangui, P.; Yao, F.Y.; Mazzaferro, V.; Toso, C.; Akamatsu, N.; Durand, F.; Ijzermans, J.; Polak, W.; Zheng, S.; et al. Liver Transplantation for Hepatocellular Carcinoma. Working Group Report from the ILTS Transplant Oncology Consensus Conference. *Transplantation* **2020**, *104*, 1136–1142. [CrossRef]

78. Lewandowski, R.J.; Kulik, L.M.; Riaz, A.; Senthilnathan, S.; Mulcahy, M.F.; Ryu, R.K.; Ibrahim, S.M.; Sato, K.T.; Baker, T.; Miller, F.H.; et al. A comparative analysis of transarterial downstaging for hepatocellular carcinoma: Chemoembolization versus radioembolization. *Am. J. Transplant.* **2009**, *9*, 1920–1928. [CrossRef] [PubMed]

79. Sonbol, M.B.; Riaz, I.B.; Naqvi, S.A.A.; Almquist, D.R.; Mina, S.; Almasri, J.; Shah, S.; Almader-Douglas, D.; Uson Junior, P.L.S.; Mahipal, A.; et al. Systemic Therapy and Sequencing Options in Advanced Hepatocellular Carcinoma: A Systematic Review and Network Meta-analysis. *JAMA Oncol.* **2020**, *6*, e204930. [CrossRef] [PubMed]

80. Finn, R.S.; Qin, S.; Ikeda, M.; Galle, P.R.; Ducreux, M.; Kim, T.Y.; Kudo, M.; Breder, V.; Merle, P.; Kaseb, A.O.; et al. Atezolizumab plus Bevacizumab in Unresectable Hepatocellular Carcinoma. *N. Engl. J. Med.* **2020**, *382*, 1894–1905. [CrossRef]

81. Lencioni, R.; Llovet, J.M. Modified RECIST (mRECIST) assessment for hepatocellular carcinoma. *Semin. Liver Dis.* **2010**, *30*, 52–60. [CrossRef]

82. Bargellini, I.; Vignali, C.; Cioni, R.; Petruzzi, P.; Cicorelli, A.; Campani, D.; De Simone, P.; Filipponi, F.; Bartolozzi, C. Hepatocellular carcinoma: CT for tumor response after transarterial chemoembolization in patients exceeding Milan criteria–selection parameter for liver transplantation. *Radiology* **2010**, *255*, 289–300. [CrossRef] [PubMed]

83. Kim, D.J.; Clark, P.J.; Heimbach, J.; Rosen, C.; Sanchez, W.; Watt, K.; Charlton, M.R. Recurrence of hepatocellular carcinoma: Importance of mRECIST response to chemoembolization and tumor size. *Am. J. Transplant.* **2014**, *14*, 1383–1390. [CrossRef] [PubMed]

84. Roberts, J.P.; Venook, A.; Kerlan, R.; Yao, F. Hepatocellular carcinoma: Ablate and wait versus rapid transplantation. *Liver Transplant.* **2010**, *16*, 925–929. [CrossRef] [PubMed]

85. Halazun, K.J.; Patzer, R.E.; Rana, A.A.; Verna, E.C.; Griesemer, A.D.; Parsons, R.F.; Samstein, B.; Guarrera, J.V.; Kato, T.; Brown, R.S., Jr.; et al. Standing the test of time: Outcomes of a decade of prioritizing patients with hepatocellular carcinoma, results of the UNOS natural geographic experiment. *Hepatology* **2014**, *60*, 1957–1962. [CrossRef] [PubMed]

86. Heimbach, J.K.; Kulik, L.M.; Finn, R.S.; Sirlin, C.B.; Abecassis, M.M.; Roberts, L.R.; Zhu, A.X.; Murad, M.H.; Marrero, J.A. AASLD guidelines for the treatment of hepatocellular carcinoma. *Hepatology* **2018**, *67*, 358–380. [CrossRef] [PubMed]

87. Mehta, N.; Dodge, J.L.; Grab, J.D.; Yao, F.Y. National Experience on Down-Staging of Hepatocellular Carcinoma Before Liver Transplant: Influence of Tumor Burden, Alpha-Fetoprotein, and Wait Time. *Hepatology* **2020**, *71*, 943–954. [CrossRef] [PubMed]

88. Mazzaferro, V.; Citterio, D.; Bhoori, S.; Bongini, M.; Miceli, R.; De Carlis, L.; Colledan, M.; Salizzoni, M.; Romagnoli, R.; Antonelli, B.; et al. Liver transplantation in hepatocellular carcinoma after tumour downstaging (XXL): A randomised, controlled, phase 2b/3 trial. *Lancet Oncol.* **2020**, *21*, 947–956. [CrossRef]

89. Forner, A.; Reig, M.; Bruix, J. Hepatocellular carcinoma. *Lancet* **2018**, *391*, 1301–1314. [CrossRef]

90. Volk, M.L.; Vijan, S.; Marrero, J.A. A novel model measuring the harm of transplanting hepatocellular carcinoma exceeding Milan criteria. *Am. J. Transplant.* **2008**, *8*, 839–846. [CrossRef] [PubMed]

91. Mazzaferro, V. Squaring the circle of selection and allocation in liver transplantation for HCC: An adaptive approach. *Hepatology* **2016**, *63*, 1707–1717. [CrossRef]

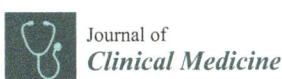

Journal of
Clinical Medicine

Review

COVID-19 in Liver Transplant Recipients: A Systematic Review

Chiara Becchetti [1,2,*], Sarah Gabriela Gschwend [1], Jean-François Dufour [1,2] and Vanessa Banz [1]

[1] University Clinic for Visceral Surgery and Medicine, Inselspital, Bern University Hospital, University of Bern, 3010 Bern, Switzerland; sarah.gschwend@students.unibe.ch (S.G.G.); jf.dufour@lasource.ch (J.-F.D.); Vanessa.BanzWuethrich@insel.ch (V.B.)
[2] Hepatology, Department of Biomedical Research, University of Bern, 3010 Bern, Switzerland
* Correspondence: chiara.becchetti@insel.ch

Abstract: Liver transplant (LT) recipients are considered a vulnerable population amidst the COVID-19 pandemic. To date, available data have been heterogeneous and scarce. Therefore, we conducted a systematic literature review identifying English-language articles published in PubMed between November 2019 and 30 May 2021. We aimed to explore three areas: (1) outcome and clinical course; (2) immunological response after COVID-19 in LT recipients; and (3) vaccination response. After systematic selection, 35, 4, and 5 articles, respectively, were considered suitable for each area of analysis. Despite the heterogeneity of the reports included in this study, we found that gastrointestinal symptoms were common in LT recipients. The outcome of the LT population was not per se worse compared to the general population, although careful management of immunosuppressive therapy is required. While a complete therapy discontinuation is not encouraged, caution needs to be taken with use of mycophenolate mofetil (MMF), favoring tacrolimus (TAC) use. Although data conflicted about acquired immunity after SARS-CoV-2 infection, vaccine immunogenicity appeared to be low, suggesting that the level of surveillance should be kept high in this population.

Keywords: solid organ transplantation; liver injury; immunosuppressant; SARS-CoV-2; humoral response; vaccination

Citation: Becchetti, C.; Gschwend, S.G.; Dufour, J.-F.; Banz, V. COVID-19 in Liver Transplant Recipients: A Systematic Review. *J. Clin. Med.* **2021**, *10*, 4015. https://doi.org/10.3390/jcm10174015

Academic Editor: Pierluigi Toniutto

Received: 31 July 2021
Accepted: 1 September 2021
Published: 5 September 2021

Publisher's Note: MDPI stays neutral with regard to jurisdictional claims in published maps and institutional affiliations.

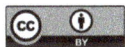
1. Introduction

Severe acute respiratory syndrome coronavirus 2 (SARS-CoV-2) has first been identified in Wuhan city, Hubei Province, China as the pathogen responsible for several cases of severe pneumonia during November 2019, subsequently defined by the World Health Organization (WHO) as Coronavirus disease 2019 (COVID-19). Typical symptoms of COVID-19 include fever, cough, dyspnea, fatigue, myalgia, gastrointestinal manifestations, and impairment of smell and/or taste [1–3]. The course of the disease ranges from asymptomatic or mild [4] to severe manifestations, mainly with respiratory features, leading to respiratory insufficiency, acute respiratory distress syndrome (ARDS), and in some cases to death. Age, male gender, and comorbidities have been established as risk factors for a more severe course of the disease and for mortality [5,6].

Since March 2020, COVID-19 has spread worldwide, has been declared a pandemic by the WHO, and has rapidly become a public health matter with several unmet issues. As of 16 July 2021, there were over 188 million confirmed cases and over 4 million reported deaths worldwide [7].

While knowledge on disease evolution, risk factors, clinical manifestations, and optimal management of affected individuals is progressively increasing, treatment guidelines are difficult to standardize when taking into account specific categories of patients. In this regard, solid organ transplant (SOT) recipients, and among them, liver transplant (LT) patients, may represent a potentially high-risk population. Concerns have been raised regarding immunosuppression therapy, including SARS-CoV-2-associated liver injury [8] and a possible impairment of the immunological response.

187

In December 2020, encouraging results on the safety and efficacy profile of the first anti-SARS-CoV-2 vaccines were published [9,10], paving the way for a large-scale vaccination campaign. However, most special populations were excluded from the pivotal studies of these vaccines, and therefore, real-life observations on efficacy and safety are necessary.

Data regarding the management of immunosuppression therapy in LT recipients affected by COVID-19, as well as information on the course of the disease, outcome, and immunological response both to the infection and vaccination, remain scarce.

The aim of this review was therefore to analyze and summarize the published literature concerning LT recipients with COVID-19.

2. Materials and Methods

A systematic literature review was conducted identifying PubMed English-language articles published between November 2019 and 30 May 2021.

We structured our search on three areas, using different MeSH terms. First, we aimed to analyze outcome and clinical course in LT recipients; second, we aimed to analyze immunological response after COVID-19 in LT recipients; and third, we aimed to analyze vaccination response.

For the first purpose, the MeSH terms used were "COVID-19" (and related terms: 2019 novel coronavirus, SARS-CoV-2 infection, 2019-nCoV infection) AND "liver transplant" (and related terms: orthotopic liver transplant (OLT), hepatic transplant, liver transplantation, solid organ transplant).

For the second purpose, the MeSH terms used were "COVID-19" (and related terms) AND "liver transplant" (and related terms) AND "humoral response" (and related terms: serology, immune response, T-cell response).

For the third purpose, the MeSH terms used were "liver transplant" (and related terms) AND "COVID-19 vaccines".

Original articles, case reports, case series, commentaries, letters to the editor, and review articles were considered. Additional articles were considered on the basis of the reference lists of the included studies. Two reviewers independently evaluated titles and abstracts for inclusion. Only well-characterized adult transplant recipients were included. Articles with known duplications were excluded. When feasible, information on LT recipients summarized in mixed cohorts of SOT patients were extracted and analyzed. Systematic selection was performed according to the Preferred Reporting Items for Systematic Reviews and Meta-Analyses (PRISMA) [11]. Data extraction was conducted independently by two researchers (SGG and CB), using the text, tables, and figures of the original published articles. Independently, the overall quality was also evaluated and graded according to the Newcastle–Ottawa scale (NOS) for assessing the quality of the observational studies and converting the results to the Agency for Health Care Research and Quality (AHRQ) standards (good, fair, and poor) where applicable. When disagreement was present, an open discussion led to a final consensus. All the reported patients' demographic and clinical characteristics, baseline immunosuppressant medications and modifications during the course of the infection, need for intensive care unit (ICU) and/or mechanical ventilation (MV), and outcome were collected. A meta-analysis to investigate association between baseline characteristics, immunosuppression, and outcomes was not performed because of the lack of sufficient data and the high heterogeneity between the different studies. For the second and third aims, we collected the data regarding the type of assay used to assess immunity and the type of vaccines applied. The principal measures used were the median, mean, standard deviation, and incidence as pooled results.

3. Results

3.1. Study Selection

For the first aim, 820 papers met the research criteria applied, of which 76 articles were considered suitable for evaluation. Preliminary reports subsequently published as extended analyses were considered duplications and therefore not included in the final analysis. In addition, data duplication for survey-based studies could not be completely ruled out. Therefore, we restricted our final selection to 35 articles, including a total of 1076 patients. No randomized control trials were found, and only two studies were prospectively designed; the remaining 33 articles were retrospective studies, case reports or case series, editorials, or letters to the editor. Five studies reached "good quality" according to the NOS converted in the AHRQ standards. One study reached "fair quality", and the other studies were rated as "poor quality". The selection process followed the PRISMA guidelines and is summarized in Figure 1.

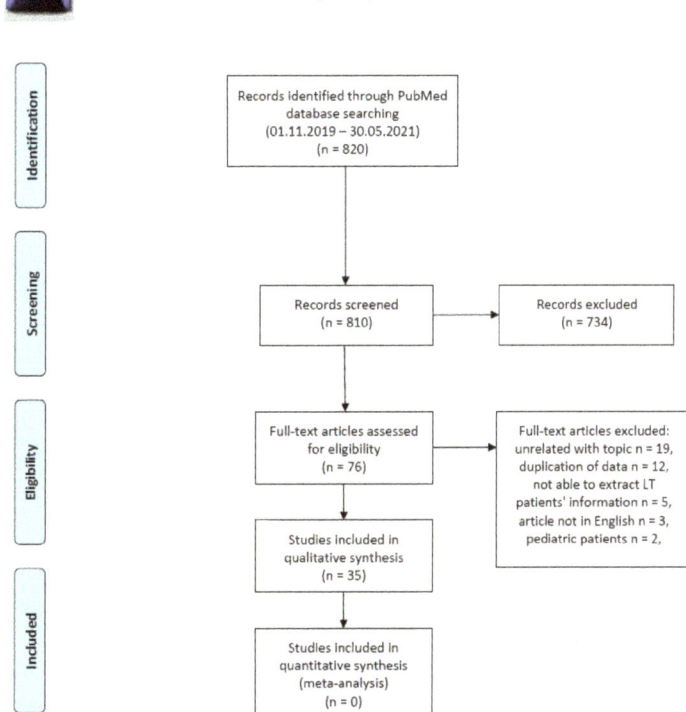

Figure 1. Flow diagram of the systematic literature search according to the PRISMA statement.

For the second and the third aims, 18 and 19 papers met the research criteria applied, respectively. Of these, four and five articles respectively were considered suitable for evaluation. No randomized control trials were found. Only two studies were prospectively designed; the remaining articles were retrospective studies, case reports or case series, editorials, or letters to the editor.

3.2. Study Population Characteristics, Clinical Course, and Management of Immunosuppression

Overall, 1076 patients were pooled. Mean age was 54.5 ± 12.1 years, with male gender being prevalent ($n = 553$, 66.8%). Extensive information on comorbidities was available in 30 papers. Diabetes mellitus type 2, arterial hypertension, and obesity were present in 38.6%, 43.5%, and 16.0% of patients, respectively. A history of previous neoplasia was described in three reports, identifying 23 out of 832 patients (2.8%). In the majority of patients, infection with SARS-CoV-2 occurred 79.7 months after LT. The demographic characteristics and main outcomes are summarized in Table 1.

Table 1. General characteristics of the included studies.

First Author	Country	Number of Patients (m/f)	Mean/Median Age	Comorbidities, n (%)	Outcome	
Alconchel et al. [12]	Spain	3 (1/2)	64 (61–68)	Hypertension 2 (67) Diabetes 1 (33) Stroke 1 (33) Hypothyroidism 1 (33) Hypertension 8 (47) Diabetes 9 (53)	CFR ICU ARDS	67% 100% 33%
Becchetti et al. [13]	Europe	17 (12/5)	Median 61 (IQR 26)	Cardiovascular disease 8 (47) CKD 7 (41) Obesity 5 (29) Respiratory disease 2 (12) Cancer 8 (47) Hypertension 111 (46) Diabetes 94 (39)	CFR ICU ARDS	24% 12% 18%
Belli et al. [14]	Europe	243 (171/72)	63 (55–69)	Cardiovascular disease 17 (7) CKD 49 (20) Obesity 46 (19) Respiratory disease 25 (10) Other 43 (18)	CFR ICU ARDS	20% 15% NA
Bösch et al. [15]	Germany	SOT 7; of them, 2 LT (1/1)	42 (18–65)	Hypertension 2 (100) CKD 1 (50)	CFR ICU ARDS	0% 0% NA
Choudhury et al. [16]	India	6 (6/–)	46 (38–52)	Hypertension 3 (50) Diabetes 3 (50) CKD 1 (17) Hypothyroidism 1 (17) Hypertension 64 (58)	CFR ICU ARDS	0% 17% NA
Colmenero et al. [17]	Spain	111 (79/32)	Median 65 (IQR 11)	Diabetes 53 (48) Cardiovascular disease 22 (20) Respiratory disease 13 (12) Cardiovascular disease 1 (50)	Mortality rate ICU ARDS	18% 11% NA
Dale et al. [18]	USA	2 (–/2)	62 (58–65)	Respiratory disease 1 (50) Rheumatoid arthritis 1 (50) Psoriatic arthritis 1 (50) Diabetes 9 (75)	CFR ICU ARDS	0% 100% NA
Dhampalwar et al. [19]	India	12 (11/1)	54 (45–63)	Hypertension 4 (33) Metabolic syndrome 1 (8) Chronic rejection 1 (8)	CFR ICU ARDS	8% NA NA

Table 1. *Cont.*

First Author	Country	Number of Patients (m/f)	Mean/Median Age	Comorbidities, *n* (%)	Outcome
Eslami et al. [20]	Iran	1 (m)	69	CKD	CFR 100% ICU 100% ARDS NA
Felldin et al. [21]	Sweden	SOT 53; of them 8 LT and 3 kidney–LT (4/7)	60 (27–72)	Hypertension 1 (9) Diabetes 6 (55) Cardiovascular disease 1 (9) CKD 2 (18) Obesity 2 (18) Respiratory disease 2 (18) Hypothyroidism 1 (9) Sarcoidosis 1 (9) Polymyalgia rheumatica 1 (9) Psychosis 1 (9) Cancer 1 (9) Hypertension Diabetes	CFR 9% ICU NA ARDS NA
Fung et al. [22]	USA	SOT 10; of them, 1 LT (f)	80	Cardiovascular disease CKD Respiratory disease Hypothyroidism Dementia	CFR 0% ICU No ARDS No
Hadi et al. [23]	USA	2307 SOT; of them, 240 LT (NA) Control group 2289 (1399/890)	NA for LT Control group 55	LT: NA Control group: Hypertension 2213 (92) Diabetes 1420 (62) Cardiovascular disease 1020 (45) Respiratory disease 633 (28)	LT: CFR NA ICU 10% ARDS NA Control group: CFR 6% ICU 9% ARDS NA
Hann et al. [24]	UK	3 (2/1)	61 (47–69)	Hypertension 2 (67) Diabetes 3 (100) CKD 2 (67) Obesity 1 (33) Other 1 (33)	CFR 33% ICU NA ARDS NA

Table 1. Cont.

First Author	Country	Number of Patients (m/f)	Mean/Median Age	Comorbidities, n (%)	Outcome
Hatami et al. [25]	Iran	1 (f)	30	Hypothyroidism	CFR 0%; ICU NA; ARDS NA
Hayashi et al. [26]	Japan	1 (m)	20	NA	CFR 0%; ICU No; ARDS No
Huang et al. [27]	China	1 (m)	59	HBV	CFR 100%; MV Yes; ARDS NA
Jamir et al. [28]	India	1 (m)	49	Obesity	CFR 0%; ICU 100%; ARDS NA
Kates et al. [29]	USA	SOT 4; of them, 1 LT (m)	67	Cirrhosis of allograft 1 (100)	CFR 0%; ICU Yes; ARDS NA
Kolonko et al. [30]	Poland	SOT 4; of them, 1 LT (m)	53	Ulcerative colitis 1 (100)	CFR 0%; ICU No; ARDS NA
Liu et al. [31]	China	1 (m)	50	NA	CFR 0%; ICU 0%; ARDS NA
Mansoor et al. [32]	USA	LT 125 (82/43) Control group 125 (85/40)	LT 57 (SD +/−19) Control group 60 (SD +/−15)	LT: Hypertension 29 (23) Diabetes 20 (16) CKD 24 (19) Respiratory disease <10 (<8) Heart failure <10 (<8) Ischemic heart disease <10 (<8) Control group: Hypertension 23 (18) Diabetes 20 (16) CKD 26 (21) Respiratory disease <10 (<8) Heart failure <10 (<8) Ischemic heart disease <10 (<8)	LT: CFR <8%; ICU <8%; ARDS NA; Control group: CFR <8%; ICU 9%; ARDS NA

Table 1. *Cont.*

First Author	Country	Number of Patients (m/f)	Mean/Median Age	Comorbidities, *n* (%)	Outcome	
Mathiasen et al. [33]	Denmark	1 (f)	58	Hypertension Obesity Hyperlipidemia Hypertension 2 (67) Cardiovascular disease 1 (33)	CFR ICU ARDS	0% 0% NA
Mehta et al. [34]	USA	SOT 11; of them, 3 LT (2/1)	65 (62–68)	Diabetes 1 (33) Obesity 2 (67) HIV 3 (100) HCV 3 (100)	CFR ICU ARDS	0% 0% NA
Modi et al. [35]	USA	1 (m)	32	HIV	CFR ICU ARDS	0% 0% NA
Niknam et al. [36]	Iran	2 (1/1)	53 (46–60)	Diabetes 1 (50)	CFR ICU ARDS CFR	0% NA 0% 0%
Nikoupour et al. [37]	Iran	1 (m)	35	Ulcerative colitis 1 (100)	ICU ARDS CFR	0% NA 0%
Prieto et al. [38]	Spain	1 (m)	52	Cardiovascular disease 1 (100)	ICU ARDS CFR	No NA 0%
Qin et al. [39]	China	1 (m)	37	NA	ICU ARDS	NA NA
Rabiee et al. [40]	USA	112 (61/51)	Median 61 (IQR 20)	Hypertension 59 (53) Diabetes 51 (46) Cardiovascular disease 15 (13) Obesity 26 (23) Respiratory disease 18 (16) Metabolic syndrome 22 (20) Cancer 7 (6) HIV 1 (1) Hypertension 5 (63) Diabetes 2 (25)	CFR ICU ARDS	22% 27% NA
Rauber et al. [41]	Germany	8 (NA)	57 (26–70)	Cardiovascular disease 1 (13) CKD 4 (50) Obesity 2 (25)	CFR ICU ARDS	0% 0% NA

Table 1. *Cont.*

First Author	Country	Number of Patients (m/f)	Mean/Median Age	Comorbidities, *n* (%)	Outcome	
Sessa et al. [42]	France	1 (m)	58	Hypertension	CFR	0%
					ICU	0%
					ARDS	NA
Terrabuio et al. [43]	Brazil	4 (1/3)	52 (42–62)	Hypertension 1 (25)	CFR	0%
				Diabetes 1 (25)	ICU	0%
				Obesity 2 (50)	ARDS	NA
				Chronic rejection 1 (25)		
				Crohn's disease 1 (25)		
Waisberg et al. [44]	Brazil	5 (4/1)	60 (34–69)	Hypertension 3 (60)	CFR	40%
				Diabetes 1 (20)	ICU	NA
				Cardiovascular disease 1 (20)	ARDS	NA
				Obesity 2 (40)		
				Respiratory disease 1 (20)		
Webb et al. [45]	International	LT 151 (102/49) Control group 627 (329/298)	LT Median 60 (IQR 47–66) Control group 73 (IQR 55–84)	LT:	LT:	
				Hypertension 63 (42)	CFR	19%
				Diabetes 65 (43)	ICU	28%
				Cardiovascular disease 22 (15)	ARDS	NA
				Obesity 44 (29)		
				Respiratory disease 8 (5)		
				Cancer 8 (5)		
				Control group:	Control group:	
				Hypertension 241 (38)	CFR	27%
				Diabetes 144 (23)	ICU	8%
				Cardiovascular disease 202 (32)	ARDS	NA
				Obesity 158 (25)		
				Respiratory disease 160 (26)		
				Cancer 92 (15)		
				Stroke 73 (12)		
Wei et al. [46]	China	1 (m)	61	NA	CFR	0%
					ICU	NA
					ARDS	NA

Abbreviations: ICU: intensive care unit; ARDS: acute respiratory distress syndrome; HBV: hepatitis B virus; HIV: human immunodeficiency virus; HCV: hepatitis C virus; SOT: solid organ transplantation; LT: liver transplant; NA: not applicable; CKD: chronic kidney insufficiency; IQR: interquartile range; CFR: case fatality rate.

Regarding the incidence of COVID-19 infections in LT recipients, only the SETH cohort provided data, showing that the incidence of COVID-19 in liver transplant recipients compared to the general population (837.41 cases/ 105 patients vs. 311.93 cases/ 105 people) was almost double [17].

On the other hand, the COVID-LT cohort recorded 57 confirmed SARS-CoV-2 infections out of 11,790 patients in regular follow-ups, resulting in an incidence of 483.46 cases/ 105 patients [13]. Another report from Germany documented, using either serology or PCR-swab test, present or past SARS-CoV-2 infection in 3.7% of their LT recipients during the study period (May and August 2020) [41].

The most frequently described clinical presentation was fever (61.4%), followed by cough (58.6%) and dyspnea (36.2%). Webb et al. [45] reported general "respiratory symptoms", which were experienced by the 77% of the LT recipients included in the study. Gastrointestinal symptoms including vomiting, diarrhea, nausea, and abdominal pain were strongly represented (159/569 patients, 27.9%). In the aforementioned study, the proportion of patients with gastrointestinal symptoms was higher among LT recipients compared to the nontransplant cohort (30% vs. 12%, $p < 0.0001$), whereas no significant difference was observed with respect to respiratory symptoms. On the same line, Belli et al. [14] found diarrhea as the presenting symptom in 55 LT recipients, corresponding to 22.6%.

Concerning immunosuppression therapy, data on basal immunosuppression (IS) therapy and on subsequent management during the course of infection was available for 33 and 29 studies, respectively. The data are summarized in Table 2.

Table 2. Information regarding immunosuppressant regimen and its modification in during COVID-19.

First Author	Number of Patients	Baseline IS, n (%)	Modification IS	Type of Modification
Alconchel et al. [12]	3	TAC + steroid, 1 (33) TAC + MMF + steroid, 2 (67)	Yes	TAC reduction 33% MMF withdrawal and TAC reduction 33% MMF withdrawal 33%
Becchetti et al. [13]	17	**Single agent** Cys, 1 (6) TAC, 4 (24) Everolimus, 1 (6) MMF, 2 (12) **Combination** CNIs + MMF, 7 (41) CNIs + steroids, 2 (12)	Yes	Reduction 29% Withdrawal 18%
Belli et al. [14]	243	**Single agent** Cys, 13 (5) Cys + MMF, 9 (4) Cys + steroid, 3 (1) Cys + MMF + steroid, 4 (2) TAC, 54 (22) TAC + MMF, 52 (21) TAC + mTORi, 12 (5) TAC + steroid, 27 (11) TAC + MMF + steroid, 15 (6) MMF, 24 (10) MMF + mTORi, 10 (4) MMF + steroid, 3 (1) mTORi, 11 (5) mTORi + steroid, 2 (1) Steroid, 2 (1)	Yes	CNIs withdrawal 7% CNIs reduction 16% Antimetabolites withdrawal 14% mTORi withdrawal 4% Other 2%
Bösch et al. [15]	SOT 7; of them, 2 LT	Everolimus + MMF, 1 (50) MMF, 1 (50)	Yes	MMF withdrawal 50%
Choudhury et al. [16]	6	TAC, 2 (33) TAC + MMF, 2 (33) Steroid, 1 (17) Everolimus, 1 (17)	Yes	TAC and MMF withdrawal and start steroids (17) TAC +and MMF withdrawal and start steroids (17) TAC withdrawal and start steroids (33) Several adjustments (17)

Table 2. *Cont.*

First Author	Number of Patients	Baseline IS, n (%)	Modification IS	Type of Modification
Colmenero et al. [17]	111	**Single agent** CNIs, 24 (31) **Combination** CNIs + MMF, 29 (26) CNIs + Everolimus, 9 (8) MMF +/− Everolimus, 37 (33)	NA	NA
Dale et al. [18]	2	TAC + steroid, 1 (50) TAC + MMF + steroid, 1 (50)	Yes	Prednisone reduction 100% (perioperative)
Dhampalwar et al. [19]	12	TAC-based, 10 (83) Cys-based, 1 (8) Everolimus-based, 1 (8) (Not available data on MMF)	Yes	MMF reduction in most patients
Eslami et al. [20]	1	TAC + steroid	No	(perioperative)
Felldin et al. [21]	SOT 53; of them, 8 LT and 3 kidney–LT	TAC, 3 (27) TAC + steroid, 1 (9) TAC + MMF 2 (18) TAC + MMF + steroid, 3 (27) TAC + AZA, 1 (9) TAC + steroid + MTX, 1 (9)	Yes	MMF withdrawal 27% MMF reduction 9% MTX withdrawal 9% TAC reduction 9%
Fung et al. [22]	1	TAC + MMF	No	-
Hann et al. [24]	3	TAC + AZA + steroid, 3 (100)	NA	NA
Hatami et al. [25]	1	TAC	Yes	TAC withdrawal
Hayashi et al. [26]	1	TAC	No	
Huang et al. [27]	1	TAC + MMF	Yes	Reduction of 50% (drug-drug interaction) MMF withdrawal
Jamir et al. [28]	1	TAC + MMF + steroid	Yes	Steroids i.v.
Kates et al. [29]	SOT 4; of them, 1 LT	Cys	No	
Kolonko et al. [30]	SOT 4; of them, 1 LT	TAC + MMF + steroid	Yes	MMF withdrawal 100%
Liu et al. [31]	1	TAC	Yes	TAC withdrawal Steroids i.v.
Mathiasen et al. [33]	1	TAC + MMF	No	-
Mehta et al. [34]	SOT 11; of them, 3 LT	TAC + steroid, 1 (33) TAC + MMF 1 (33) TAC + MMF + steroid, 1 (33)	Yes	TAC and MMF withdrawal 33%
Modi et al. [35]	1	TAC + MMF + steroid	Yes	MMF withdrawal TAC reduction

Table 2. *Cont.*

First Author	Number of Patients	Baseline IS, *n* (%)	Modification IS	Type of Modification
Niknam et al. [36]	2	TAC + MMF + steroid, 2 (100)	Yes	MMF reduction 100%
Nikoupour et al. [37]	1	Tac + MMF + steroid	Yes	MMF reduction
Prieto et al. [38]	1	Basiliximab + MMF + TAC + steroid	Yes	Several adjustments (perioperative)
Qin et al. [39]	1	TAC + steroid	Yes	Several adjustments (perioperative)
Rabiee et al. [40]	112	TAC, 103 (92); MMF, 56 (50); Steroid, 34 (30); Cys, 7 (6); mTOR inhibitors, 4 (4); AZA, 1 (1); TAC, 1 (13)	Yes	**Patients with liver injury** (ALT > 2×ULN) n = 81; MMF withdrawal 33%; TAC reduction 26%; TAC withdrawal 5%
Rauber et al. [41]	8	TAC + MMF, 4 (50); TAC + mTORi, 1 (13); Cys, 1 (13); mTORi, 1 (13)	NA	-
Sessa et al. [42]	1	TAC	No	-
Terrabuio et al. [43]	4	TAC + MMF + steroid, 3 (75); TAC + AZA, 1 (25)	Yes	MMF withdrawal and steroid reduction 50%; MMF withdrawal and steroid increase 25%; MMF withdrawal and TAC reduction 25%; Reduction 40%
Waisberg et al. [44]	5	NA for LT	Yes	Withdrawal 20%; Increase 20% (ACR) (all perioperative)
Wei et al. [46]	1	TAC	Yes	TAC withdrawal

Abbreviations: AZA: azathioprine; CNI: calcineurin inhibitors; Cys: cyclosporine; TAC: tacrolimus; MMF: mycophenolate mofetil; mTORi: mammalian target of rapamycin inhibitor; SOT: solid organ transplantation; LT: liver transplant; NA: not applicable; MTX: methotrexate.

In the study by Colmenero et al. [17] patients receiving MMF or in whom an attempt was made to completely withdraw immunosuppression were more prevalent in the severe COVID-19 group (*p* = 0.014, and *p* = 0.016 respectively). Conversely, tacrolimus-based immunosuppression was more frequent in the nonsevere COVID-19 group, albeit without statistical significance (*p* = 0.113). Similar findings regarding calcineurin inhibitor (CNIs)-based regimens were observed in the COVID-LT study, where the continuation of CNIs therapy after COVID-19 diagnosis was higher among survivors (64% vs. 42.8%) [47]. Indeed, in the study of Belli et al. [14], after multivariable analysis, the use of TAC was confirmed to be independently associated with a reduced mortality risk (HR, 0.55; 95% CI, 0.31–0.99). Additionally, in the Spanish cohort, survival curves illustrated the negative prognostic impact of MMF, particularly at doses higher than 1000 mg/day. In agreement with this finding, in patients receiving full-dose of MMF at baseline (i.e., 2000 mg/day), complete drug withdrawal showed a trend towards reduced severe COVID-19 (41.7% vs. 69.2%, *p* = 0.16) [17].

Overall, 375 out of 1064 (35.2%) patients were managed in an outpatient setting, whereas 64.8% were hospitalized. Of the hospitalized patients, 158/689 (22.9%) were admitted to an ICU. Death was reported in 135 cases. In the COVID-LT study, case fatality was estimated at 12% (95% CI 5–24%), which increased to 17% (95% CI 7–32%) among hospitalized patients [13], whereas Rabiee and coauthors found a 22.3% case fatality rate [40]. In the study by Webb and coauthors [45], case fatality was 19% (vs. the 27% reported for the comparison cohort, *p* = 0.046), with the propensity-score-matched analysis showing that LT did not significantly increase the risk of death in patients with SARS-CoV-2 infection (absolute risk difference 1.4% (95% CI 7.7–10.4)). Colmenero et al. [17] described a mortality rate of 18% among LT patients.

In Webb et al., multivariate analyses showed that factors significantly associated with death were: increased age (OR 1.06 (95% CI 1.01–1.11) per 1 year increase, *p* = 0.031), presence of nonliver cancer (OR 18.30 (1.96–170.75); *p* = 0.011), and higher baseline serum creatinine (OR 1.57 (1.05–2.36) per 1 mg/dL increase) *p* = 0.028) [45]. Results derived from the multivariate analysis performed within the SETH cohort study identified the following independent predictors: Charlson comorbidity index (relative risk (RR) = 1.28 (95% CI 1.05–1.56), male gender (RR = 2.49; 95% CI 1.14–5.41), dyspnea at diagnosis (RR = 7.25; 95% CI 2.95–17.82), and baseline immunosuppression containing MMF (RR = 3.94; 95% CI 1.59–9.74) [17]. Belli et al. reported risk factors associated with worse prognosis including advanced age (>70 vs. <60 years, HR 4.16; 95% CI 1.78–9.73) and the use of TAC [14].

Despite theoretically higher levels of immunosuppression, only the report by Belli et al. [14] mentioned time since LT as an independent factor associated with poor outcome in univariate analysis. On the other hand, Colmenero et al. [17] showed that the time from LT had no impact on the risk of suffering from severe COVID, a finding that was confirmed by Webb et al. [45], who reported no association between death and time since LT.

Lastly, Rabiee et al. showed that the incidence of acute liver injury (defined by ALT 2-5x ULN) was not higher in LT recipients when compared to age- and gender-matched nontransplant patients with chronic liver disease and COVID-19 (47.5% vs. 34.6%; *p* = 0.037). The presence of liver injury during COVID-19 in LT recipients was significantly associated with mortality (OR 6.91 (95% CI: 1.68–28.48), *p* = 0.007) and ICU admission (OR 7.93 (95% CI: 1.75–35.69), *p* = 0.007) [40]. In the US study of Hadi et al., considering only LT recipients, only 18 patients (7.5%) experienced the composite outcome including mechanical ventilation and death at 30 days. This rate was lower when compared to that for recipients of other organ transplants [23].

3.3. Immunological Response after COVID-19 in LT Recipients

Regarding the immunological response after SARS-CoV-2 infection in LT patients, only four studies were considered, including a total of 91 LT recipients. However, all of these studies examined different types of tests/assays directed toward different targets, and data could not always be extrapolated to LT recipients alone, as shown in Table 3, making a pooled analysis not feasible.

Table 3. Summary of the included studies concerning immunological response of LT recipients after COVID-19.

First Author	Country	Number of Patients	Type of Test	Type of Assay	Main Conclusions
Zilla et al. [50]	USA	SOT 3; of them, 1 LT and 1 kidney–LT	Anti-SARS-CoV-2 (S1 subunit) IgA and IgG	EUROIMMUN®	Delayed serological response and worst outcome
Burack et al. [51]	USA	SOT 70; of them, 14 LT	Anti-SARS-CoV-2 (antinucleocapsid antigen) IgM, IgG, and IgA	Roche Elecsys®	80% of liver transplant recipients turned positive
Favà et al. [49]	Spain	SOT 28; of them, 5 LT	Anti-SARS-CoV-2 IgM and IgG + T cell responses	MaglumiTM 2019 (Snibe Diagnostic®) + AID® Gmbh	SOT and immunocompetent patients achieved a similarly robust serological and functional T cell immune response, albeit with a certain delay.
Caballeros-Marcos et al. [48]	Spain	71 LT	Anti-SARS-CoV-2 (antinucleocapsid antigen) IgG	Abbott ARCHITECT i2000®	LT recipients, compared to immunocompetent patients, showed a lower incidence of antinucleocapsid IgG antibodies at 3 months and at 6 months.

Abbreviations: SOT: solid organ transplantation; LT: liver transplant.

Caballero-Marcos et al. [48] showed a decline over time of IgG-antinucleocapsid, with lower incidence at 3 months (77.4% vs. 100%, $p < 0.001$) and at 6 months (63.4% vs. 90.1%, $p < 0.001$) when compared with a matched cohort of immunocompetent subjects. A more comprehensive analysis performed in 28 SOT patients (of which five were LT patients) of the immunological response, which also considered T-cell responses, showed that the overall response was not impaired in the SOT patients. However, when the humoral response was considered alone, there was some delay in mounting a response compared to the immunocompetent control group [49].

3.4. COVID-19 Vaccine Immunogenicity in LT Recipients

Regarding response to COVID-19 vaccines, we considered five studies. Overall, the studies included 269 LT recipients (Table 4). However, analogously to those regarding the immunological response after COVID-19, the included studies considered different types of tests/assays, and data could not always be extrapolated to LT recipients alone, making comparisons difficult. Two studies evaluated side effects after receiving one dose of mRNA-1273 or BNT162b2 vaccine or two doses of BNT162b2 vaccine. Both studies showed local and systemic side effects in proportions comparable to those in pivotal studies for RNA vaccines.

Table 4. Summary of the included study concerning vaccination against SARS-CoV-2 response in LT recipients.

First Author	Country	Number of Patients	Type of Vaccine	Type of Assay	Side Effect	Main Conclusions
Boyarsky et al. [54]	USA	SOT 658; of them, 129 LT	mRNA-1273 (Moderna) 307 SOT BNT162b2 (Pfizer-BioNTech) 342 SOT	Anti-SARS-CoV-2 (S1 subunit) IgA and IgG (EUROIMMUN®) and Anti-SARS-CoV-2 (antinucleocapsid antigen) IgM, IgG, and IgA (Roche Elecsys®)	–	Humoral response to 2 doses of mRNA SARS-CoV-2 vaccine among SOT was present, although participants without a response after dose 1 had generally low antibody levels. Poor humoral response was associated with use of antimetabolite immunosuppression.
Boyarsky et al. [56]	USA	SOT 187; of them, 26 LT	mRNA-1273 (Moderna) 94 SOT BNT162b2 (Pfizer-BioNTech) 93 SOT	–	**Local reactions:** pain (61%) swelling (16%) **Systemic reactions:** fever (4%) chills (9%) fatigue (38%) headache (32%) myalgias (15%)	SOT patients, after 1 dose of vaccine, experienced typically minimal perivaccine reactogenicity similar to reported rates in non-SOT patients.
Mazzola et al. [52]	France	SOT 143; of them, 56 LT	BNT162b2 (Pfizer-BioNTech)	Anti-SARS-CoV-2 (Receptor Binding Domain of S1) IgG (Abbott Alinity i®)	**Local reactions:** pain (26%) **Systemic reactions:** fatigue (14%) headache (6%)	Low antibody response 28 days after 2 doses of vaccine among SOT recipients, with 28.6% of seroconversion, particularly for kidney and heart SOT.
Miele et al. [55]	Italy	SOT 16; of them, 4 LT	BNT162b2 (Pfizer-BioNTech)	Anti-SARS-CoV-2 spike protein (S1/S2) (DiaSorin®) and ex vivo IFN-γ-ELISpot assay (Mabtech®)	–	Humoral and T-cell responses were significantly lower in SOT recipients than in immunocompetent group.
Rabinowich et al. [53]	Israel	80 LT	BNT162b2 (Pfizer-BioNTech)	Anti-SARS-CoV-2 (antinucleocapsid antigen) IgG (Abbott ARCHITECT i2000®) and anti-spike protein (S1/S2) (DiaSorin®)	–	Positive serology was observed in only 47.5% ($p < 0.001$) of LT recipients. Predictors for negative response among LT recipients were older age, lower estimated glomerular filtration rate, and treatment with high-dose steroids and mycophenolate mofetil.

Abbreviations: SOT: solid organ transplantation; LT: liver transplant.

Concerning immunogenicity, four studies, although using different assays, evaluated the humoral response recording seroconversion rates between 29 and 50% [52,53]. Two studies emphasized that the use of antimetabolites as immunosuppression was a risk factor for reduced serum conversion rates [53,54]. Only one study also analyzed T-cell response, which was described as reduced [55], and only one of the included studies considered only LT recipients [53].

4. Discussion

At the beginning of the COVID-19 pandemic, SOT recipients, including LT recipients, were considered a vulnerable population, raising the question as to whether they would be at particular risk for severe disease and graft injury given their immunocompromised state and high prevalence of metabolic comorbidities. The aim of our study was to systematically pool all the available literature on this topic. We found that middle-aged men with metabolic comorbidities were the main target for the infection. Even though respiratory problems represented the main clinical feature in LT patients, a high percentage of gastrointestinal symptoms were also reported. Approximately 70% of LT patients with SARS-CoV-2 infection were hospitalized. Modification/reduction of IS was common, particularly for MMF, although complete withdrawal of all IS was rarely observed. With respect to outcome, a case fatality rate ranging between 12 and 22% was described in the major reports accessible for this analysis. Interestingly, when compared to the control population, outcomes were not worse in the LT recipient group.

There seems to be a difference in the immune response to the SARS-CoV-2 infection and the immune response as acquired by vaccination. In the first case, the data conflict, but if we consider the response mediating the neutralizing activity (anti-spike protein IgG and T-cell mediated), it seems that there is a similar response, albeit probably slightly delayed, in LT recipients compared to immunocompetent subjects. On the other hand, vaccine-induced immunogenicity seems to be defective.

Although a considerable number of patients were included in the present study, the quality of the manuscripts analyzed makes it difficult to consolidate associations and predictive factors regarding COVID-19 and the LT population.

The epidemiological distribution of the disease is superimposable to that of the general population [2,57], with COVID-19 being mainly prevalent in middle-aged males.

Recently, new findings have highlighted how obesity [58], diabetes type II [59], and arterial hypertension [60] are associated with a more severe course of COVID-19 and hence a poorer outcome. Despite the high prevalence of these metabolic conditions in LT recipients [61,62] and more specifically in the present cohort, this did not seem to negatively affect the prognosis of the current study population.

Interestingly, the presence of gastrointestinal complaints (28%) was considerably higher among LT recipients. A recent review on gastrointestinal symptoms in COVID-19 [63] showed a high heterogeneity in incidence (ranging between 3 and 79%), with other large cohorts of patients reporting rates of gastrointestinal symptoms between 5 and 15% [60,64]. It is widely accepted that SARS-CoV-2 enters host mucosal cells via the cell receptor angiotensin-converting enzyme-2 (ACE-2) and the transmembrane serine protease 2 (TMPRSS2), which are also highly expressed in the absorptive enterocytes from the ileum and colon [65]. Once the virus enters the enterocytes, it can start replication and its cytopathic effect [66]. The gut microbiome can be significantly altered by SARS-CoV-2 through several mechanisms (e.g., proinflammatory cytokines, perturbation in the gut–lung axis, medications, changing ratio of pathogenic organisms) leading to clinical manifestations such as diarrhea and vomiting [67]. LT patients are also known to have an extremely vulnerable gut microbiomes [68,69], and immunosuppressive fluctuation in trough level can interfere with gut flora stability [70]. Furthermore, it was observed that patients with digestive symptoms, probably not recognized from the outset as symptoms associated with COVID-19, had a significantly longer time from onset to admission than patients without digestive symptoms (9.0 days vs. 7.3 days, $p = 0.013$) [71]. Interestingly, a recent study aiming to analyze the gut inflammatory response in immunocompetent subjects infected with SARS-CoV-2 highlighted the absence of a proinflammatory response in the gastrointestinal tract despite detection of SARS-CoV-2. Additionally, this study showed reduced mortality in patients with COVID-19 presenting with GI symptoms. Therefore, the authors speculated on a potential role of the gastrointestinal tract in attenuating SARS-CoV-2-associated inflammation [72].

In the current cohort, the mortality rate and case-fatality rate did not seem to exceed those expected in the general population. Indeed, the hypothesis that LT is a possible associated factor for a pejorative outcome could not be confirmed. However, of note was the high rate of hospitalization, with 64.8% of LT recipients being admitted to a ward and 22.9% of such patients requiring intensive care. This may of course reflect a certain selection bias, with more LT recipients being hospitalized per se. Additionally, one must keep in mind that during the first wave, there were many logistical difficulties, which probably led to an underdiagnosis of asymptomatic or paucisymptomatic cases [73].

With regard to the management of immunosuppression, not all the information can be extrapolated, as most studies have had descriptive designs. The different nature of the immunosuppressive regimens adopted, often multiple, and the modification of these regimens during the course of infection make it difficult to provide any clear guidelines to this respect. However, it seems that a complete discontinuation of IS therapy was very rare and limited to extremely severe cases. Unfortunately, complete cessation of IS was not associated with improved prognosis [17] and should therefore only be considered as a last resort in selected cases.

In the Spanish cohort, patients receiving MMF were more prevalent in the severe COVID-19 group. Baseline immunosuppression containing MMF was identified as an independent predictor of mortality, whereas the withdrawal of IS was not. However, data on modifications in immunosuppressive therapy during the infection were not extensively available in this study [17] and reduction or discontinuation of MMF was recommended by the guidelines shared by experts at the beginning of the pandemic [74]. Therefore, whether the impact on outcome is attributable to the MMF itself or to its reduction/discontinuation remains objects of further investigation. In a preclinical setting, MMF showed promising results against Middle East respiratory syndrome (MERS); however, in vivo studies suggested that its use is likely to cause more harm than benefit against coronavirus (CoV) infection [75]. Bearing in mind that MMF acts on activated lymphocytes with a cytostatic effect [76] and that SARS-CoV-2 has a cytotoxic effect on the same target [77], these synergistic effects may represent an additional risk factor and worsen the prognosis of LT patients taking MMF.

In Belli et al. [14], TAC was found to protect against worse outcomes in COVID-19 LT recipients. In vitro experiments have shown that TAC, and CNIs in general, are capable of inhibiting human CoV growth, mainly by acting on the cyclophilin pathway [78]. Additionally, by modulating T-cell activation, CNIs may act on reducing the deleterious effect of the COVID-19 late inflammatory phase [79].

Concerning the immunological response to SARS-CoV-2 infection, contrasting results were seen. However, most of the studies considered analyzed only the humoral response and in particular used an assay, the antinucleocapsid test, more suitable to evaluate preexisting exposure to the virus than to assess protective efficacy. Indeed, these antibodies have low or no neutralizing activity [80]. On the other hand, the analysis of the T-cell-mediated response in LT recipients showed similar results compared to that for immunocompetent subjects. Further studies are therefore necessary that take into account the complexity of the immune response in vivo and of the interplay among native, humoral, and T-cell immunity.

In contrast, all studies evaluating vaccine immunity have demonstrated reduced immunogenicity of LT recipients, and SOT recipients in general. It is possible, as pointed out by Mazzola et al. [52], that this reduced response is more evident in other SOT recipients, such as those for kidney or heart SOTs, than in LT recipients. In this line, the serum conversion data of the only cohort that included only LT recipients were actually higher than the average of the other studies, which included mixed cohorts. A deterrent role could be played again by more sustained immunosuppression (with dual or triple regimens) and by the use of antimetabolites [53]. Reduced immunogenicity in LT recipients has already been demonstrated with other respiratory virus (e.g., influenza) vaccines [81], suggesting that more than the standard dose may be needed to achieve protective immunogenicity [82].

Several limitations affected the current study, mainly because of the high heterogeneity and quality of the majority of the studies considered, leading in several cases to incomplete information. Therefore, more than a few research questions remain open and will need future investigation (Figure 2).

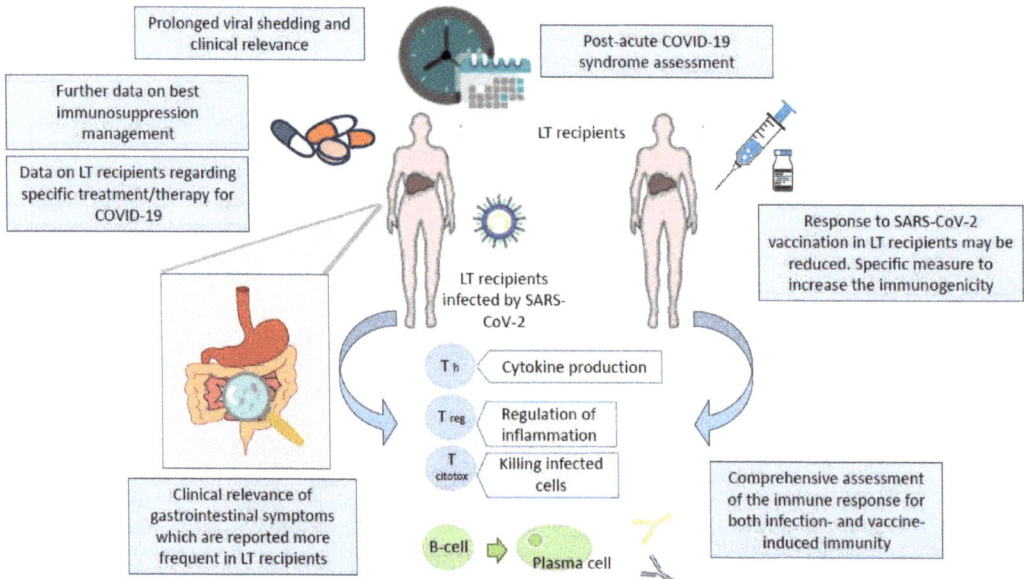

Figure 2. Graphical representation of the key unresolved issues for SARS-CoV-2 infection in LT recipients.

5. Conclusions

Despite the heterogeneity of the reports included in this study, we are able to show that the middle-aged man with metabolic comorbidities represents the main target of COVID-19 among LT recipients, as is the case in nontransplanted patients. Gastrointestinal symptoms are very common in LT recipients with COVID-19, and particular attention should be paid to these complaints as a surrogate marker for COVID-19, even in the absence of fever or respiratory problems. The outcome of the LT population is nevertheless similar to that of the general population. This is, in part, also likely due to a more cautious management of immunosuppressive therapy, paying particular attention to the use of MMF and TAC while discouraging the complete discontinuation of all immunosuppression. LT recipients should be vaccinated, and great attention to protective measures should be maintained in these individuals even after a regular course of vaccination.

Author Contributions: C.B. contributed to this paper with conception, literature review, statistical analysis, writing the manuscript, critical revision, and editing. S.G.G. participated in drafting and literature review. V.B. and J.-F.D. contributed with critical revision and editing. All authors have read and agreed to the published version of the manuscript.

Funding: Chiara Becchetti received financial support from the Stiftung für Leberkrankheiten.

Data Availability Statement: Not applicable.

Conflicts of Interest: The funders had no role in the design of the study; in the collection, analyses, or interpretation of data; in the writing of the manuscript, or in the decision to publish the results.

References

1. Zhou, P.; Yang, X.-L.; Wang, X.-G.; Hu, B.; Zhang, L.; Zhang, W.; Si, H.-R.; Zhu, Y.; Li, B.; Huang, C.-L.; et al. A pneumonia outbreak associated with a new coronavirus of probable bat origin. *Nature* **2020**, *579*, 270–273. [CrossRef]
2. Suleyman, G.; Fadel, R.A.; Malette, K.M.; Hammond, C.; Abdulla, H.; Entz, A.; Demertzis, Z.; Hanna, Z.; Failla, A.; Dagher, C.; et al. Clinical Characteristics and Morbidity Associated with Coronavirus Disease 2019 in a Series of Patients in Metropolitan Detroit. *JAMA Netw. Open* **2020**, *3*, e2012270. [CrossRef] [PubMed]
3. Mao, L.; Jin, H.; Wang, M.; Hu, Y.; Chen, S.; He, Q.; Chang, J.; Hong, C.; Zhou, Y.; Wang, D.; et al. Neurologic Manifestations of Hospitalized Patients with Coronavirus Disease 2019 in Wuhan, China. *JAMA Neurol.* **2020**, *77*, 683–690. [CrossRef] [PubMed]
4. Hu, Z.; Song, C.; Xu, C.; Jin, G.; Chen, Y.; Xu, X.; Ma, H.; Chen, W.; Lin, Y.; Zheng, Y.; et al. Clinical characteristics of 24 asymptomatic infections with COVID-19 screened among close contacts in Nanjing, China. *Sci. China Life Sci.* **2020**, *63*, 706–711. [CrossRef] [PubMed]
5. Loomba, R.S.; Aggarwal, G.; Aggarwal, S.; Flores, S.; Villarreal, E.G.; Farias, J.S.; Lavie, C.J. Disparities in case frequency and mortality of coronavirus disease 2019 (COVID-19) among various states in the United States. *Ann. Med.* **2021**, *53*, 151–159. [CrossRef]
6. Palaiodimos, L.; Kokkinidis, D.G.; Li, W.; Karamanis, D.; Ognibene, J.; Arora, S.; Southern, W.N.; Mantzoros, C.S. Severe obesity, increasing age and male sex are independently associated with worse in-hospital outcomes, and higher in-hospital mortality, in a cohort of patients with COVID-19 in the Bronx, New York. *Metabolism* **2020**, *108*, 154262. [CrossRef]
7. Available online: https://www.who.int (accessed on 1 June 2021).
8. Bertolini, A.; Van De Peppel, I.P.; Bodewes, F.A.; Moshage, H.; Fantin, A.; Farinati, F.; Fiorotto, R.; Jonker, J.W.; Strazzabosco, M.; Verkade, H.J.; et al. Abnormal Liver Function Tests in Patients with COVID-19: Relevance and Potential Pathogenesis. *Hepatology* **2020**, *72*, 1864–1872. [CrossRef]
9. Polack, F.P.; Thomas, S.J.; Kitchin, N.; Absalon, J.; Gurtman, A.; Lockhart, S.; Perez, J.L.; Marc, G.P.; Moreira, E.D.; Zerbini, C.; et al. Safety and Efficacy of the BNT162b2 mRNA Covid-19 Vaccine. *N. Engl. J. Med.* **2020**, *383*, 2603–2615. [CrossRef]
10. Sadoff, J.; Le Gars, M.; Shukarev, G.; Heerwegh, D.; Truyers, C.; de Groot, A.M.; Stoop, J.; Tete, S.; Van Damme, W.; Leroux-Roels, I.; et al. Interim Results of a Phase 1–2a Trial of Ad26.COV2.S Covid-19 Vaccine. *N. Engl. J. Med.* **2021**, *384*, 1824–1835. [CrossRef]
11. Shamseer, L.; Moher, D.; Clarke, M.; Ghersi, D.; Liberati, A.; Petticrew, M.; Shekelle, P.; Stewart, L.A.; the PRISMA-P Group. Preferred reporting items for systematic review and meta-analysis protocols (PRISMA-P) 2015: Elaboration and explanation. *BMJ* **2015**, *349*, g7647. [CrossRef]
12. Alconchel, F.; Cascales-Campos, P.A.; Pons, J.A.; Martínez, M.; Valiente-Campos, J.; Gajownik, U.; Ortiz, M.L.; Martínez-Alarcón, L.; Parrilla, P.; Robles, R.; et al. Severe COVID-19 after liver transplantation, surviving the pitfalls of learning on-the-go: Three case reports. *World J. Hepatol.* **2020**, *12*, 870–879. [CrossRef] [PubMed]
13. Becchetti, C.; Zambelli, M.F.; Pasulo, L.; Donato, M.F.; Invernizzi, F.; Detry, O.; Dahlqvist, G.; Ciccarelli, O.; Morelli, M.C.; Fraga, M.; et al. COVID-19 in an international European liver transplant recipient cohort. *Gut* **2020**, *69*, 1832–1840. [CrossRef]
14. Belli, L.S.; Fondevila, C.; Cortesi, P.A.; Conti, S.; Karam, V.; Adam, R.; Coilly, A.; Ericzon, B.G.; Loinaz, C.; Cuervas-Mons, V.; et al. Protective Role of Tacrolimus, Deleterious Role of Age and Comorbidities in Liver Transplant Recipients with Covid-19: Results From the ELITA/ELTR Multi-center European Study. *Gastroenterology* **2021**, *160*, 1151–1163.e3. [CrossRef] [PubMed]
15. Bösch, F.; Börner, N.; Kemmner, S.; Lampert, C.; Jacob, S.; Koliogiannis, D.; Stangl, M.; Michel, S.; Kneidinger, N.; Schneider, C.; et al. Attenuated early inflammatory response in solid organ recipients with COVID-19. *Clin. Transplant.* **2020**, *34*, e14027. [CrossRef]
16. Choudhury, A.; Reddy, G.S.; Venishetty, S.; Pamecha, V.; Shasthry, S.M.; Tomar, A.; Mitra, L.G.; Prasad, V.S.T.; Mathur, R.P.; Bhattacharya, D.; et al. COVID-19 in Liver Transplant Recipients—A Series with Successful Recovery. *J. Clin. Transl. Hepatol.* **2020**, *8*, 1–7. [CrossRef] [PubMed]
17. Colmenero, J.; Rodríguez-Perálvarez, M.; Salcedo, M.; Arias-Milla, A.; Muñoz-Serrano, A.; Graus, J.; Nuño, J.; Gastaca, M.; Bustamante-Schneider, J.; Cachero, A.; et al. Epidemiological pattern, incidence, and outcomes of COVID-19 in liver transplant patients. *J. Hepatol.* **2021**, *74*, 148–155. [CrossRef]
18. Dale, M.; Sogawa, H.; Seyedsaadat, S.M.; Wolf, D.C.; Bodin, R.; Partiula, B.; Nog, R.; Latifi, R.; John, D.; Veillette, G.; et al. Successful Management of COVID-19 Infection in 2 Early Post-Liver Transplant Recipients. *Transplant. Proc.* **2021**, *53*, 1175–1179. [CrossRef]
19. Dhampalwar, S.; Saigal, S.; Choudhary, N.; Saraf, N.; Bhangui, P.; Rastogi, A.; Thiagrajan, S.; Soin, A.S. Outcomes of Coronavirus Disease 2019 in Living Donor Liver Transplant Recipients. *Liver Transplant.* **2020**, *26*, 1665–1666. [CrossRef]
20. Eslami, P.; Moradi, M.; Moghadam, A.D.; Pirsalehi, A.; Lateef, S.A.; Hadaegh, A.; Rezai, B.; Sadeghi, A.; Aghdaei, H.A.; Zali, M.R. Lethal outcome of Covid-19 pneumonia in a new liver recipient with neurological manifestation. *Gastroenterol. Hepatol. Bed Bench* **2020**, *13*, 405–409. Available online: http://www.ncbi.nlm.nih.gov/pubmed/33244386 (accessed on 1 May 2021).

21. Felldin, M.; Søfteland, J.M.; Magnusson, J.; Ekberg, J.; Karason, K.; Schult, A.; Larsson, H.; Oltean, M.; Friman, V. Initial Report From a Swedish High-volume Transplant Center After the First Wave of the COVID-19 Pandemic. *Transplantation* **2021**, *105*, 108–114. [CrossRef]
22. Fung, M.; Chiu, C.Y.; DeVoe, C.; Doernberg, S.B.; Schwartz, B.S.; Langelier, C.; Henrich, T.J.; Yokoe, D.; Davis, J.; Hays, S.R.; et al. Clinical outcomes and serologic response in solid organ transplant recipients with COVID-19: A case series from the United States. *Arab. Archaeol. Epigr.* **2020**, *20*, 3225–3233. [CrossRef]
23. Hadi, Y.B.; Naqvi, S.F.; Kupec, J.T.; Sofka, S.; Sarwari, A. Outcomes of Coronavirus Infectious Disease -19 (COVID-19) in Solid Organ Transplant Recipients: A Propensity-matched Analysis of a Large Research Network. *Transplantation* **2021**, *105*, 1365–1371. [CrossRef]
24. Hann, A.J.; Lembach, H.; McKay, S.C.; Perrin, M.; Isaac, J.; Oo, Y.H.; Mutimer, D.; Mirza, D.F.; Hartog, H.; Perera, T. Controversies regarding shielding and susceptibility to COVID-19 disease in liver transplant recipients in the United Kingdom. *Transpl. Infect. Dis.* **2020**, *22*, 13352. [CrossRef]
25. Hatami, B.; Moghadam, P.K.; Zali, M. Presentation of COVID-19 in a liver transplant recipient. *Gastroenterol. Hepatol. Bed Bench* **2020**, *13*, 396–399. Available online: http://www.ncbi.nlm.nih.gov/pubmed/33244384 (accessed on 1 May 2021). [PubMed]
26. Hayashi, K.; Ito, Y.; Yamane, R.; Yoshizaki, M.; Matsushita, K.; Kajikawa, G.; Kozawa, T.; Mizutani, T.; Shimizu, Y.; Nagano, K.; et al. The case of a liver-transplant recipient with severe acute respiratory syndrome coronavirus 2 infection who had a favorable outcome. *Clin. J. Gastroenterol.* **2021**, *14*, 842–845. [CrossRef] [PubMed]
27. Huang, J.; Zheng, K.I.; George, J.; Gao, H.; Wei, R.; Yan, H.; Zheng, M. Fatal outcome in a liver transplant recipient with COVID-19. *Arab. Archaeol. Epigr.* **2020**, *20*, 1907–1910. [CrossRef] [PubMed]
28. Jamir, I.; Lohia, P.; Pande, R.K.; Setia, R.; Singhal, A.K.; Chaudhary, A.A. Convalescent plasma therapy and remdesivir duo successfully salvaged an early liver transplant recipient with severe COVID-19 pneumonia. *Ann. Hepato-Biliary-Pancreat. Surg.* **2020**, *24*, 526–532. [CrossRef]
29. Kates, O.S.; Fisher, C.E.; Stankiewicz-Karita, H.C.; Shepherd, A.K.; Church, E.C.; Kapnadak, S.G.; Lease, E.D.; Riedo, F.X.; Rakita, R.M.; Limaye, A.P. Earliest cases of coronavirus disease 2019 (COVID-19) identified in solid organ transplant recipients in the United States. *Arab. Archaeol. Epigr.* **2020**, *20*, 1885–1890. [CrossRef]
30. Kolonko, A.; Dudzicz, S.; Wiecek, A.; Król, R. COVID-19 infection in solid organ transplant recipients: A single-center experience with patients immediately after transplantation. *Transpl. Infect. Dis.* **2021**, *23*, e13381. [CrossRef] [PubMed]
31. Liu, B.; Wang, Y.; Zhao, Y.; Shi, H.; Zeng, F.; Chen, Z. Successful treatment of severe COVID-19 pneumonia in a liver transplant recipient. *Arab. Archaeol. Epigr.* **2020**, *20*, 1891–1895. [CrossRef]
32. Mansoor, E.; Perez, A.; Abou-Saleh, M.; Sclair, S.N.; Cohen, S.; Cooper, G.S.; Mills, A.; Schlick, K.; Khan, A. Clinical Characteristics, Hospitalization, and Mortality Rates of Coronavirus Disease 2019 Among Liver Transplant Patients in the United States: A Multicenter Research Network Study. *Gastroenterology* **2021**, *160*, 459–462.e1. [CrossRef] [PubMed]
33. Mathiasen, V.D.; Oversoe, S.K.; Ott, P.; Jensen-Fangel, S.; Leth, S. Recovery of Moderate Coronavirus Disease 2019 in a Liver Transplant Recipient on Continued Immunosuppression: A Case Report. *Transplant. Proc.* **2020**, *52*, 2703–2706. [CrossRef]
34. Mehta, S.A.; Rana, M.M.; Motter, J.D.; Small, C.B.; Pereira, M.R.; Stosor, V.; Elias, N.; Haydel, B.; Florman, S.; Odim, J.; et al. Incidence and Outcomes of COVID-19 in Kidney and Liver Transplant Recipients With HIV: Report from the National HOPE in Action Consortium. *Transplantation* **2021**, *105*, 216–224. [CrossRef]
35. Modi, A.R.; Koval, C.E.; Taege, A.J.; Esfeh, J.M.; Eghtesad, B.; Menon, K.N.; Quintini, C.; Miller, C. Coronavirus disease 2019 in an orthotopic liver transplant recipient living with human immunodeficiency virus. *Transpl. Infect. Dis.* **2020**, *22*, e13351. [CrossRef] [PubMed]
36. Niknam, R.; Malek-Hosseini, S.A.; Hashemieh, S.S.; Dehghani, M. COVID-19 in Liver Transplant Patients: Report of 2 Cases and Review of the Literature. *Int. Med Case Rep. J.* **2020**, *13*, 317–321. [CrossRef]
37. Nikoupour, H.; Arasteh, P.; Gholami, S.; Nikeghbalian, S. Liver transplantation and COVID-19: A case report and cross comparison between two identical twins with COVID-19. *BMC Surg.* **2020**, *20*, 1–3. [CrossRef]
38. Prieto, M.; Gastaca, M.; Ruiz, P.; Ventoso, A.; Palomares, I.; Íguez-Álvarez, R.J.R.; Salvador, P.; Bustamante, J.; Valdivieso, A.A. A case of COVID-19 immediately after liver transplantation: Not only bad news. *Ann. Hepato-Biliary-Pancreat. Surg.* **2020**, *24*, 314–318. [CrossRef] [PubMed]
39. Qin, J.; Wang, H.; Qin, X.; Zhang, P.; Zhu, L.; Cai, J.; Yuan, Y.; Li, H. Perioperative Presentation of COVID-19 Disease in a Liver Transplant Recipient. *Hepatology* **2020**, *72*, 1491–1493. [CrossRef] [PubMed]
40. Rabiee, A.; Sadowski, B.; Adeniji, N.; Perumalswami, P.V.; Nguyen, V.; Moghe, A.; Latt, N.L.; Kumar, S.; Aloman, C.; Catana, A.M.; et al. Liver Injury in Liver Transplant Recipients with Coronavirus Disease 2019 (COVID-19): U.S. Multicenter Experience. *Hepatology* **2020**, *72*, 1900–1911. [CrossRef]
41. Rauber, C.; Tiwari-Heckler, S.; Pfeiffenberger, J.; Mehrabi, A.; Lund, F.; Gath, P.; Mieth, M.; Merle, U.; Rupp, C. SARS-CoV-2 Seroprevalence and Clinical Features of COVID-19 in a German Liver Transplant Recipient Cohort: A Prospective Serosurvey Study. *Transplant. Proc.* **2021**, *53*, 1112–1117. [CrossRef] [PubMed]
42. Sessa, A.; Mazzola, A.; Lim, C.; Atif, M.; Pappatella, J.; Pourcher, V.; Scatton, O.; Conti, F. COVID-19 in a liver transplant recipient: Could iatrogenic immunosuppression have prevented severe pneumonia? A case report. *World J. Gastroenterol.* **2020**, *26*, 7076–7084. [CrossRef]

43. Terrabuio, D.R.B.; Haddad, L.; Ducatti, L.; Gouveia, L.; Rocha-Santos, V.; Ferreira, R.M.T.; Darce, G.F.; Cardoso, A.J.A.; Carrilho, F.J.; Andraus, W.; et al. Insights in the approach of long-term liver transplant recipients with COVID-19. *Transpl. Infect. Dis.* **2021**, *23*, e13424. [CrossRef] [PubMed]

44. Waisberg, D.R.; Abdala, E.; Nacif, L.S.; Haddad, L.B.; Ducatti, L.; Santos, V.R.; Gouveia, L.N.; Lazari, C.S.; Martino, R.B.; Pinheiro, R.S.; et al. Liver transplant recipients infected with SARS-CoV-2 in the early postoperative period: Lessons from a single center in the epicenter of the pandemic. *Transpl. Infect. Dis.* **2020**, e13418. [CrossRef]

45. Webb, G.J.; Marjot, T.; Cook, J.A.; Aloman, C.; Armstrong, M.J.; Brenner, E.J.; Catana, M.-A.; Cargill, T.; Dhanasekaran, R.; García-Juárez, I.; et al. Outcomes following SARS-CoV-2 infection in liver transplant recipients: An international registry study. *Lancet Gastroenterol. Hepatol.* **2020**, *5*, 1008–1016. [CrossRef]

46. Wei, L.; Liu, B.; Zhao, Y.; Chen, Z. Prolonged shedding of SARS-CoV-2 in an elderly liver transplant patient infected by COVID-19: A case report. *Ann. Palliat. Med.* **2021**, *10*, 7003–7007. [CrossRef] [PubMed]

47. Rodriguez-Peralvarez, M.; Salcedo, M.; Colmenero, J.; Pons, J.A. Modulating immunosuppression in liver transplant patients with COVID-19. *Gut* **2021**, *70*, 1412–1414. [CrossRef] [PubMed]

48. Caballero-Marcos, A.; Salcedo, M.; Alonso-Fernández, R.; Rodríguez-Perálvarez, M.; Olmedo, M.; Morales, J.G.; Cuervas-Mons, V.; Cachero, A.; Loinaz-Segurola, C.; Iñarrairaegui, M.; et al. Changes in humoral immune response after SARS-CoV-2 infection in liver transplant recipients compared to immunocompetent patients. *Arab. Archaeol. Epigr.* **2021**, *21*, 2876–2884. [CrossRef]

49. Favà, A.; Donadeu, L.; Sabé, N.; Pernin, V.; González-Costello, J.; Lladó, L.; Meneghini, M.; Charmetant, X.; García-Romero, E.; Cachero, A.; et al. SARS-CoV-2-specific serological and functional T cell immune responses during acute and early COVID-19 convalescence in solid organ transplant patients. *Arab. Archaeol. Epigr.* **2021**, *21*, 2749–2761. [CrossRef]

50. Zilla, M.L.; Keetch, C.; Mitchell, G.; McBreen, J.; Shurin, M.R.; E Wheeler, S. SARS-CoV-2 Serologic Immune Response in Exogenously Immunosuppressed Patients. *J. Appl. Lab. Med.* **2021**, *6*, 486–490. [CrossRef]

51. Burack, D.; Pereira, M.R.; Tsapepas, D.S.; Harren, P.; Farr, M.A.; Arcasoy, S.; Cohen, D.J.; Mohan, S.; Emond, J.C.; Hod, E.A.; et al. Prevalence and predictors of SARS-CoV-2 antibodies among solid organ transplant recipients with confirmed infection. *Arab. Archaeol. Epigr.* **2021**, *21*, 2254–2261. [CrossRef]

52. Mazzola, A.; Todesco, E.; Drouin, S.; Hazan, F.; Marot, S.; Thabut, D.; Varnous, S.; Soulié, C.; Barrou, B.; Marcelin, A.-G.; et al. Poor Antibody Response After Two Doses of Severe Acute Respiratory Syndrome Coronavirus 2 (SARS-CoV-2) Vaccine in Transplant Recipients. *Clin. Infect. Dis.* **2021**. [CrossRef]

53. Rabinowich, L.; Grupper, A.; Baruch, R.; Ben-Yehoyada, M.; Halperin, T.; Turner, D.; Katchman, E.; Levi, S.; Houri, I.; Lubezky, N.; et al. Low immunogenicity to SARS-CoV-2 vaccination among liver transplant recipients. *J. Hepatol.* **2021**, *75*, 435–438. [CrossRef] [PubMed]

54. Boyarsky, B.J.; Werbel, W.A.; Avery, R.K.; Tobian, A.A.R.; Massie, A.B.; Segev, D.L.; Garonzik-Wang, J.M. Antibody Response to 2-Dose SARS-CoV-2 mRNA Vaccine Series in Solid Organ Transplant Recipients. *JAMA* **2021**, *325*, 2204–2206. [CrossRef] [PubMed]

55. Miele, M.; Busà, R.; Russelli, G.; Sorrentino, M.C.; Di Bella, M.; Timoneri, F.; Mularoni, A.; Panarello, G.; Vitulo, P.; Conaldi, P.G.; et al. Impaired anti-SARS-CoV-2 humoral and cellular immune response induced by Pfizer-BioNTech BNT162b2 mRNA vaccine in solid organ transplanted patients. *Arab. Archaeol. Epigr.* **2021**, *21*, 2919–2921. [CrossRef]

56. Boyarsky, B.J.; Ou, M.T.; Greenberg, R.S.; Teles, A.T.; Werbel, W.A.; Avery, R.K.; Massie, A.B.; Segev, D.L.; Garonzik-Wang, J.M. Safety of the First Dose of SARS-CoV-2 Vaccination in Solid Organ Transplant Recipients. *Transplantation* **2021**, *105*, e56–e57. [CrossRef] [PubMed]

57. Li, L.-Q.; Huang, T.; Wang, Y.-Q.; Wang, Z.-P.; Liang, Y.; Huang, T.-B.; Zhang, H.-Y.; Sun, W.; Wang, Y. COVID-19 patients' clinical characteristics, discharge rate, and fatality rate of meta-analysis. *J. Med. Virol.* **2020**, *92*, 577–583. [CrossRef] [PubMed]

58. Hussain, A.; Mahawar, K.; Xia, Z.; Yang, W.; El-Hasani, S. RETRACTED: Obesity and mortality of COVID-19. Meta-analysis. *Obes. Res. Clin. Pract.* **2020**, *14*, 295–300. [CrossRef]

59. Kumar, A.; Arora, A.; Sharma, P.; Anikhindi, S.A.; Bansal, N.; Singla, V.; Khare, S.; Srivastava, A. Is diabetes mellitus associated with mortality and severity of COVID-19? A meta-analysis. *Diabetes Metab. Syndr. Clin. Res. Rev.* **2020**, *14*, 535–545. [CrossRef]

60. Li, X.; Xu, S.; Yu, M.; Wang, K.; Tao, Y.; Zhou, Y.; Shi, J.; Zhou, M.; Wu, B.; Yang, Z.; et al. Risk factors for severity and mortality in adult COVID-19 inpatients in Wuhan. *J. Allergy Clin. Immunol.* **2020**, *146*, 110–118. [CrossRef] [PubMed]

61. Watt, K.D.; Charlton, M.R. Metabolic syndrome and liver transplantation: A review and guide to management. *J. Hepatol.* **2010**, *53*, 199–206. [CrossRef]

62. Becchetti, C.; Dirchwolf, M.; Banz, V.; Dufour, J.-F. Medical management of metabolic and cardiovascular complications after liver transplantation. *World J. Gastroenterol.* **2020**, *26*, 2138–2154. [CrossRef]

63. Tian, Y.; Rong, L.; Nian, W.; He, Y. Review article: Gastrointestinal features in COVID-19 and the possibility of faecal transmission. *Aliment. Pharmacol. Ther.* **2020**, *51*, 843–851. [CrossRef]

64. Mao, R.; Qiu, Y.; He, J.-S.; Tan, J.-Y.; Li, X.-H.; Liang, J.; Shen, J.; Zhu, L.-R.; Chen, Y.; Iacucci, M.; et al. Manifestations and prognosis of gastrointestinal and liver involvement in patients with COVID-19: A systematic review and meta-analysis. *Lancet Gastroenterol. Hepatol.* **2020**, *5*, 667–678. [CrossRef]

65. Zhang, H.; Kang, Z.; Gong, H.; Xu, D.; Wang, J.; Li, Z.; Li, Z.; Cui, X.; Xiao, J.; Zhan, J.; et al. Digestive system is a potential route of COVID-19: An analysis of single-cell coexpression pattern of key proteins in viral entry process. *Gut* **2020**, *69*, 1010–1018. [CrossRef]

66. Xiao, F.; Tang, M.; Zheng, X.; Liu, Y.; Li, X.; Shan, H. Evidence for Gastrointestinal Infection of SARS-CoV-2. *Gastroenterology* **2020**, *158*, 1831–1833.e3. [CrossRef]
67. Perisetti, A.; Goyal, H.; Gajendran, M.; Boregowda, U.; Mann, R.; Sharma, N. Prevalence, Mechanisms, and Implications of Gastrointestinal Symptoms in COVID-19. *Front. Med.* **2020**, *7*, 588711. [CrossRef] [PubMed]
68. Bajaj, J.S.; Kakiyama, G.; Cox, I.J.; Nittono, H.; Takei, H.; White, M.; Fagan, A.; Gavis, E.A.; Heuman, D.M.; Gilles, H.C.; et al. Alterations in gut microbial function following liver transplant. *Liver Transplant.* **2018**, *24*, 752–761. [CrossRef]
69. Sun, L.; Yang, Y.-S.; Qu, W.; Zhu, Z.-J.; Wei, L.; Ye, Z.-S.; Zhang, J.-R.; Sun, X.-Y.; Zeng, Z.-G. Gut microbiota of liver transplantation recipients. *Sci. Rep.* **2017**, *7*, 3762. [CrossRef]
70. Jiang, J.-W.; Ren, Z.-G.; Lu, H.-F.; Zhang, H.; Li, A.; Cui, G.-Y.; Jia, J.-J.; Xie, H.-Y.; Chen, X.-H.; He, Y.; et al. Optimal immunosuppressor induces stable gut microbiota after liver transplantation. *World J. Gastroenterol.* **2018**, *24*, 3871–3883. [CrossRef] [PubMed]
71. Pan, L.; Mu, M.; Yang, P.; Sun, Y.; Wang, R.; Yan, J.; Li, P.; Hu, B.; Wang, J.; Hu, C.; et al. Clinical Characteristics of COVID-19 Patients With Digestive Symptoms in Hubei, China: A Descriptive, Cross-Sectional, Multicenter Study. *Am. J. Gastroenterol.* **2020**, *115*, 766–773. [CrossRef]
72. Livanos, A.E.; Jha, D.; Cossarini, F.; Gonzalez-Reiche, A.S.; Tokuyama, M.; Aydillo, T.; Parigi, T.L.; Ladinsky, M.S.; Ramos, I.; Dunleavy, K.; et al. Intestinal Host Response to SARS-CoV-2 Infection and COVID-19 Outcomes in Patients with Gastrointestinal Symptoms. *Gastroenterology* **2021**, *160*, 2435–2450.e34. [CrossRef]
73. Krantz, S.G.; Rao, A.S.S. Level of underreporting including underdiagnosis before the first peak of COVID-19 in various countries: Preliminary retrospective results based on wavelets and deterministic modeling. *Infect. Control. Hosp. Epidemiol.* **2020**, *41*, 857–859. [CrossRef]
74. Fix, O.K.; Hameed, B.; Fontana, R.J.; Kwok, R.M.; McGuire, B.M.; Mulligan, D.C.; Pratt, D.S.; Russo, M.W.; Schilsky, M.L.; Verna, E.C.; et al. Clinical Best Practice Advice for Hepatology and Liver Transplant Providers during the COVID-19 Pandemic: AASLD Expert Panel Consensus Statement. *Hepatology* **2020**, *72*, 287–304. [CrossRef]
75. Russell, B.; Moss, C.; George, G.; Santaolalla, A.; Cope, A.; Papa, S.; Van Hemelrijck, M. Associations between immune-suppressive and stimulating drugs and novel COVID-19—A systematic review of current evidence. *Ecancermedicalscience* **2020**, *14*, 1022. [CrossRef] [PubMed]
76. Allison, A.C.; Eugui, E.M. Mycophenolate mofetil and its mechanisms of action. *Immunopharmacology* **2000**, *47*, 85–118. [CrossRef]
77. Wang, F.; Nie, J.; Wang, H.; Zhao, Q.; Xiong, Y.; Deng, L.; Song, S.; Ma, Z.; Mo, P.; Zhang, Y. Characteristics of Peripheral Lymphocyte Subset Alteration in COVID-19 Pneumonia. *J. Infect. Dis.* **2020**, *221*, 1762–1769. [CrossRef] [PubMed]
78. Ma-Lauer, Y.; Zheng, Y.; Malesevic, M.; Von Brunn, B.; Fischer, G.; Von Brunn, A. Influences of cyclosporin A and non-immunosuppressive derivatives on cellular cyclophilins and viral nucleocapsid protein during human coronavirus 229E replication. *Antivir. Res.* **2020**, *173*, 104620. [CrossRef] [PubMed]
79. Willicombe, M.; Thomas, D.; McAdoo, S. COVID-19 and Calcineurin Inhibitors: Should They Get Left Out in the Storm? *J. Am. Soc. Nephrol.* **2020**, *31*, 1145–1146. [CrossRef] [PubMed]
80. Galipeau, Y.; Greig, M.; Liu, G.; Driedger, M.; Langlois, M.-A. Humoral Responses and Serological Assays in SARS-CoV-2 Infections. *Front. Immunol.* **2020**, *11*, 610688. [CrossRef]
81. Natori, Y.; Shiotsuka, M.; Slomovic, J.; Hoschler, K.; Ferreira, V.; Ashton, P.; Rotstein, C.; Lilly, L.; Schiff, J.; Singer, L.; et al. A Double-Blind, Randomized Trial of High-Dose vs Standard-Dose Influenza Vaccine in Adult Solid-Organ Transplant Recipients. *Clin. Infect. Dis.* **2017**, *66*, 1698–1704. [CrossRef] [PubMed]
82. Kamar, N.; Abravanel, F.; Marion, O.; Couat, C.; Izopet, J.; Del Bello, A. Three Doses of an mRNA Covid-19 Vaccine in Solid-Organ Transplant Recipients. *N. Engl. J. Med.* **2021**, *385*, 661–662. [CrossRef] [PubMed]

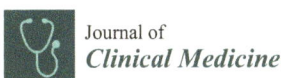

Journal of
Clinical Medicine

Review

New Indications for Liver Transplantation

Alberto Zanetto, Sarah Shalaby, Martina Gambato, Giacomo Germani, Marco Senzolo, Debora Bizzaro , Francesco Paolo Russo and Patrizia Burra *

Multivisceral Transplant Unit, Department of Surgery Oncology and Gastroenterology, University of Padova, Via Giustiniani 2, 35128 Padova, Italy; alberto.zanetto@yahoo.it (A.Z.); sarahshalaby18@gmail.com (S.S.); martina.gambato@gmail.com (M.G.); germani.giacomo@gmail.com (G.G.); marcosenzolo@hotmail.com (M.S.); debora.bizzaro@gmail.com (D.B.); francescopaolo.russo@unipd.it (F.P.R.)
* Correspondence: burra@unipd.it

Abstract: Liver transplantation (LT) is an important therapeutic option for the treatment of several liver diseases. Modern LT is characterized by remarkable improvements in post-transplant patient survival, graft survival, and quality of life. Thanks to these great improvements, indications for LT are expanding. Nowadays, clinical conditions historically considered exclusion criteria for LT, have been considered new indications for LT, showing survival advantages for patients. In this review, we provide an updated overview of the principal newer indications for LT, with particular attention to alcoholic hepatitis, acute-on-chronic liver failure (ACLF), cholangiocarcinoma and colorectal cancer metastases.

Keywords: alcoholic hepatitis; acute-on-chronic liver failure; cholangiocarcinoma; colorectal cancer metastases

Citation: Zanetto, A.; Shalaby, S.; Gambato, M.; Germani, G.; Senzolo, M.; Bizzaro, D.; Russo, F.P.; Burra, P. New Indications for Liver Transplantation. *J. Clin. Med.* **2021**, *10*, 3867. https://doi.org/10.3390/jcm10173867

Academic Editors: Pierluigi Toniutto and Hidekazu Suzuki

Received: 30 July 2021
Accepted: 27 August 2021
Published: 28 August 2021

Publisher's Note: MDPI stays neutral with regard to jurisdictional claims in published maps and institutional affiliations.

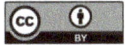
1. Introduction

Since the first procedure performed in 1963, liver transplantation (LT) has become an important therapeutic option for the treatment of inborn metabolic disorders, acute liver failure, end-stage chronic liver disease, and primary hepatic cancers [1].

Over the past several decades LT has continued to grow and evolve with huge improvements in surgical techniques, organ preservation and procurement, and immunosuppression. Therefore, the modern LT is characterized by remarkable improvements in post-transplant patient survival, graft survival, and quality of life. Thanks to these ever-increasing improvements in overall survival, with one-year graft and patient survival nowadays around 90% [2], indications for LT are expanding, also as a result of a better understanding of liver diseases and innovative therapies.

Nowadays, clinical conditions historically considered exclusion criteria for LT, such as severe alcoholic hepatitis (AH), acute-on-chronic liver failure (ACLF), colorectal cancer metastases and cholangiocarcinoma are now considered new indications for LT, showing survival advantages for patients. In this review, we provide an updated overview of these newer indications for LT (Figure 1).

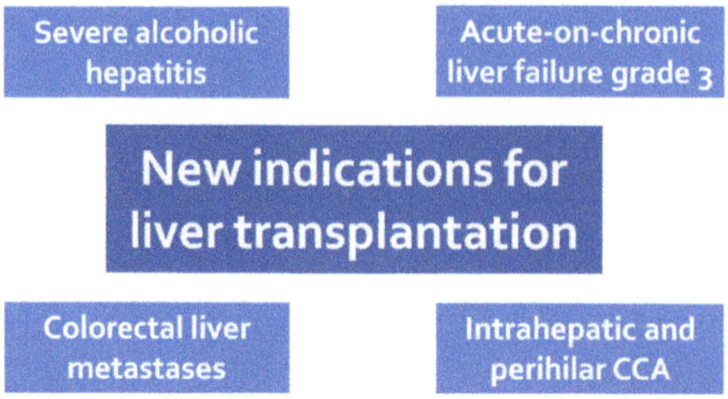

Figure 1. New indications for liver transplantation. *Controversial* indications include severe alcoholic hepatitis and ACLF grade 3. *Questionable* indications include non-hepatocellular carcinoma liver cancer, and liver metastases from colorectal cancer. CCA: cholangiocarcinoma; ACLF: acute-on-chronic liver failure.

2. Alcoholic Hepatitis

Worldwide, alcohol-related liver disease (ALD) is one of the most prevalent liver diseases and the second most frequent indication for LT [3], representing around 30% of all primary LT procedures in Europe and approximately 25% in the USA [4,5].

The first cornerstone in the treatment of patients with ALD is abstinence from alcohol. An adequate time of abstinence may decrease hepatic fibrosis, reduce the risk of progression to cirrhosis, improve the prognosis of cirrhotic patients and reduce the mortality [6–8]. Abstinence is important, but usually it cannot reverse advanced ALD and in many cases the only definitive treatment for ALD is LT. Despite the fact post-LT outcomes and survival rates are analogous with those of other etiologies [4], ALD is still judged a controversial indication for LT. The discussion is generated mainly by the opinion that ALD is a self-inflicted disease, and by the possible risk of harmful effects to the graft after alcohol relapse [9]. In the majority of transplant programs, a period of 6-month of abstinence ("six-month rule") is a compulsory condition to consider a patient eligible for LT. This rule has a double scope: first, to avoid LT in those patients in whom liver function and general clinical status will improve after alcohol removal, second to identify patients at higher risk of relapse after LT.

Nevertheless, the role of the pre-LT extent of abstinence as a predictor of alcohol relapse post-LT has not been clearly confirmed and the enforceability of this rule is still controversial [10]. Indeed, in a systematic review including 22 studies, in only two of them the six months of alcohol abstinence was predictive of post-LT relapse [11]. Furthermore, the ideal period of abstinence pre-LT is still controversial, although there are data confirming that a shorter prelisting abstinence period is associated with a faster post-LT relapse [12].

In recent years, an alarming increase in incidence of hospitalization for AH and mortality rates has been observed both in the US [13] and in Europe [14]. AH presents with fatigue, anorexia, nausea, jaundice, mild-to-moderate increase of transaminases, hyperbilirubinemia, hypoalbuminemia, elevation of neutrophils and prothrombin time (PT) prolongation [3]. The most used validated prognostic scoring system is the Maddrey Discriminant Function (MDF). Usually AH is defined by a MDF >32 [15]. The role of pharmacological treatments, especially corticosteroids, in patients with AH is still debated, with studies demonstrating efficacy in improving survival [16–18] and others showing a negligible effect on reducing mortality [19,20]. In patients not responding to medical therapy the prognosis is very poor, with a 6-month mortality rate of 75%.

In accordance with the "six-month rule", AH patients are ineligible for LT at most transplant centers. Nonetheless, there is growing evidence that, in selected patients after the first episode of AH not responding to medical therapy, LT represents an effective treatment [21,22]. it was demonstrated that the post-LT outcomes are good, with survival rates significantly higher compared to not transplanted patients with AH not responding to steroid therapy [23–25].

Like with ALD cirrhotic LT recipients some ethical and social concerns remain. These are mostly originated by the public opinion that a graft is afforded to patients who were actively consuming alcohol immediately previous to admission on the waiting list, with higher risk of post-LT alcohol relapse. However, the existing data on LT in these patients demonstrate that relapse rates are analogous to those observed in patients with ALD that respected the "6-month rule", if a rigorous and appropriate selection process is applied [23–25].

Multiple arguments for either "tight" or "loose" selection criteria have been proposed for LT in AH [26]. One major argument for tight selection is that current models for predicting survival without LT are not adequately precise for use in an individual patient, which implies not only that some patients will be subjected to LT unnecessarily, but also that others will be denied a potentially lifesaving LT. Additionally, most criteria for listing rely on clinical judgment, which may vary across different centers, thus leading to inequity of access to LT. On the other hand, real-life patients with AH undergoing LT often present with ACLF and a high risk of short-term mortality, thus making unnecessary LT very rare. Furthermore, a careful selection of patients at the first event of liver decompensation has repeatedly yielded excellent outcomes and low risk of relapse [26].

Like other indications for LT, further refinement of selection criteria is expected to evolve gradually over time. However, without the establishment of national and international agreement on criteria for admitting in waiting list and transplanting patients with AH, a high variability persists in terms of admittance to LT for those patients, with disparities that are manifest also at a national level with a potential inequality among patients with the same clinical conditions [27].

Data reporting good outcomes of early LT in selected patients were published in the last years. In the study by Mathurin et al. [23], 26 patients with AH with no response to corticosteroids were subjected to early LT as rescue therapy, after a strict multidisciplinary selection process. Survival after 6 and 24 months post-LT were significantly higher than in matched not transplanted controls (77% vs. 23%). Alcohol relapse was detected up to three years after LT in about 10% of patients.

A US study, published by Im et al. [28] confirmed the good outcomes of early LT in 94 patients with AH, in whom the 6-month survival rate was higher compared with matched not transplanted patients (89% vs. 11%). Alcohol relapse was diagnosed in only one recipient at 180 days after LT. Similarly, in a retrospective study published by Lee et al. [29], cumulative patient survival percentages after LT for AH were 94% and 84% at 1 year and 3 years, respectively After LT, 72% were abstinent, 18% had occasionally relapses, and 11% had sustained alcohol intake.

In Italy, Germani et al. coordinated the first Italian experience in a pilot study on early LT for AH from four different LT centers. Among those centers, the coordinating center is the Multivisceral Transplant Unit of Padua University Hospital. The inclusion criteria were AH, as a first episode of decompensation in chronic liver disease and no responses to medical therapies, but more importantly, the patient should have been socially integrated and have supportive family members, with psychiatric assessment and addiction profile and no comorbidities [30]. Preliminary data coming from Padua Liver Transplant center demonstrated a significantly higher survival rate amongst patients who underwent early LT compared to non-responding patients who were denied early LT.

The Spanish Society of Liver Transplantation has recently published a consensus statement on the potential expansion of indications for LT including patients with a first episode of severe AH not responding to medical therapy [31], whereas no specific guidelines or position statements have been published with this regards in Germany. In UK a pilot program for LT in patients with severe AH was developed. Over a 3-year period 20 patients aged between 18 and 40 years were evaluated, but none underwent LT, mainly due to the extremely stringent criteria for listing and the need for unanimity among members of the transplant panel [27].

The most significant concern in patients actively drinking before admission, is the post-LT risk of relapse. In the already mentioned landmark paper [23], about 10% of patients had a relapse up to three years after LT. This could be important not only from the "single-patient" perspective, but also for the possible negative effects on donation rate. Nevertheless, a recent multicenter survey suggests that organ donation was not negatively influenced by the early LT for AH [32]. Given the complexity of the selection and management of patients with AH, a multidisciplinary approach, involving various stakeholders including transplant hepatologists and transplant surgeons, but also psychiatrists, psychologists, and addiction specialists is becoming compulsory to accurately evaluate LT candidates [33,34]. The SALT prognostic score, developed including four objective pre-LT variables, was proposed in order to foresee the risk of sustained alcohol intake after early LT for AH assisting in the selection of patient candidates for early LT or in advising controls post-LT [35].

The psychosocial assessment of LT candidates and the evaluation of social background, including the presence of an active and effective support by the family, are essential parts of the pre-transplant evaluation process. In fact, the transplant outcome is undoubtedly influenced also by psychosocial and behavioral issues along with the usual medical factors [36]. This concept is even more important in the context of early LT where the psychosocial assessment is essential for the establishment of the real probability of long-term abstinence. Indeed, alcohol abuse is frequently associated with depression, personality disorders and other psychiatric disease, that can affect the post-transplant outcome of these patients [37,38].

To ensure to the LT candidates for AH the best long-term outcomes, globally accepted clinical and psychosocial selection criteria should be identified [39]. Very strict criteria should be explored for the early LT in this setting, as indicated in an Italian position statement [34]. Notably, a transparent and direct interaction between clinicians and society, based on the concept of no "a priori" exclusion to the evaluation for LT in the case of AH is essential.

3. Acute-On-Chronic Liver Failure (ACLF)

ACLF is a clinical syndrome characterized by acute decompensation (AD) of chronic liver disease, development of organ failures and systemic inflammation, and high risk of short-term mortality (>15% at 28 day) [40–43]. Development of ACLF in patients with chronic liver disease results from various precipitating factors that vary according to geographical regions: alcoholic hepatitis and bacterial infections in the West and relapse of chronic HBV infection in the East [44]. In approximately 40–50% of the cases, however, development of ACLF is not associated with identifiable triggers and current hypothesis in these cases is that metabolites from gut bacteria or translocation of DAMPs from leaky gut (or a combination of both) may be involved and trigger inflammation which in turn leads to organ dysfunction/failure [44]. There is no specific treatment for patients with ACLF, and current management include treatment of associated complications/precipitating factors and organ support. In patients with ACLF due to one or more specific factors (i.e., bacterial infections, alcoholic hepatitis, bleeding events, drug-induced liver injury), early identification of trigger factor(s) and specific treatments are important though it's unclear whether this can really prevent worsening of ACLF [40]. All patients with ACLF should be preferably managed in a tertiary care center and by a multidisciplinary team including transplant hepatologists, ICU doctors, and transplant surgeons. General management of patients with ACLF and their complications should follow current guidelines for management of critically ill patients with cirrhosis [45]. Patients should be monitored frequently and evaluated serially for potential transfer to intensive care unit. Each organ dysfunction shall be treated specifically in order to prevent a stage in which multiorgan failure occurs and all treatments eventually become futile [45].

Per current consensus, severity of ACLF is defined by number of organ failures, and is not surprising that patients with three or more organ failures have increased risk of mortality compared with those with one or two organ failures. Specifically, patients with ≥3 organ failures have grade 3 ACLF (ACLF 3), and 28-day mortality in these patients approaches 80% [40]. Given such a high risk of death and the lack of alternative medical treatments, LT may be the only viable option in certain patients with ACLF [46,47]. Yet, selection of patients suitable for LT, prioritization of candidates during wait-list time, and best timing for LT in ACLF remain problematic [48]. Here, we discuss the current knowledge and the main open issues regarding LT in patients with ACLF, particularly those with ACLF 3.

3.1. Wait-List Priority in Patients with ACLF Awaiting LT: Beyond MELD-Based Allocation

ACLF is a rapidly progressive syndrome with a variable course [49,50]. On the one hand, it is important to identify patients with potential for full recovery, in whom LT would be unnecessary and not beneficial; on the other, one has to identify those at higher risk for progression, in whom development of either sepsis or irreversible organ failures can compromise eligibility for LT and post-transplant outcomes [41]. In these patients, the therapeutic window for LT is significantly narrow and unexpected clinical deterioration may determine removal of candidates from the waiting list [51].

Unfortunately, the discrimination between these groups remains unclear. The Model for End-Stage Liver Disease (MELD) score, that is used to estimate wait-list mortality and guide organ allocation in patients with cirrhosis awaiting LT, is not appropriate to predict survival in candidates with ACLF [52]. In fact, MELD does not reflect severity of hepatic encephalopathy and respiratory/circulatory failures, which are major drivers of mortality in ACLF [40–42]. Also, it does not include biomarkers of systemic inflammation, such as white blood cells and levels of C reactive protein, which reflect severity of ACLF and correlate with survival [53].

In a retrospective analysis based on the United Network for Organ Sharing (UNOS) database and including approximately 100,000 patients, Sundaram and coworkers demonstrated that the risk of death in ACLF 3 was 44% even if their MELD score was <25, and was greater than that in advanced patients as defined by a MELD >35 but without ACLF [53]. In an independent cohort including 71,894 veterans with decompensated cirrhosis, Hernaez et al. found that in those with ACLF the probability of 90-day mortality was significantly higher than the one predicted by MELD-Na alone [54]. In a third, large retrospective analysis including patients from the UNOS registry between 2002 and 2014, those with ACLF 3 (n = 5099) had a significantly higher risk of death at 14 days than those listed for acute liver failure (n = 3377), regardless of MELD-Na [55]. Taken together, these studies indicate that in ACLF patients, particularly grade 3 ACLF, an early discussion about LT should be initiated independent of their MELD status.

Whether a combination of MELD score and grade of ACLF could be the optimal strategy to assess wait-list priority in patients with ACLF has not yet been thoroughly investigated. To this end, in a large, retrospective study including 18,416 candidates with ACLF from UNOS registry, Abdallah showed that the severity of ACLF and MELD score interacted synergistically in anticipating the risk of mortality at 90-day, and that the effect of ACLF grade was relatively more relevant at lower (i.e., ≤25) levels of MELD [56]. A new prognostic tool integrating MELD score and grade of ACLF was therefore proposed to mitigate disparities regarding organ allocation in ACLF, particularly for candidates with a MELD score ≤ 25 [56]. If these results will be confirmed in prospective cohorts, it is plausible that a combination of MELD score and ACLF grade will become the next standard to assess priority of candidates with ACLF.

In conclusion, there is a strong need to improve the MELD-based allocation to mitigate wait-list mortality in candidates with ACLF [47,57]. Innovative scores are supposed to capture recipient factors (number and severity of organ failures), global patient's status and performance (sarcopenia and frailty), and chronic associated conditions (comorbidities).

This could lead to a more personalized approach regarding management of wait-list priority in ACLF and would ultimately improve patient's survival and LT outcomes [58].

3.2. Benefit of Liver Transplantation in Patients with ALCF Grade 3

Patients with ACLF 3 have a 28-day LT-free survival of 20% [40–42]. Considering such a high risk of death, LT is a potentially life-saving treatment for the vast majority of these patients. Preliminary data, however, suggested that post-transplant survival in ACLF 3 might be lower than that in recipients transplanted for decompensated cirrhosis [59]. Hence, the question rose as to which all patients with ACLF, independent of ACLF grade, could be considered for transplantation [57].

Results from other studies, on the other hand, indicated good survival 1-year after LT [53,60–62]. Sundaram et al. retrospectively analyzed the UNOS database for the years 2004–2017 [63]. In total, 56,801 patients received LT and 54.6% had no ACLF, 15.4% had ACLF 1, 15.9% had ACLF 2, and 14.1% had ACLF 3. Interestingly, survival at 1-year post-LT was comparable between patients with ACLF 3 and those with grade 0–2, and that was above 80% in all groups [63]. More interestingly, although patients with ACLF 3 had lower long-term survival compared with those with grade 0–2, 68% of patients who received LT for ACLF 3 were alive 5 years after transplantation, which would justify both the transplant benefit in these patients, set at >50% 5-year after LT [64], and the acceptable utility of donor grafts. Comparable findings were reported by multicenter cohort studies from Europe [49,60,65] and by one recent study from Asia that first evaluated the outcomes of living donor LT for the treatment of ACLF [66]. In this study, including 321 candidates with high MELD score who underwent living donor LT, survival at 5-year was comparable between patients with and without ACLF (72% versus 81.82%), and 1 year-survival in ACLF 3 was comparable with that of grade 1 and 2 (76% vs. 85% vs. 93%; $p = 0.2$) [66]. Taken together, these studies indicate that ACLF grade 3 is not an absolute contraindication for LT, and that satisfactory outcomes can be achieved provided there is a good selection of candidates.

To this end, new methods to improve assessment of LT eligibility in these patients are eagerly awaited, that is to evaluate whether an individual patient has become "too sick to be transplanted" [58,67]. The fact that no patient with ACLF and severe respiratory failure in the CANONIC trial underwent LT indicated that this condition was considered an absolute contraindication for LT in ACLF [49]. Two large multicenter studies from US [53,68] indicated the following factors to be associated with higher risk of death post transplantation: need for mechanical ventilation at transplant, levels of lactate >4 mmol/L before transplantation, pre-transplant white blood cells count within normal limits, older age of recipient, and transplantation of marginal-grafts. The combination of three different organ supports (dialysis, vasoactive drugs, and mechanical ventilation) has been proposed as a potential criterion to withhold LT [51], however it may also prevent transplantation in a significant number of subjects with potentially favourable outcome. In fact, other factors may affect severity of organ failures and therefore the chance to perform a successful LT. This includes indications for organ support (i.e., ventilation for severe respiratory dysfunction vs. grade IV encephalopathy) and intensity (dose of vasoactives) and/or duration (i.e., 2–3 vs. >7 days) of organs support.

Given the increasing number of LTs performed in patients with ACLF worldwide, a better understanding of how to define too-sick-to transplant patients and thereby avoid "futile" transplantations is urgently needed [58]. Not only it is important to confirm whether LT in ACLF 3 confers a significant survival benefit, but also whether is associated with an improved quality of life [69]. For example, pre-transplant acute kidney injury (AKI), that is commonly observed in cirrhosis and ACLF [70–72], is a major predictor of post-LT chronic kidney disease (CKD) and need for replacement therapy [73]. Although the burden of CKD after LT in ACLF 1 may not be substantially increased [74], more specific results regarding patients with ACLF 3 are lacking. Long-term data regarding quality of life after LT for ACLF are awaited and may help to improve selection criteria and management of candidates with ACLF both before and after LT [75,76].

3.3. Timing of LT: The Earlier the Better?

One major challenge in candidates with ACLF is to assess the appropriate timing for LT. Given their high risk of death, one would expect that "as soon as possible" could lead to the greatest transplant benefit. In support of this assumption, in a landmark analysis of UNOS database, Sundaram and Jalan demonstrated that patients with ACLF who received LT within 30 days within listing had higher survival at 1-year than those who were transplanted thereafter (83% vs. 79%, respectively; $p = 0.03$) [53]. The same study demonstrated that LT within 30 days could significantly improve survival in patients who underwent LT on machinal ventilation (77% vs. 72%; $p = 0.03$). Comparable results were described in the CANONIC trial where survival at 6 months in patients with ACLF 2 and 3 who underwent LT within 28 days was 81% compared with 10% in those treated with medical therapy [49].

Yet, other evidence suggested that the benefits of early LT have to be balanced against benefits conferred by resolution of organ failures. In a retrospective trial including 98 candidates with ACLF who received LT, the 37 who had improvement of ACLF grade prior to transplantation had a significantly better survival compared with controls with no improvement [61]. Similar results were reported by Sundaram in a larger study from UNOS data [77]. The authors included 3636 candidates with ACLF 3 who received LT within 28 days of listing. Of these patients, 24.5% recovered to either no ACLF or grade 1 or 2 ACLF, whereas 75.5% remained with ACLF 3 at time of surgery. Interestingly, survival at 1 year was 82% in patients who underwent LT with ACLF 3 and 88% in patients recovering to ACLF 0–2 ($p < 0.001$). Furthermore, the probability of survival of ACLF 0–2 who worsened to ACLF 3 was significantly lower than in patients who remained at ACLF 0–2 (84% vs. 90%; $p < 0.001$). However, <25% of candidates with ACLF 3 at enlisting were able to achieve a lower grade of ACLF [77]. Hence, while in principle it would be optimal to undergo LT upon recovering of organ failures, this appears not doable in the major part of patients with ACLF 3.

In summary, in candidates awaiting LT for ACLF 3, two major variables need to be balanced to assess the best timing for transplantation, that is on one hand the individual patient's risk of progression and death on the waiting list, on the other whether there is any chance to postpone transplantation with the goal of waiting for ALCF to improve prior to LT [43,58].

4. Colorectal Liver Metastases and Liver Transplantation

Colorectal carcinoma (CRC) shows an incidence of about 700 per million population in Western countries and the liver is involved in approximately 70% of patients with colorectal metastases [78]. Currently, the only potentially curative treatment is represented by surgical resection of metastases [79], with a median 5-year survival of 30–40% compared to only 5% in those non-resected [79,80]. Despite the recent advancements in surgical techniques, only ~20% of patients are resectable at diagnosis [81] and the disease often recurs within 3 years of resection [82]. Percutaneous radiological treatments such as ablative treatments (radiofrequency, microwave and cryosurgical ablation, transcatheter intra-arterial therapy), hepatic arterial infusion chemotherapy, transarterial embolization and chemoembolization, and radioembolization with yttrium 90 can be applied to achieve tumor resectability. Even though it has been demonstrated that interventional radiology contributes to the improvement of overall survival rates [83,84], its role in the curative intent is still marginal. Palliative chemotherapy remains the main option for patients non candidable for surgery. Even though the initiation of first-line chemotherapy in selected patients with good performance status, no KRAS or BRAF mutations, and left-sided tumors prolongs median overall survival [85–89], prognosis remains poor and only ~10% of them survive up to 5 years [86,90]. Interestingly, recent clinical trials show an improvement of median survival with modern chemotherapy including the use of bevacizumab/EGFR antibodies, from 6 months to 2 years [85,91,92].

In this context, LT has been explored as an option to remove all viable disease in those patients with disease spread limited to the liver, which are not elegible for resection due to the low remnant liver volume [93,94]. In the past, several attempts were performed obtaining 5-year overall survivals <20% [95]. Due to these poor results and organ shortages, active colorectal liver metastasis remained a contraindication for LT thereafter. Nonetheless, the majority of these patients were disease-free at death, which was due to transplant-related complications instead. A prospective study from Norway a few years ago (the SECA-I study) has renewed focus for this potentially curative option. Patients included in this study had completed surgical resection of the primary tumor, had a good performance status, and received LT after at least 6 weeks of chemotherapy. The estimated 1, 3 and 5-year overall survival after LT were 95%, 68% and 60%, respectively. The median follow-up was 27 months (range 8–60 months) and disease-free survival was 35% at 1 year. The candidates with the best prognosis were those with presence of colorectal liver metastasis at diagnosis, pN0, pretransplant maximal CCR diameter <5.5 cm, levels of carcinoembryonic antigen (CEA) <80 mg/L, response or stable disease on chemotherapy, and >2 years from diagnosis to LT [93]. The 5-year overall survival rate of these patients with favorable prognostic factors was similar to that of patients transplanted for hepatocellular carcinoma (HCC) following the Milan criteria [96,97]. Interestingly overall survival was much longer when compared to disease-free survival. As a matter of facts, most recurrences in CRC patients were slowly-growing lung metastases amenable to treatment, regardless of immunosuppression [98,99], which is not the case for HCC-recurrence after LT. As a reinforcement to these results, LT was demonstrated to produce longer 5-year overall survival rates when compared to chemotherapy in patients non amenable to surgical resection of liver metastastases when data from the SECA-I study were compared to those of the NORDIC VII trial (56% vs. 9%, respectively) [88].

Following the SECA-I study, Toso et al. reported the results of 12 patients with colorectal liver metastases undergoing LT, confirming 1-, 3- and 5-year overall survival rates of 83%, 62%, and 50%, respectively, and disease-free survivals of 56%, 38% and 38% at 1, 3 and 5 years, respectively [94]. The time from diagnosis to LT appeared to have a high impact on survival rates, suggesting a natural selection of those tumors with more favorable characteristics. The authors suggested that a minimum of 12–24 months should be applied as a selection criterion during the evaluation for LT of these patients. In the recently published open label randomized controlled SECA-II trial, the application of more strict selection criteria led to a significant raise of overall survival after LT (1 and 5 years were 100% and 83%, respectively), with a median follow-up of 36 months (range 5–60 months) [100]. As a matter of fact, patients included in the SECA-II study showed better pre-LT prognostic factors and more favorable tumor biology (lower number of metastatic lesions, size of largest liver lesions, CEA levels, and recurrence risk scores) than SECA-I patients. Nevertheless, the burden of the disease was considerable at the time of LT in both cohorts.

Even though patients that were included had different tumoral characteristics and underwent different treatments before LT, it is becoming clear that it represents a valid option for curative intent in the context of colorectal liver metastases, offering the possibility of long-term overall survival to highly-selected patients with extensive disease. Data and experience are still limited, however several clinical trials are coming through (NCT 04161092, NCT 03494946, NCT 04616495, NCT 04874259). The major aim is to refine selection criteria in order to raise overall survival rates close to those of patients undergoing LT as a standard of care. Moreover, one multicentre Italian trial based in Milan (NCT 03803436) is aiming to assess the efficacy of LT compared with a matched cohort of patients included in another trial involving chemotherapy plus anti-EGFR. Among others, another element which needs to be evaluated is the possibility to add adjuvant chemotherapy after LT, considering possible graft toxicity. In this regard, the TRANSMET Trial from France (NCT 02597348) is currently comparing the survival rates between standard of care chemotherapy and LT plus adjuvant chemotherapy [101]. Another major challenge is related to the paucity of liver grafts, challenging the approval of new oncological indications. The recruitment of patients in LT trials is currently limited to a minimum percentage of the total amount of transplants per center, aiming to not impact the waiting time for other waitlisted patients. One of the suggested strategies is the use of marginal grafts, as patients with CRC rarely present at LT with either portal hypetension, end stage liver disease or deterioration of other organs functionality and thus could be more easily matched with these donors [100]. Another alternative to increase the donor pool is represented by the RAPID-protocol, which involves a two-stage hepatectomy followed by LT using a left-lateral split graft and delayed total hepatectomy [102]. Three trials, one in our center (NCT04865471), one in Oslo, Norway (NCT 02215889) and one in Jena, Germany (NCT 03488953) are currently evaluating this option. Additionally, a protocol started in Toronto (Canada), is also evaluating the option of living donor LT in patients with CRC (NCT 02864485).

5. Cholangiocarcinoma and Liver Transplantation

Cholangiocarcinoma (CCA) is one of the most frequent primary liver cancers, second only to HCC. It can be classified in three subtypes: intrahepatic (iCCA), perihilar (pCCA) and distal extrahepatic (eCCA) cholangiocarcinoma. In all three subtypes the current gold standard for treatment is surgical resection [103]. Extensive surgery protocols have been established [104], however radical surgical resection can be achieved in <50% of patients due to insufficient remnant liver and difficulties in vascular reconstructions [104]. However, in many cases, complete surgical resection cannot be achieved [105]. Moreover, CCA frequently presents with local vascular infiltration, and primary sclerosing cholangitis (PSC) associated CCA is often considered as unresectable due to the underlying liver disease and predisposition to skip lesions [106]. Radiological treatments, such as intra-arterial therapies, ablation, radioembolization and brachytherapy (iodine-125 seed implantation) are used as locoregional oncological, palliative, and bridging to surgery in patients with unresectable or recurrent CCA after hepatectomy [107,108], however with no curative potential. Within this frame, [106]. LT has been suggested as a potential curative treatment for those patients presenting with non-resectable pCCA and more recently for patients with "very early" iCCA, since it ideally allows radical resection and eradication underlying PSC when associated. Patients included in clinical trials were free from extrahepatic metastases, vascular or lymphnodes invasion. Even though the initial experiences discouraged many centers to pursue this goal [109], a few groups kept on offering LT to these patients, improving selection criteria and treatment protocols. Eventually some impressive survival data were produced leading to internationally re-evaluate LT as a curative option [109] as a treatment for nonresectable CCA, particularly in those countries suffering from graft shortages.

5.1. Intrahepatic Cholangiocarcinoma (iCCA)

ICCA is a subtype of CCA that arises from the intrahepatic biliary tract, which can be divided into mass-forming, periductal-infiltrating, intraductal, and undefined subtypes, depending on macroscopic growth patterns. The incidence of iCCA has been increasing in the last decades, particularly among cirrhotic patients [110]. Despite surgical advances, long-term outcomes of liver resections remain poor, with a 5-year overall survival of 40% and very high prevalence of postoperative morbidity [111–113]. Additionally, in >50% of patients the disease recurs, typically within 24 months after resection [114]. Even though iCCA is still widely considered a contraindication to LT, there is still a quite high percentage of grafts showing incidental tumors at explant pathology (1–3.3% of all LT) [115,116], as it still represents a diagnostical challenge. Retrospective data from these accidentally transplanted iCCA demonstrated an acceptable 5-year overall- and recurrence free-survivals in cirrhotic patients with "very early" iCCA (<2 cm), [117–119]. This led to reconsider LT as a potentially curative option in this context. Moreover, the 2 cm cut-off has been challenged by De Martin et al. who showed comparable survival rates after LT for iCCA of <2 cm and those of 2.1–3 cm [120]. As a matter of fact, in this study the only independent variable associated with tumoral recurrence was its differentiation, which, when available, reduces the impact of tumor size for prognosis. On the other hand, iCCA features are still often underestimated during pre-LT diagnostic evaluation, leading to higher recurrence rates and worse post-LT survival when compared to HCC [121]. Thus, careful consideration of potential higher aggressiveness of the tumor needs to be born in mind, especially in the context of PSC. Independent predictors of post-LT recurrence and survival include microvascular, perineural or lymphovascular invasion, multifocality, poor differentiation, infiltrative subtype, lack of neo- or adjuvant treatments [120,122]. In the noncirrhotic population, Lunsford et al. recently showed a 50% recurrence-free survival, and 83% 5-year overall survival following LT in six patients with locally advanced, unresectable iCCA [123]. Inclusion criteria were solitary tumor >2 cm or multifocal disease confined to the liver without evidence of macrovascular or lymph node involvement and sustained response to neoadjuvant gemcitabine-based chemotherapy. Neither tumor volume nor multifocality affected the incidence of disease recurrence after LT. This neoadjuvant protocol has also been proven successful in downstaging iCCA to surgical resections, which still remains the gold standard of treatment for iCCA. In this scenario, LT could be kept as an option to those remaining non-resectable despite the neoadjuvant treatment [124]. Validation of these findings in ongoing clinical trials may change the current exclusion of patients with iCCA from transplant programs, and the identification of the best selection criteria could further implement long term results (NCT 04195503, NCT 02878473, NCT04556214). For now, iCCA remains a contraindication for LT outside of clinical trials. Ongoing studies are evaluating the role of mutations in KRAS, fibroblast growth factor receptor and VEGF expression and dysregulated immune checkpoints [124]. Therefore it has been proposed to sequence the whole genome to facilitate the individuation of new therapeutic targets.

5.2. Perihilar Cholangiocarcinoma (pCCA)

PCCA is a subtype of CCA that arises anywhere from the second-order biliary ducts to above the site of cystic duct origin; it can have exophytic (mass-forming) and intraductal growth patterns. PCCA is one of the current challenges for hepatic surgery, which still represents the first-line treatment for this malignancy in case of localized disease [125]. Achievement of curative intent often requires implementation of surgery with neo- or adjuvant chemo and radiotherapies [126,127]. Still <20% of pCCA are amenable of surgery at diagnosis, due to the innate propensity of this tumor for the invasion of the adjacent vessels. For non-resectable patients, chemotherapy offers a minimal extension of survival which, in any case, remains <1 year [128,129], with a progression-free survival of 5 months [130,131]. Additionally, frequently pCCA arises from underlying PSC, which limits the possibility of resection [132]. LT has been considered as it can theoretically maximize resection margins and remove the underlying parenchymal liver disease when present. The first reports in the 1990s gave disappointing 28% 5-year survival and a 51% recurrence rate with LT alone, which withheld transplant centers from accepting this as [132]. LT can theoretically maximize resection margins and cure the underlying parenchymal liver disease. The early experience in the 1990s with LT alone gave disappointing 28% 5-year survival and a 51% recurrence rate for pCCA, which deterred transplant centers from accepting this oncological indication [122]. However, in these studies no selection criteria was imposed, treatment arms did not distinguish between pCCA and iCCA and neo- or adjuvant treatment where not included in the treatment protocols. Therefore, despite these dismal initial results, the University of Nebraska and the Mayo Clinic kept on working on this program until they established a successful multimodality protocol for unresectable pCCA preliminary to LT [133–135]. The so called "Mayo Clinic Protocol" includes external beam radiation, combined with intravenous 5-fluorouracil, followed by intraluminal brachytherapy and oral capecitabine. After this a routine exploratory laparoscopic staging is performed to confirm the absence of extrahepatic disease lymphonodal localizations prior to LT. By adopting this protocol, Heimbach et al. were able to obtain a 5-year survival exceeding 80% after LT in those patients with solitary tumors including nonresectable ones <3 cm in radial diameter not extending below the cystic duct, without evidence of lymph node metastases, and in those pCCA associated to PSC [135]. Similar results were confirmed in 12 large-volume transplant centers in the US, which reported a median 5-years disease-free survival rates of 65% [135]. Similar results were confirmed in 12 large-volume transplant centers in the US, which reported 5-years disease-free survival rates of 65% [136]. During the years it became evident that those patients with early disease had improved outcomes following LT [137–139], and that neoadjuvant chemoradiotherapy followed by LT offered the best outcomes for patients selected following the Mayo Clinic criteria [140–142]. Moreover, Mandel et al. demonstrated that patients selected for LT with these criteria reach a significant better survival compared to those not respecting them (59% versus 21% at 5-years) [143]. Thus, the "Mayo Clinic Protocol" has been gradually adopted, confirming 5-year survival rates of approximately 65–70% across different transplant centers [136,144–146]. These results, similar to those obtained in patients transplanted for HCC, led the United Network for Organ Sharing (UNOS) to allow the assignment of a Model for End-Stage Liver Disease (MELD) score exception to patients with unresectable pCCA or arising in the setting of PSC, for accessing LT [136,147]. However, concerns regarding organ allocation, waiting times, and the intensity of the neoadjuvant protocol have been limiting the spread of this indication in clinical practice. As for now, the guidelines of the European Association for the Study of the Liver recommend LT for pCCA to be limited to centers with clinical research protocols employing strict selection of patients and adjuvant or neoadjuvant therapy [10]. Still several patients drop out from the waiting list due to tumoral progression and its related complications, positive laparoscopy or inability to tolerate chemotherapy prior to LT. As demonstrated by a recent observational study, the estimated 82% 5-year survival rate precipitated to 58% on intention to treat analysis, since 46% of patients initially included did not access LT due to neoplastic progression [148]. The Mayo Clinic group reported that the risk factors for dropout of the LT waiting list due to disease progression were: CA 19.9 ≥500 U/mL, a mass ≥3 cm, malignant brushing or biopsy and a MELD score ≥20. Likewise, predictors of recurrence after LT were elevated CA 19.9, invasion of portal vein and evidence of residual tumor at explant [149]. Furthermore, the time interval between neoadjuvant therapy and LT was found to be inversely proportional to recurrence rates, which in turn correlates with tumor biology [150]. However, waiting time needs to be balanced with more pronounced fibrosis induced by prolonged radiotheraphy, hampering both staging laparoscopy and LT. Living donor LT could theoretically avoid timing issues. However ethical concerns toward living donation need to be considered as well at this stage of evidence. Ongoing and future studies will probably better address these issues and further refine treatment protocols [151]. A group at Washington University are currently recruiting for a prospective study which aims to assess whether highly selected patients still require neoadjuvant chemoradiation (NCT 00301379). Moreover, the use of sirolimus will be explored in a pilot trial (NCT 01888302). The rationale of giving sirolimus with gemcitabine and cisplatin is that it may be useful for patients with high risk of CCA recurrence after LT or either surgery. The results of these and other ongoing trials (NCT01549795, NCT02178280, NCT 04378023, NCT02232932) will be of great interest.

6. Conclusions

The LT scenario is undoubtedly evolving rapidly, with a plethora of new indications that could give hope for a better life for a large number of patients. However, these newer indications increase the pressure in an already difficult context of organ shortage. Strategies are therefore needed to increase the pool of transplantable organs that aim to ensure the balance between new indications and available resources. Moreover, it is mandatory to optimize the patients' selection criteria to guarantee transplant advantages and achieve adequate patient and graft survival. Specialized surgeons, oncologists, hepatologists and radiologists should collaborate in a multi-disciplinary transplant team to ensure

J. Clin. Med. **2021**, *10*, 3867

proper work-up and minimize the risks for these patients. Finally, the new scenario of transplants makes it essential to review and standardize the allocation systems and ethical considerations across countries to ensure the same treatment options for all patients.

Author Contributions: A.Z., S.S., M.G., G.G., M.S., D.B. writing—original draft preparation, F.P.R., P.B. writing—review and editing. All authors have read and agreed to the published version of the manuscript.

Funding: This research received no external funding.

Acknowledgments: The Authors are grateful to the Marina Minnaja Foundation for co-founding the research grant of A.Z., S.S. and D.B.

Conflicts of Interest: The authors declare no conflict of interest.

References

1. Starzl, T.E.; Marchioro, T.L.; Porter, K.A.; Brettschneider, L. Homotransplantation of the liver. *Transplantation* **1967**, *5*, 790–803. [CrossRef]
2. Adam, R.; Karam, V.; Cailliez, V.; Grady, J.G.O.; Mirza, D.; Cherqui, D.; Klempnauer, J.; Salizzoni, M.; Pratschke, J.; Jamieson, N.; et al. 2018 Annual Report of the European Liver Transplant Registry (ELTR)—50-Year Evolution of Liver Transplantation. *Transplant. Int.* **2018**, *31*, 1293–1317. [CrossRef]
3. Mathurin, P.; Bataller, R. Trends in the management and burden of alcoholic liver disease. *J. Hepatol.* **2015**, *62*, S38–S46. [CrossRef]
4. Burra, P.; Senzolo, M.; Adam, R.; Delvart, V.; Karam, V.; Germani, G.; Neuberger, J. Liver transplantation for alcoholic liver disease in Europe: A study from the ELTR (European Liver Transplant Registry). *Am. J. Transplant.* **2010**, *10*, 138–148. [CrossRef] [PubMed]
5. Singal, A.K.; Guturu, P.; Hmoud, B.; Kuo, Y.F.; Salameh, H.; Wiesner, R.H. Evolving frequency and outcomes of liver transplantation based on etiology of liver disease. *Transplantation* **2013**, *95*, 755–760. [CrossRef] [PubMed]
6. Mehta, G.; Macdonald, S.; Cronberg, A.; Rosselli, M.; Khera-Butler, T.; Sumpter, C.; Al-Khatib, S.; Jain, A.; Maurice, J.; Charalambous, C.; et al. Short-term abstinence from alcohol and changes in cardiovascular risk factors, liver function tests and cancer-related growth factors: A prospective observational study. *BMJ Open* **2018**, *8*, e020673. [CrossRef] [PubMed]
7. Lackner, C.; Spindelboeck, W.; Haybaeck, J.; Douschan, P.; Rainer, F.; Terracciano, L.; Haas, J.; Berghold, A.; Bataller, R.; Stauber, R.E. Histological parameters and alcohol abstinence determine long-term prognosis in patients with alcoholic liver disease. *J. Hepatol.* **2017**, *66*, 610–618. [CrossRef] [PubMed]
8. Kirpich, I.A.; McClain, C.J.; Vatsalya, V.; Schwandt, M.; Phillips, M.; Falkner, K.C.; Zhang, L.; Harwell, C.; George, D.T.; Umhau, J.C. Liver Injury and Endotoxemia in Male and Female Alcohol-Dependent Individuals Admitted to an Alcohol Treatment Program. *Alcohol. Clin. Exp. Res.* **2017**, *41*, 747–757. [CrossRef]
9. Neuberger, J. Transplantation for alcoholic liver disease: A perspective from Europe. *Liver Transpl. Surg.* **1998**, *4*, S51–S57.
10. European Association for the Study of the Liver. EASL Clinical Practice Guidelines: Liver transplantation. *J. Hepatol.* **2016**, *64*, 433–485. [CrossRef]
11. McCallum, S.; Masterton, G. Liver transplantation for alcoholic liver disease: A systematic review of psychosocial selection criteria. *Alcohol Alcohol.* **2006**, *41*, 358–363. [CrossRef]
12. Varma, V.; Webb, K.; Mirza, D.F. Liver transplantation for alcoholic liver disease. *World J. Gastroenterol.* **2010**, *16*, 4377–4393. [CrossRef]
13. Liangpunsakul, S. Clinical characteristics and mortality of hospitalized alcoholic hepatitis patients in the United States. *J. Clin. Gastroenterol.* **2011**, *45*, 714–719. [CrossRef]
14. Sandahl, T.D.; Jepsen, P.; Thomsen, K.L.; Vilstrup, H. Incidence and mortality of alcoholic hepatitis in Denmark 1999–2008: A nationwide population based cohort study. *J. Hepatol.* **2011**, *54*, 760–764. [CrossRef] [PubMed]
15. Maddrey, W.C.; Boitnott, J.K.; Bedine, M.S.; Weber, F.L., Jr.; Mezey, E.; White, R.I., Jr. Corticosteroid therapy of alcoholic hepatitis. *Gastroenterology* **1978**, *75*, 193–199. [CrossRef]
16. Mathurin, P.; Duchatelle, V.; Ramond, M.J.; Degott, C.; Bedossa, P.; Erlinger, S.; Benhamou, J.P.; Chaput, J.C.; Rueff, B.; Poynard, T. Survival and prognostic factors in patients with severe alcoholic hepatitis treated with prednisolone. *Gastroenterology* **1996**, *110*, 1847–1853. [CrossRef] [PubMed]
17. Mathurin, P.; Mendenhall, C.L.; Carithers, R.L.; Ramond, M.J.; Maddrey, W.C.; Garstide, P.; Rueff, B.; Naveau, S.; Chaput, J.C.; Poynard, T. Corticosteroids improve short-term survival in patients with severe alcoholic hepatitis (AH): Individual data analysis of the last three randomized placebo controlled double blind trials of corticosteroids in severe AH. *J. Hepatol.* **2002**, *36*, 480–487. [CrossRef]
18. Ramond, M.J.; Poynard, T.; Rueff, B.; Mathurin, P.; Theodore, C.; Chaput, J.C.; Benhamou, J.P. A randomized trial of prednisolone in patients with severe alcoholic hepatitis. *N. Engl. J. Med.* **1992**, *326*, 507–512. [CrossRef]

19. Rambaldi, A.; Saconato, H.H.; Christensen, E.; Thorlund, K.; Wetterslev, J.; Gluud, C. Systematic review: Glucocorticosteroids for alcoholic hepatitis—A Cochrane Hepato-Biliary Group systematic review with meta-analyses and trial sequential analyses of randomized clinical trials. *Aliment. Pharmacol. Ther.* **2008**, *27*, 1167–1178. [CrossRef]

20. Thursz, M.R.; Richardson, P.; Allison, M.; Austin, A.; Bowers, M.; Day, C.P.; Downs, N.; Gleeson, D.; MacGilchrist, A.; Grant, A.; et al. Prednisolone or pentoxifylline for alcoholic hepatitis. *N. Engl. J. Med.* **2015**, *372*, 1619–1628. [CrossRef]

21. Burra, P.; Germani, G. Transplantation for acute alcoholic hepatitis. *Clin. Liver Dis.* **2017**, *9*, 141–143. [CrossRef]

22. Burra, P.; Bizzaro, D.; Forza, G.; Feltrin, A.; Volpe, B.; Ronzan, A.; Feltrin, G.; Carretta, G.; D'Amico, F.; Cillo, U.; et al. Severe acute alcoholic hepatitis: Can we offer early liver transplantation? *Minerva Gastroenterol.* **2021**, *67*, 23–25. [CrossRef] [PubMed]

23. Mathurin, P.; Moreno, C.; Samuel, D.; Dumortier, J.; Salleron, J.; Durand, F.; Castel, H.; Duhamel, A.; Pageaux, G.P.; Leroy, V.; et al. Early Liver Transplantation for Severe Alcoholic Hepatitis. *N. Engl. J. Med.* **2011**, *365*, 1790–1800. [CrossRef]

24. Weeks, S.R.; Sun, Z.; McCaul, M.E.; Zhu, H.; Anders, R.A.; Philosophe, B.; Ottmann, S.E.; Garonzik Wang, J.M.; Gurakar, A.O.; Cameron, A.M. Liver Transplantation for Severe Alcoholic Hepatitis, Updated Lessons from the World's Largest Series. *J. Am. Coll. Surg.* **2018**, *226*, 549–557. [CrossRef] [PubMed]

25. Lee, B.P.; Mehta, N.; Platt, L.; Gurakar, A.; Rice, J.P.; Lucey, M.R.; Im, G.Y.; Therapondos, G.; Han, H.; Victor, D.W.; et al. Outcomes of Early Liver Transplantation for Patients With Severe Alcoholic Hepatitis. *Gastroenterology* **2018**, *155*, 422–430. [CrossRef] [PubMed]

26. Im, G.Y.; Neuberger, J. Debate on Selection Criteria for Liver Transplantation for Alcoholic Hepatitis: Tighten or Loosen? *Liver Transpl.* **2020**, *26*, 916–921. [CrossRef]

27. Thursz, M.; Allison, M. Liver transplantation for alcoholic hepatitis: Being consistent about where to set the bar. *Liver Transpl.* **2018**, *24*, 733–734. [CrossRef]

28. Im, G.Y.; Kim-Schluger, L.; Shenoy, A.; Schubert, E.; Goel, A.; Friedman, S.L.; Florman, S.; Schiano, T.D. Early Liver Transplantation for Severe Alcoholic Hepatitis in the United States—A Single-Center Experience. *Am. J. Transplant.* **2016**, *16*, 841–849. [CrossRef]

29. Lee, B.P.; Chen, P.H.; Haugen, C.; Hernaez, R.; Gurakar, A.; Philosophe, B.; Dagher, N.; Moore, S.A.; Li, Z.P.; Cameron, A.M. Three-year Results of a Pilot Program in Early Liver Transplantation for Severe Alcoholic Hepatitis. *Ann. Surg.* **2017**, *265*, 20–27. [CrossRef]

30. Germani, G.; Angrisani, D.; Addolorato, G.; Merli, M.; Mazzarelli, C.; Tarli, C. Liver transplantation for severe alcoholic hepatitis:a multicentre Italian study. *Am. J. Transplant.* **2021**. submitted.

31. Rodríguez-Perálvarez, M.; Gómez-Bravo, M.; Sánchez-Antolín, G.; De la Rosa, G.; Bilbao, I.; Colmenero, J. Expanding Indications of Liver Transplantation in Spain: Consensus Statement and Recommendations by the Spanish Society of Liver Transplantation. *Transplantation* **2021**, *105*, 602–607. [CrossRef] [PubMed]

32. Stroh, G.; Rosell, T.; Dong, F.; Forster, J. Early Liver Transplantation for Patients With Acute Alcoholic Hepatitis: Public Views and the Effects on Organ Donation. *Am. J. Transplant.* **2015**, *15*, 1598–1604. [CrossRef] [PubMed]

33. EASL Clinical Practice Guidelines: Management of alcohol-related liver disease. *J. Hepatol.* **2018**, *69*, 154–181. [CrossRef]

34. Burra, P.; Belli, L.S.; Corradini, S.G.; Volpes, R.; Marzioni, M.; Giannini, E.; Toniutto, P. Common issues in the management of patients in the waiting list and after liver transplantation. *Dig. Liver Dis.* **2017**, *49*, 241–253. [CrossRef] [PubMed]

35. Lee, B.P.; Vittinghoff, E.; Hsu, C.; Han, H.S.; Therapondos, G.; Fix, O.K.; Victor, D.W.; Dronamraju, D.; Im, G.Y.; Voigt, M.D.; et al. Predicting Low Risk for Sustained Alcohol Use After Early Liver Transplant for Acute Alcoholic Hepatitis: The Sustained Alcohol Use Post-Liver Transplant Score. *Hepatology* **2019**, *69*, 1477–1487. [CrossRef]

36. Maldonado, J.R. Why It is Important to Consider Social Support When Assessing Organ Transplant Candidates? *Am. J. Bioeth.* **2019**, *19*, 1–8. [CrossRef]

37. Walter, M.; Scholler, G.; Moyzes, D.; Hildebrandt, M.; Neuhaus, R.; Danzer, G.; Klapp, B.F. Psychosocial prediction of abstinence from ethanol in alcoholic recipients following liver transplantation. *Transplant. Proc.* **2002**, *34*, 1239–1241. [CrossRef]

38. Bottesi, G.; Granziol, U.; Forza, G.; Volpe, B.; Feltrin, A.; Battermann, F.; Cavalli, C.; Cillo, U.; Gerosa, G.; Fraiese, A.; et al. The Psychosocial Assessment of Transplant Candidates: Inter-Rater Reliability and Predictive Value of the Italian Stanford Integrated Psychosocial Assessment for Transplantation (SIPAT). *Psychosomatics* **2020**, *61*, 127–134. [CrossRef] [PubMed]

39. Donckier, V.; Lucidi, V.; Gustot, T.; Moreno, C. Ethical considerations regarding early liver transplantation in patients with severe alcoholic hepatitis not responding to medical therapy. *J. Hepatol.* **2014**, *60*, 866–871. [CrossRef]

40. Moreau, R.; Jalan, R.; Gines, P.; Pavesi, M.; Angeli, P.; Cordoba, J.; Durand, F.; Gustot, T.; Saliba, F.; Domenicali, M.; et al. Acute-on-chronic liver failure is a distinct syndrome that develops in patients with acute decompensation of cirrhosis. *Gastroenterology* **2013**, *144*, 1426–1437. [CrossRef]

41. O'Leary, J.G.; Reddy, K.R.; Garcia-Tsao, G.; Biggins, S.W.; Wong, F.; Fallon, M.B.; Subramanian, R.M.; Kamath, P.S.; Thuluvath, P.; Vargas, H.E.; et al. NACSELD acute-on-chronic liver failure (NACSELD-ACLF) score predicts 30-day survival in hospitalized patients with cirrhosis. *Hepatology* **2018**, *67*, 2367–2374. [CrossRef] [PubMed]

42. Sarin, S.K.; Choudhury, A.; Sharma, M.K.; Maiwall, R.; Al Mahtab, M.; Rahman, S.; Saigal, S.; Saraf, N.; Soin, A.S.; Devarbhavi, H.; et al. Acute-on-chronic liver failure: Consensus recommendations of the Asian Pacific association for the study of the liver (APASL): An update. *Hepatol. Int.* **2019**, *13*, 353–390. [CrossRef]

43. Ferrarese, A.; Feltracco, P.; Barbieri, S.; Cillo, U.; Burra, P.; Senzolo, M. Outcome of critically ill cirrhotic patients admitted to the ICU: The role of ACLF. *J. Hepatol.* **2019**, *70*, 801–803. [CrossRef]

44. Hernaez, R.; Solà, E.; Moreau, R.; Ginès, P. Acute-on-chronic liver failure: An update. *Gut* **2017**, *66*, 541–553. [CrossRef]

45. Nadim, M.K.; Durand, F.; Kellum, J.A.; Levitsky, J.; O'Leary, J.G.; Karvellas, C.J.; Bajaj, J.S.; Davenport, A.; Jalan, R.; Angeli, P.; et al. Management of the critically ill patient with cirrhosis: A multidisciplinary perspective. *J. Hepatol.* **2016**, *64*, 717–735. [CrossRef] [PubMed]

46. Abdallah, M.A.; Waleed, M.; Bell, M.G.; Nelson, M.; Wong, R.; Sundaram, V.; Singal, A.K. Systematic review with meta-analysis: Liver transplant provides survival benefit in patients with acute on chronic liver failure. *Aliment. Pharmacol. Ther.* **2020**, *52*, 222–232. [CrossRef]

47. Trebicka, J.; Sundaram, V.; Moreau, R.; Jalan, R.; Arroyo, V. Liver Transplantation for Acute-on-Chronic Liver Failure: Science or Fiction? *Liver Transpl.* **2020**, *26*, 906–915. [CrossRef] [PubMed]

48. Toniutto, P.; Zanetto, A.; Ferrarese, A.; Burra, P. Current challenges and future directions for liver transplantation. *Liver Int.* **2017**, *37*, 317–327. [CrossRef]

49. Gustot, T.; Fernandez, J.; Garcia, E.; Morando, F.; Caraceni, P.; Alessandria, C.; Laleman, W.; Trebicka, J.; Elkrief, L.; Hopf, C.; et al. Clinical Course of acute-on-chronic liver failure syndrome and effects on prognosis. *Hepatology* **2015**, *62*, 243–252. [CrossRef] [PubMed]

50. Piano, S.; Tonon, M.; Vettore, E.; Stanco, M.; Pilutti, C.; Romano, A.; Mareso, S.; Gambino, C.; Brocca, A.; Sticca, A.; et al. Incidence, predictors and outcomes of acute-on-chronic liver failure in outpatients with cirrhosis. *J. Hepatol.* **2017**, *67*, 1177–1184. [CrossRef] [PubMed]

51. Putignano, A.; Gustot, T. New concepts in acute-on-chronic liver failure: Implications for liver transplantation. *Liver Transpl.* **2017**, *23*, 234–243. [CrossRef]

52. Mookerjee, R.P. Prognosis and Biomarkers in Acute-on-Chronic Liver Failure. *Semin. Liver Dis.* **2016**, *36*, 127–132. [CrossRef] [PubMed]

53. Sundaram, V.; Jalan, R.; Wu, T.; Volk, M.L.; Asrani, S.K.; Klein, A.S.; Wong, R.J. Factors Associated with Survival of Patients With Severe Acute-On-Chronic Liver Failure Before and After Liver Transplantation. *Gastroenterology* **2019**, *156*, 1381–1391.e3. [CrossRef] [PubMed]

54. Hernaez, R.; Liu, Y.; Kramer, J.R.; Rana, A.; El-Serag, H.B.; Kanwal, F. Model for end-stage liver disease-sodium underestimates 90-day mortality risk in patients with acute-on-chronic liver failure. *J. Hepatol.* **2020**, *73*, 1425–1433. [CrossRef] [PubMed]

55. Sundaram, V.; Shah, P.; Wong, R.J.; Karvellas, C.J.; Fortune, B.E.; Mahmud, N.; Kuo, A.; Jalan, R. Patients With Acute on Chronic Liver Failure Grade 3 Have Greater 14-Day Waitlist Mortality Than Status-1a Patients. *Hepatology* **2019**, *70*, 334–345. [CrossRef]

56. Abdallah, M.A.; Kuo, Y.F.; Asrani, S.; Wong, R.J.; Ahmed, A.; Kwo, P.; Terrault, N.; Kamath, P.S.; Jalan, R.; Singal, A.K. Validating a novel score based on interaction between ACLF grade and MELD score to predict waitlist mortality. *J. Hepatol.* **2021**, *74*, 1355–1361. [CrossRef]

57. Zaccherini, G.; Weiss, E.; Moreau, R. Acute-on-chronic liver failure: Definitions, pathophysiology and principles of treatment. *JHEP Rep.* **2021**, *3*, 100176. [CrossRef]

58. Burra, P.; Samuel, D.; Sundaram, V.; Duvoux, C.; Petrowsky, H.; Terrault, N.; Jalan, R. Limitations of current liver donor allocation systems and the impact of newer indications for liver transplantation. *J. Hepatol.* **2021**, *75*, S178–S190. [CrossRef] [PubMed]

59. Levesque, E.; Winter, A.; Noorah, Z.; Daures, J.P.; Landais, P.; Feray, C.; Azoulay, D. Impact of acute-on-chronic liver failure on 90-day mortality following a first liver transplantation. *Liver Int.* **2017**, *37*, 684–693. [CrossRef]

60. Artru, F.; Louvet, A.; Ruiz, I.; Levesque, E.; Labreuche, J.; Ursic-Bedoya, J.; Lassailly, G.; Dharancy, S.; Boleslawski, E.; Lebuffe, G.; et al. Liver transplantation in the most severely ill cirrhotic patients: A multicenter study in acute-on-chronic liver failure grade 3. *J. Hepatol.* **2017**, *67*, 708–715. [CrossRef] [PubMed]

61. Huebener, P.; Sterneck, M.R.; Bangert, K.; Drolz, A.; Lohse, A.W.; Kluge, S.; Fischer, L.; Fuhrmann, V. Stabilisation of acute-on-chronic liver failure patients before liver transplantation predicts post-transplant survival. *Aliment. Pharmacol. Ther.* **2018**, *47*, 1502–1510. [CrossRef]

62. Thuluvath, P.J.; Thuluvath, A.J.; Hanish, S.; Savva, Y. Liver transplantation in patients with multiple organ failures: Feasibility and outcomes. *J. Hepatol.* **2018**, *69*, 1047–1056. [CrossRef] [PubMed]

63. Sundaram, V.; Mahmud, N.; Perricone, G.; Katarey, D.; Wong, R.J.; Karvellas, C.J.; Fortune, B.E.; Rahimi, R.S.; Maddur, H.; Jou, J.H.; et al. Longterm Outcomes of Patients Undergoing Liver Transplantation for Acute-on-Chronic Liver Failure. *Liver Transpl.* **2020**, *26*, 1594–1602. [CrossRef] [PubMed]

64. Linecker, M.; Krones, T.; Berg, T.; Niemann, C.U.; Steadman, R.H.; Dutkowski, P.; Clavien, P.A.; Busuttil, R.W.; Truog, R.D.; Petrowsky, H. Potentially inappropriate liver transplantation in the era of the "sickest first" policy—A search for the upper limits. *J. Hepatol.* **2018**, *68*, 798–813. [CrossRef]

65. Finkenstedt, A.; Nachbaur, K.; Zoller, H.; Joannidis, M.; Pratschke, J.; Graziadei, I.W.; Vogel, W. Acute-on-chronic liver failure: Excellent outcomes after liver transplantation but high mortality on the wait list. *Liver Transpl.* **2013**, *19*, 879–886. [CrossRef]

66. Moon, D.B.; Lee, S.G.; Kang, W.H.; Song, G.W.; Jung, D.H.; Park, G.C.; Cho, H.D.; Jwa, E.K.; Kim, W.J.; Ha, T.Y.; et al. Adult Living Donor Liver Transplantation for Acute-on-Chronic Liver Failure in High-Model for End-Stage Liver Disease Score Patients. *Am. J. Transplant.* **2017**, *17*, 1833–1842. [CrossRef] [PubMed]

67. Weiss, E.; Saner, F.; Asrani, S.K.; Biancofiore, G.; Blasi, A.; Lerut, J.; Durand, F.; Fernandez, J.; Findlay, J.Y.; Fondevila, C.; et al. When Is a Critically Ill Cirrhotic Patient Too Sick to Transplant? Development of Consensus Criteria by a Multidisciplinary Panel of 35 International Experts. *Transplantation* **2021**, *105*, 561–568. [CrossRef] [PubMed]

68. Artzner, T.; Michard, B.; Weiss, E.; Barbier, L.; Noorah, Z.; Merle, J.C.; Paugam-Burtz, C.; Francoz, C.; Durand, F.; Soubrane, O.; et al. Liver transplantation for critically ill cirrhotic patients: Stratifying utility based on pretransplant factors. *Am. J. Transplant.* **2020**, *20*, 2437–2448. [CrossRef]

69. Goosmann, L.; Buchholz, A.; Bangert, K.; Fuhrmann, V.; Kluge, S.; Lohse, A.W.; Huber, S.; Fischer, L.; Sterneck, M.R.; Huebener, P. Liver transplantation for acute-on-chronic liver failure predicts post-transplant mortality and impaired long-term quality of life. *Liver Int.* **2020**, *41*, 574–584. [CrossRef]

70. Arora, V.; Maiwall, R.; Rajan, V.; Jindal, A.; Muralikrishna Shasthry, S.; Kumar, G.; Jain, P.; Sarin, S.K. Terlipressin Is Superior to Noradrenaline in the Management of Acute Kidney Injury in Acute on Chronic Liver Failure. *Hepatology* **2020**, *71*, 600–610. [CrossRef]

71. Campello, E.; Zanetto, A.; Radu, C.M.; Bulato, C.; Truma, A.; Spiezia, L.; Senzolo, M.; Garcia-Tsao, G.; Simioni, P. Acute kidney injury is associated with increased levels of circulating microvesicles in patients with decompensated cirrhosis. *Dig. Liver Dis.* **2021**. [CrossRef]

72. Zanetto, A.; Rinder, H.M.; Campello, E.; Saggiorato, G.; Deng, Y.; Ciarleglio, M.; Wilson, F.P.; Senzolo, M.; Gavasso, S.; Bulato, C.; et al. Acute Kidney Injury in Decompensated Cirrhosis Is Associated With Both Hypo-coagulable and Hyper-coagulable Features. *Hepatology* **2020**, *72*, 1327–1340. [CrossRef] [PubMed]

73. Durand, F.; Francoz, C.; Asrani, S.K.; Khemichian, S.; Pham, T.A.; Sung, R.S.; Genyk, Y.S.; Nadim, M.K. Acute Kidney Injury After Liver Transplantation. *Transplantation* **2018**, *102*, 1636–1649. [CrossRef] [PubMed]

74. Marciano, S.; Mauro, E.; Giunta, D.; Torres, M.C.; Diaz, J.M.; Bermudez, C.; Gutierrez-Acevedo, M.N.; Narvaez, A.; Ortiz, J.; Dirchwolf, M.; et al. Impact of acute-on-chronic liver failure on post-transplant survival and on kidney outcomes. *Eur. J. Gastroenterol. Hepatol.* **2019**, *31*, 1157–1164. [CrossRef]

75. Burra, P.; De Bona, M. Quality of life following organ transplantation. *Transpl. Int.* **2007**, *20*, 397–409. [CrossRef]

76. Burra, P.; Ferrarese, A.; Feltrin, G. Quality of life and adherence in liver transplant recipients. *Minerva Gastroenterol. Dietol.* **2018**, *64*, 180–186. [CrossRef]

77. Sundaram, V.; Kogachi, S.; Wong, R.J.; Karvellas, C.J.; Fortune, B.E.; Mahmud, N.; Levitsky, J.; Rahimi, R.S.; Jalan, R. Effect of the clinical course of acute-on-chronic liver failure prior to liver transplantation on post-transplant survival. *J. Hepatol.* **2020**, *72*, 481–488. [CrossRef] [PubMed]

78. Riihimäki, M.; Hemminki, A.; Sundquist, J.; Hemminki, K. Patterns of metastasis in colon and rectal cancer. *Sci. Rep.* **2016**, *6*, 29765. [CrossRef]

79. Hackl, C.; Gerken, M.; Loss, M.; Klinkhammer-Schalke, M.; Piso, P.; Schlitt, H.J. A population-based analysis on the rate and surgical management of colorectal liver metastases in Southern Germany. *Int. J. Colorectal Dis.* **2011**, *26*, 1475–1481. [CrossRef]

80. Kanas, G.P.; Taylor, A.; Primrose, J.N.; Langeberg, W.J.; Kelsh, M.A.; Mowat, F.S.; Alexander, D.D.; Choti, M.A.; Poston, G. Survival after liver resection in metastatic colorectal cancer: Review and meta-analysis of prognostic factors. *Clin. Epidemiol.* **2012**, *4*, 283–301. [CrossRef]

81. Kopetz, S.; Chang, G.J.; Overman, M.J.; Eng, C.; Sargent, D.J.; Larson, D.W.; Grothey, A.; Vauthey, J.N.; Nagorney, D.M.; McWilliams, R.R. Improved survival in metastatic colorectal cancer is associated with adoption of hepatic resection and improved chemotherapy. *J. Clin. Oncol.* **2009**, *27*, 3677–3683. [CrossRef]

82. Nordlinger, B.; Sorbye, H.; Glimelius, B.; Poston, G.J.; Schlag, P.M.; Rougier, P.; Bechstein, W.O.; Primrose, J.N.; Walpole, E.T.; Finch-Jones, M.; et al. Perioperative FOLFOX4 chemotherapy and surgery versus surgery alone for resectable liver metastases from colorectal cancer (EORTC 40983): Long-term results of a randomised, controlled, phase 3 trial. *Lancet Oncol.* **2013**, *14*, 1208–1215. [CrossRef]

83. Kallini, J.R.; Gabr, A.; Abouchaleh, N.; Ali, R.; Riaz, A.; Lewandowski, R.J.; Salem, R. New Developments in Interventional Oncology Liver Metastases From Colorectal Cancer. *Cancer J.* **2016**, *22*, 373–380. [CrossRef] [PubMed]

84. Andres, A.; Majno, P.; Terraz, S.; Morel, P.; Roth, A.; Rubbia-Brandt, L.; Schiffer, E.; Ris, F.; Toso, C. Management of patients with colorectal liver metastasis in eleven questions and answers. *Expert Rev. Anticancer Ther.* **2016**, *16*, 1277–1290. [CrossRef] [PubMed]

85. Van Cutsem, E.; Köhne, C.H.; Láng, I.; Folprecht, G.; Nowacki, M.P.; Cascinu, S.; Shchepotin, I.; Maurel, J.; Cunningham, D.; Tejpar, S.; et al. Cetuximab plus irinotecan, fluorouracil, and leucovorin as first-line treatment for metastatic colorectal cancer: Updated analysis of overall survival according to tumor KRAS and BRAF mutation status. *J. Clin. Oncol.* **2011**, *29*, 2011–2019. [CrossRef]

86. Masi, G.; Vasile, E.; Loupakis, F.; Cupini, S.; Fornaro, L.; Baldi, G.; Salvatore, L.; Cremolini, C.; Stasi, I.; Brunetti, I.; et al. Randomized trial of two induction chemotherapy regimens in metastatic colorectal cancer: An updated analysis. *J. Natl. Cancer Inst.* **2011**, *103*, 21–30. [CrossRef] [PubMed]

87. Douillard, J.Y.; Siena, S.; Cassidy, J.; Tabernero, J.; Burkes, R.; Barugel, M.; Humblet, Y.; Bodoky, G.; Cunningham, D.; Jassem, J.; et al. Randomized, phase III trial of panitumumab with infusional fluorouracil, leucovorin, and oxaliplatin (FOLFOX4) versus FOLFOX4 alone as first-line treatment in patients with previously untreated metastatic colorectal cancer: The PRIME study. *J. Clin. Oncol.* **2010**, *28*, 4697–4705. [CrossRef]

88. Dueland, S.; Guren, T.K.; Hagness, M.; Glimelius, B.; Line, P.D.; Pfeiffer, P.; Foss, A.; Tveit, K.M. Chemotherapy or liver transplantation for nonresectable liver metastases from colorectal cancer? *Ann. Surg.* **2015**, *261*, 956–960. [CrossRef]

89. Boeckx, N.; Koukakis, R.; Op de Beeck, K.; Rolfo, C.; Van Camp, G.; Siena, S.; Tabernero, J.; Douillard, J.Y.; André, T.; Peeters, M. Primary tumor sidedness has an impact on prognosis and treatment outcome in metastatic colorectal cancer: Results from two randomized first-line panitumumab studies. *Ann. Oncol.* **2017**, *28*, 1862–1868. [CrossRef]

90. Van Cutsem, E.; Köhne, C.H.; Hitre, E.; Zaluski, J.; Chang Chien, C.R.; Makhson, A.; D'Haens, G.; Pintér, T.; Lim, R.; Bodoky, G.; et al. Cetuximab and chemotherapy as initial treatment for metastatic colorectal cancer. *N. Engl. J. Med.* **2009**, *360*, 1408–1417. [CrossRef]

91. Glimelius, B.; Cavalli-Björkman, N. Metastatic colorectal cancer: Current treatment and future options for improved survival. Medical approach–present status. *Scand. J. Gastroenterol.* **2012**, *47*, 296–314. [CrossRef]

92. Quaranta, M.; Micelli, G.; Coviello, M.; Donadeo, A.; Lozupone, A.; Schittulli, F. Clinical usefulness of CA M26 and CA M29 in breast carcinoma. *J. Nucl. Med. Allied Sci.* **1990**, *34*, 35–38. [PubMed]

93. Hagness, M.; Foss, A.; Line, P.D.; Scholz, T.; Jørgensen, P.F.; Fosby, B.; Boberg, K.M.; Mathisen, O.; Gladhaug, I.P.; Egge, T.S.; et al. Liver transplantation for nonresectable liver metastases from colorectal cancer. *Ann. Surg.* **2013**, *257*, 800–806. [CrossRef] [PubMed]

94. Toso, C.; Pinto Marques, H.; Andres, A.; Castro Sousa, F.; Adam, R.; Kalil, A.; Clavien, P.A.; Furtado, E.; Barroso, E.; Bismuth, H. Liver transplantation for colorectal liver metastasis: Survival without recurrence can be achieved. *Liver Transpl.* **2017**, *23*, 1073–1076. [CrossRef] [PubMed]

95. Hoti, E.; Adam, R. Liver transplantation for primary and metastatic liver cancers. *Transpl. Int.* **2008**, *21*, 1107–1117. [CrossRef] [PubMed]

96. Pavel, M.C.; Fuster, J. Expansion of the hepatocellular carcinoma Milan criteria in liver transplantation: Future directions. *World J. Gastroenterol.* **2018**, *24*, 3626–3636. [CrossRef]

97. Dueland, S.; Foss, A.; Solheim, J.M.; Hagness, M.; Line, P.D. Survival following liver transplantation for liver-only colorectal metastases compared with hepatocellular carcinoma. *Br. J. Surg.* **2018**, *105*, 736–742. [CrossRef]

98. Hagness, M.; Foss, A.; Egge, T.S.; Dueland, S. Patterns of recurrence after liver transplantation for nonresectable liver metastases from colorectal cancer. *Ann. Surg. Oncol.* **2014**, *21*, 1323–1329. [CrossRef]

99. Grut, H.; Solberg, S.; Seierstad, T.; Revheim, M.E.; Egge, T.S.; Larsen, S.G.; Line, P.D.; Dueland, S. Growth rates of pulmonary metastases after liver transplantation for unresectable colorectal liver metastases. *Br. J. Surg.* **2018**, *105*, 295–301. [CrossRef]

100. Dueland, S.; Syversveen, T.; Solheim, J.M.; Solberg, S.; Grut, H.; Bjørnbeth, B.A.; Hagness, M.; Line, P.D. Survival Following Liver Transplantation for Patients With Nonresectable Liver-only Colorectal Metastases. *Ann. Surg.* **2020**, *271*, 212–218. [CrossRef] [PubMed]

101. Gorgen, A.; Muaddi, H.; Zhang, W.; McGilvray, I.; Gallinger, S.; Sapisochin, G. The New Era of Transplant Oncology: Liver Transplantation for Nonresectable Colorectal Cancer Liver Metastases. *Can. J. Gastroenterol. Hepatol.* **2018**, *2018*, 9531925. [CrossRef]

102. Line, P.D.; Hagness, M.; Berstad, A.E.; Foss, A.; Dueland, S. A Novel Concept for Partial Liver Transplantation in Nonresectable Colorectal Liver Metastases: The RAPID Concept. *Ann. Surg.* **2015**, *262*, e5–e9. [CrossRef] [PubMed]

103. Waisberg, D.R.; Pinheiro, R.S.; Nacif, L.S.; Rocha-Santos, V.; Martino, R.B.; Arantes, R.M.; Ducatti, L.; Lai, Q.; Andraus, W.; D'Albuquerque, L.C. Resection for intrahepatic cholangiocellular cancer: New advances. *Transl. Gastroenterol. Hepatol.* **2018**, *3*, 60. [CrossRef]

104. Laurent, S.; Verhelst, X.; Geerts, A.; Geboes, K.; De Man, M.; Troisi, R.; Vanlander, A.; Rogiers, X.; Berrevoet, F.; Van Vlierberghe, H. Update on liver transplantation for cholangiocarcinoma: A review of the recent literature. *Acta Gastroenterol. Belg.* **2019**, *82*, 417–420.

105. Squires, M.H.; Cloyd, J.M.; Dillhoff, M.; Schmidt, C.; Pawlik, T.M. Challenges of surgical management of intrahepatic cholangiocarcinoma. *Expert Rev. Gastroenterol. Hepatol.* **2018**, *12*, 671–681. [CrossRef] [PubMed]

106. Fung, B.M.; Tabibian, J.H. Cholangiocarcinoma in patients with primary sclerosing cholangitis. *Curr. Opin. Gastroenterol.* **2020**, *36*, 77–84. [CrossRef]

107. Li, H.; Chen, L.; Zhu, G.Y.; Yao, X.; Dong, R.; Guo, J.H. Interventional Treatment for Cholangiocarcinoma. *Front. Oncol.* **2021**, *11*, 671327. [CrossRef] [PubMed]

108. Mosconi, C.; Calandri, M.; Javle, M.; Odisio, B.C. Interventional radiology approaches for intra-hepatic cholangiocarcinoma. *Chin. Clin. Oncol.* **2020**, *9*, 8. [CrossRef]

109. Schmeding, M.; Neumann, U.P. Liver Transplant for Cholangiocarcinoma: A Comeback? *Exp. Clin. Transplant.* **2015**, *13*, 301–308. [PubMed]

110. Wu, L.; Tsilimigras, D.I.; Paredes, A.Z.; Mehta, R.; Hyer, J.M.; Merath, K.; Sahara, K.; Bagante, F.; Beal, E.W.; Shen, F.; et al. Trends in the Incidence, Treatment and Outcomes of Patients with Intrahepatic Cholangiocarcinoma in the USA: Facility Type is Associated with Margin Status, Use of Lymphadenectomy and Overall Survival. *World J. Surg.* **2019**, *43*, 1777–1787. [CrossRef] [PubMed]

111. Katayose, Y.; Rikiyama, T.; Motoi, F.; Yamamoto, K.; Yoshida, H.; Morikawa, T.; Hayashi, H.; Kanno, A.; Hirota, M.; Satoh, K.; et al. Phase I trial of neoadjuvant chemoradiation with gemcitabine and surgical resection for cholangiocarcinoma patients (NACRAC study). *Hepatogastroenterology* **2011**, *58*, 1866–1872. [CrossRef]

112. Endo, I.; Gonen, M.; Yopp, A.C.; Dalal, K.M.; Zhou, Q.; Klimstra, D.; D'Angelica, M.; DeMatteo, R.P.; Fong, Y.; Schwartz, L.; et al. Intrahepatic cholangiocarcinoma: Rising frequency, improved survival, and determinants of outcome after resection. *Ann. Surg.* **2008**, *248*, 84–96. [CrossRef] [PubMed]

113. Merath, K.; Chen, Q.; Bagante, F.; Alexandrescu, S.; Marques, H.P.; Aldrighetti, L.; Maithel, S.K.; Pulitano, C.; Weiss, M.J.; Bauer, T.W.; et al. A Multi-institutional International Analysis of Textbook Outcomes Among Patients Undergoing Curative-Intent Resection of Intrahepatic Cholangiocarcinoma. *JAMA Surg.* **2019**, *154*, e190571. [CrossRef] [PubMed]

114. Zhang, X.F.; Beal, E.W.; Bagante, F.; Chakedis, J.; Weiss, M.; Popescu, I.; Marques, H.P.; Aldrighetti, L.; Maithel, S.K.; Pulitano, C.; et al. Early versus late recurrence of intrahepatic cholangiocarcinoma after resection with curative intent. *Br. J. Surg.* **2018**, *105*, 848–856. [CrossRef]

115. Takahashi, K.; Obeid, J.; Burmeister, C.S.; Bruno, D.A.; Kazimi, M.M.; Yoshida, A.; Abouljoud, M.S.; Schnickel, G.T. Intrahepatic Cholangiocarcinoma in the Liver Explant After Liver Transplantation: Histological Differentiation and Prognosis. *Ann. Transplant.* **2016**, *21*, 208–215. [CrossRef]

116. Sapisochín, G.; Fernández de Sevilla, E.; Echeverri, J.; Charco, R. Liver transplantation for cholangiocarcinoma: Current status and new insights. *World J. Hepatol.* **2015**, *7*, 2396–2403. [CrossRef] [PubMed]

117. Sapisochín, G.; Rodríguez de Lope, C.; Gastaca, M.; Ortiz de Urbina, J.; Suarez, M.A.; Santoyo, J.; Castroagudín, J.F.; Varo, E.; López-Andujar, R.; Palacios, F.; et al. "Very early" intrahepatic cholangiocarcinoma in cirrhotic patients: Should liver transplantation be reconsidered in these patients? *Am. J. Transplant.* **2014**, *14*, 660–667. [CrossRef] [PubMed]

118. Sapisochín, G.; de Lope, C.R.; Gastaca, M.; de Urbina, J.O.; López-Andujar, R.; Palacios, F.; Ramos, E.; Fabregat, J.; Castroagudín, J.F.; Varo, E.; et al. Intrahepatic cholangiocarcinoma or mixed hepatocellular-cholangiocarcinoma in patients undergoing liver transplantation: A Spanish matched cohort multicenter study. *Ann. Surg.* **2014**, *259*, 944–952. [CrossRef]

119. Sapisochín, G.; Facciuto, M.; Rubbia-Brandt, L.; Marti, J.; Mehta, N.; Yao, F.Y.; Vibert, E.; Cherqui, D.; Grant, D.R.; Hernandez-Alejandro, R.; et al. Liver transplantation for "very early" intrahepatic cholangiocarcinoma: International retrospective study supporting a prospective assessment. *Hepatology* **2016**, *64*, 1178–1188. [CrossRef]

120. De Martin, E.; Rayar, M.; Golse, N.; Dupeux, M.; Gelli, M.; Gnemmi, V.; Allard, M.A.; Cherqui, D.; Sa Cunha, A.; Adam, R.; et al. Analysis of Liver Resection Versus Liver Transplantation on Outcome of Small Intrahepatic Cholangiocarcinoma and Combined Hepatocellular-Cholangiocarcinoma in the Setting of Cirrhosis. *Liver Transpl.* **2020**, *26*, 785–798. [CrossRef]

121. Lee, D.D.; Croome, K.P.; Musto, K.R.; Melendez, J.; Tranesh, G.; Nakhleh, R.; Taner, C.B.; Nguyen, J.H.; Patel, T.; Harnois, D.M. Liver transplantation for intrahepatic cholangiocarcinoma. *Liver Transpl.* **2018**, *24*, 634–644. [CrossRef] [PubMed]

122. Hand, F.; Hoti, E. Contemporary role of liver transplantation for the treatment of cholangiocarcinoma. *Expert Rev. Gastroenterol. Hepatol.* **2020**, *14*, 475–481. [CrossRef] [PubMed]

123. Lunsford, K.E.; Javle, M.; Heyne, K.; Shroff, R.T.; Abdel-Wahab, R.; Gupta, N.; Mobley, C.M.; Saharia, A.; Victor, D.W.; Nguyen, D.T.; et al. Liver transplantation for locally advanced intrahepatic cholangiocarcinoma treated with neoadjuvant therapy: A prospective case-series. *Lancet Gastroenterol. Hepatol.* **2018**, *3*, 337–348. [CrossRef]

124. Sapisochín, G.; Javle, M.; Lerut, J.; Ohtsuka, M.; Ghobrial, M.; Hibi, T.; Kwan, N.M.; Heimbach, J. Liver Transplantation for Cholangiocarcinoma and Mixed Hepatocellular Cholangiocarcinoma: Working Group Report From the ILTS Transplant Oncology Consensus Conference. *Transplantation* **2020**, *104*, 1125–1130. [CrossRef] [PubMed]

125. Mansour, J.C.; Aloia, T.A.; Crane, C.H.; Heimbach, J.K.; Nagino, M.; Vauthey, J.N. Hilar cholangiocarcinoma: Expert consensus statement. *HPB* **2015**, *17*, 691–699. [CrossRef] [PubMed]

126. McMasters, K.M.; Tuttle, T.M.; Leach, S.D.; Rich, T.; Cleary, K.R.; Evans, D.B.; Curley, S.A. Neoadjuvant chemoradiation for extrahepatic cholangiocarcinoma. *Am. J. Surg.* **1997**, *174*, 605–608; discussion 608–609. [CrossRef]

127. Burke, E.C.; Jarnagin, W.R.; Hochwald, S.N.; Pisters, P.W.; Fong, Y.; Blumgart, L.H. Hilar Cholangiocarcinoma: Patterns of spread, the importance of hepatic resection for curative operation, and a presurgical clinical staging system. *Ann. Surg.* **1998**, *228*, 385–394. [CrossRef]

128. Weigt, J.; Malfertheiner, P. Cisplatin plus gemcitabine versus gemcitabine for biliary tract cancer. *Expert Rev. Gastroenterol. Hepatol.* **2010**, *4*, 395–397. [CrossRef]

129. Matsuo, K.; Rocha, F.G.; Ito, K.; D'Angelica, M.I.; Allen, P.J.; Fong, Y.; Dematteo, R.P.; Gonen, M.; Endo, I.; Jarnagin, W.R. The Blumgart preoperative staging system for hilar cholangiocarcinoma: Analysis of resectability and outcomes in 380 patients. *J. Am. Coll. Surg.* **2012**, *215*, 343–355. [CrossRef]

130. Hu, J.H.; Tang, J.H.; Lin, C.H.; Chu, Y.Y.; Liu, N.J. Preoperative staging of cholangiocarcinoma and biliary carcinoma using 18F-fluorodeoxyglucose positron emission tomography: A meta-analysis. *J. Investig. Med.* **2018**, *66*, 52–61. [CrossRef]

131. Eckel, F.; Schmid, R.M. Chemotherapy and targeted therapy in advanced biliary tract carcinoma: A pooled analysis of clinical trials. *Chemotherapy* **2014**, *60*, 13–23. [CrossRef] [PubMed]

132. Rosen, C.B.; Nagorney, D.M. Cholangiocarcinoma complicating primary sclerosing cholangitis. *Semin. Liver Dis.* **1991**, *11*, 26–30. [CrossRef]

133. Sudan, D.; DeRoover, A.; Chinnakotla, S.; Fox, I.; Shaw, B., Jr.; McCashland, T.; Sorrell, M.; Tempero, M.; Langnas, A. Radiochemotherapy and transplantation allow long-term survival for nonresectable hilar cholangiocarcinoma. *Am. J. Transplant.* **2002**, *2*, 774–779. [CrossRef]

134. De Vreede, I.; Steers, J.L.; Burch, P.A.; Rosen, C.B.; Gunderson, L.L.; Haddock, M.G.; Burgart, L.; Gores, G.J. Prolonged disease-free survival after orthotopic liver transplantation plus adjuvant chemoirradiation for cholangiocarcinoma. *Liver Transpl.* **2000**, *6*, 309–316. [CrossRef]
135. Heimbach, J.K.; Gores, G.J.; Haddock, M.G.; Alberts, S.R.; Nyberg, S.L.; Ishitani, M.B.; Rosen, C.B. Liver transplantation for unresectable perihilar cholangiocarcinoma. *Semin. Liver Dis.* **2004**, *24*, 201–207. [CrossRef] [PubMed]
136. Darwish Murad, S.; Kim, W.R.; Harnois, D.M.; Douglas, D.D.; Burton, J.; Kulik, L.M.; Botha, J.F.; Mezrich, J.D.; Chapman, W.C.; Schwartz, J.J.; et al. Efficacy of neoadjuvant chemoradiation, followed by liver transplantation, for perihilar cholangiocarcinoma at 12 US centers. *Gastroenterology* **2012**, *143*, 88–98. [CrossRef] [PubMed]
137. Meyer, C.G.; Penn, I.; James, L. Liver transplantation for cholangiocarcinoma: Results in 207 patients. *Transplantation* **2000**, *69*, 1633–1637. [CrossRef] [PubMed]
138. Robles, R.; Figueras, J.; Turrión, V.S.; Margarit, C.; Moya, A.; Varo, E.; Calleja, J.; Valdivieso, A.; Valdecasas, J.C.; López, P.; et al. Spanish experience in liver transplantation for hilar and peripheral cholangiocarcinoma. *Ann. Surg.* **2004**, *239*, 265–271. [CrossRef]
139. Rizvi, S.; Khan, S.A.; Hallemeier, C.L.; Kelley, R.K.; Gores, G.J. Cholangiocarcinoma—Evolving concepts and therapeutic strategies. *Nat. Rev. Clin. Oncol.* **2018**, *15*, 95–111. [CrossRef]
140. Blechacz, B. Cholangiocarcinoma: Current Knowledge and New Developments. *Gut Liver* **2017**, *11*, 13–26. [CrossRef]
141. Welling, T.H.; Feng, M.; Wan, S.; Hwang, S.Y.; Volk, M.L.; Lawrence, T.S.; Zalupski, M.M.; Sonnenday, C.J. Neoadjuvant stereotactic body radiation therapy, capecitabine, and liver transplantation for unresectable hilar cholangiocarcinoma. *Liver Transpl.* **2014**, *20*, 81–88. [CrossRef]
142. Duignan, S.; Maguire, D.; Ravichand, C.S.; Geoghegan, J.; Hoti, E.; Fennelly, D.; Armstrong, J.; Rock, K.; Mohan, H.; Traynor, O. Neoadjuvant chemoradiotherapy followed by liver transplantation for unresectable cholangiocarcinoma: A single-centre national experience. *HPB* **2014**, *16*, 91–98. [CrossRef]
143. Mantel, H.T.; Westerkamp, A.C.; Adam, R.; Bennet, W.F.; Seehofer, D.; Settmacher, U.; Sánchez-Bueno, F.; Fabregat Prous, J.; Boleslawski, E.; Friman, S.; et al. Strict Selection Alone of Patients Undergoing Liver Transplantation for Hilar Cholangiocarcinoma Is Associated with Improved Survival. *PLoS ONE* **2016**, *11*, e0156127. [CrossRef] [PubMed]
144. Goldaracena, N.; Gorgen, A.; Sapisochin, G. Current status of liver transplantation for cholangiocarcinoma. *Liver Transpl.* **2018**, *24*, 294–303. [CrossRef] [PubMed]
145. Zilbert, N.; Sapisochin, G. Time to reconsider liver transplantation for intrahepatic cholangiocarcinoma? *Lancet Gastroenterol. Hepatol.* **2018**, *3*, 294–295. [CrossRef]
146. DeOliveira, M.L.; Kambakamba, P.; Clavien, P.A. Advances in liver surgery for cholangiocarcinoma. *Curr. Opin. Gastroenterol.* **2013**, *29*, 293–298. [CrossRef]
147. Gores, G.J.; Gish, R.G.; Sudan, D.; Rosen, C.B. Model for end-stage liver disease (MELD) exception for cholangiocarcinoma or biliary dysplasia. *Liver Transpl.* **2006**, *12*, S95–S97. [CrossRef]
148. Rea, D.J.; Heimbach, J.K.; Rosen, C.B.; Haddock, M.G.; Alberts, S.R.; Kremers, W.K.; Gores, G.J.; Nagorney, D.M. Liver transplantation with neoadjuvant chemoradiation is more effective than resection for hilar cholangiocarcinoma. *Ann. Surg.* **2005**, *242*, 451–458; discussion 458–461. [CrossRef]
149. Darwish Murad, S.; Kim, W.R.; Therneau, T.; Gores, G.J.; Rosen, C.B.; Martenson, J.A.; Alberts, S.R.; Heimbach, J.K. Predictors of pretransplant dropout and posttransplant recurrence in patients with perihilar cholangiocarcinoma. *Hepatology* **2012**, *56*, 972–981. [CrossRef]
150. Heimbach, J.K.; Gores, G.J.; Haddock, M.G.; Alberts, S.R.; Pedersen, R.; Kremers, W.; Nyberg, S.L.; Ishitani, M.B.; Rosen, C.B. Predictors of disease recurrence following neoadjuvant chemoradiotherapy and liver transplantation for unresectable perihilar cholangiocarcinoma. *Transplantation* **2006**, *82*, 1703–1707. [CrossRef] [PubMed]
151. Tan, E.K.; Taner, T.; Heimbach, J.K.; Gores, G.J.; Rosen, C.B. Liver Transplantation for Peri-hilar Cholangiocarcinoma. *J. Gastrointest. Surg.* **2020**, *24*, 2679–2685. [CrossRef] [PubMed]

MDPI

St. Alban-Anlage 66

4052 Basel

Switzerland

Tel. +41 61 683 77 34

Fax +41 61 302 89 18

www.mdpi.com

Journal of Clinical Medicine Editorial Office

E-mail: jcm@mdpi.com

www.mdpi.com/journal/jcm

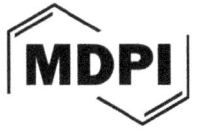